The spondylarthritides

Dose schedules are being continually revised and new side effects recognized. Oxford University Press makes no representation, express or implied, that the drug dosages in this book are correct. For these reasons the reader is strongly urged to consult the pharmaceutical company's printed instructions before administering any of the drugs recommended in this book.

The spondylarthritides

Edited by

Andrei Calin

Consultant Rheumatologist
Royal National Hospital for Rheumatic Diseases,
Bath, UK

and

Joel D. Taurog

Professor of Internal Medicine,
William M. and Guy Burnett Professor for Arthritis Research
Harold C. Simmons Arthritis Research Center,
University of Texas Southwestern Medical Center,
Dallas, Texas, USA

OXFORD NEW YORK TOKYO

OXFORD UNIVERSITY PRESS
1998

Oxford University Press, Great Clarendon Street, Oxford OX2 6DP

Oxford New York
Athens Auckland Bangkok Bogota Bombay Buenos Aires
Calcutta Cape Town Dar es Salaam Delhi Florence Hong Kong
Instanbul Karachi Kuala Lumpur Madras Madrid Melbourne
Mexico City Nairobi Paris Singapore Taipei Tokyo Toronto Warsaw
and associated companies in
Berlin Ibadan

Oxford is a trade mark of Oxford University Press

Published in the United States
by Oxford University Press Inc., New York

A catalogue record for this book is available from the British Library

Library of Congress Cataloging in Publication Data

The spondylarthritides/edited by Andrei Calin and Joel D. Taurog.
(Oxford medical publications)
Includes bibliographical references and index.
1. Ankylosing spondylitis. I. Calin, Andrei. II. Taurog, Joel D. III. Series.
[DNLM: 1. Spondylitis, Ankylosing. WE 725 S7628 1998]
RC935.S67S65 1998 616.7′3—dc21 97–25516

ISBN 0 19 262749 X

Typeset by EXPO Holdings, Malaysia

Printed in Great Britain by
Bookcraft (Bath) Ltd
Midsomer Norton, Avon

Preface

Some of the authors of this publication were participants in a multi-authored book on the spondylarthropathies edited by one of us, published in 1984. Since then, major advances in all aspects of this field have occurred. This new book is an attempt to provide a current, in-depth survey of the spondylarthropathies, from peptides to patients to populations, that we hope will be a resource for the many professionals who deal with these disorders. Many of the authors are rheumatologists who have established their own separate niches in the study and investigation of these disorders. Their efforts are complemented by those of the authors from other disciplines, and the individual chapters rest overall on a solid foundation of expertise.

It has been a quarter of a century since the discovery of the association of the spondylarthropathies with HLA-B27. The speed and accuracy of diagnosis of these disorders has improved dramatically since 1973, and this period has also seen the emergence of patients' societies in countries throughout the world, as indicated in Chapter 17. Nonetheless, it is sobering that the molecular basis for this striking genetic association is still not known, despite the elucidation during these 25 years of a detailed understanding of the structure, function, and population genetics of MHC molecules. It is also sobering that the therapy of the spondylarthropathies remains largely inadequate. We remain optimistic, however, that continued clinical, molecular, and epidemiologic investigation will eventually lead to rational and effective therapy and prevention for these disorders, and we hope that this book will make a useful contribution to this effort.

We wish to thank the authors of the individual chapters for producing timely and conscientious reviews of their topics. We also wish to acknowledge the many colleagues who have provided helpful comments and suggestions. We thank the staff of Oxford University Press for their support and assistance in the production of this book. In addition to the usual difficulties in producing a multi-authored book, they have also had to contend with the variations in the spelling of *spondylarthropathy* by the various authors. After much deliberation and consultation with learned authorities, they have made the Solomonic decision to publish all of the variations.

We also gratefully thank our respective secretaries, Ms. Liz Alexander and Ms. Sherry Fariss, for cheerfully and efficiently laboring many long hours in the service of this book.

Bath, UK
Dallas, TX, USA
October 1997

Andre Calin
Joel D. Taurog

Dedication

To our families and patients.

Contents

Contributors

Ulrich Böcker Postdoctoral Research Fellow, Division of Digestive Diseases, University of North Carolina, Chapel Hill, NC, USA

Jürgen Braun Senior Lecturer, Department of Medicine, Division of Nephrology and Rheumatology, Klinikum Benjamin Franklin, Free University of Berlin, Berlin, Germany

Matthew Brown Arthritis and Rheumatism Council Clinical Scientist; Honorary Consultant in Rheumatology, Nuffield Orthopaedic Centre NHS Trust, Oxford, UK

Andrei Calin Consultant Rheumatologist, Royal National Hospital for Rheumatic Diseases, Bath, England

M. L. Cuéllar Instructor, Section of Rheumatology, Department of Medicine, Louisiana State University School of Medicine, New Orleans, LA, USA

Luis R. Espinoza Professor and Chief, Section of Rheumatology, Department of Medicine, Louisiana State University School of Medicine, New Orleans, LA, USA

Kaisa Granfors National Public Health Institute, Turku, Finland

L. Gail Kennedy Research Assistant, Department of Social Medicine, University of Bristol, Bristol, UK

Muhammad Asim Khan Professor of Medicine, Case Western Reserve University, Cleveland, OH, USA

Marjatta Leirisalo-Repo Consultant Rheumatologist, Department of Medicine, Helsinki University Central Hospital, Helsinki, Finland

Herman Mielants Professor of Rheumatology, Department of Rheumatology, University Hospital, Gent, Belgium

Ross E. Petty Professor and Head, Division of Rheumatology, Department of Paediatrics, University of British Columbia, Vancouver, British Columbia, Canada

Fergus J. Rogers Director of the National Ankylosing Spondylitis Society (NASS), London, UK, and President of the Ankylosing Spondylitis International Federation (ASIF)

James T. Rosenbaum Professor of Medicine, Ophthalmology, and Cell Biology, Casey Eye Institute, Oregon Health Sciences University, Portland, OR, USA

Alan M. Rosenberg Professor and Head, Department of Paediatrics and Head, Section of Paediatric Rheumatology, University of Saskatchewan, Saskatoon, Saskatchewan, Canada

R. Balfour Sartor Professor of Medicine, Microbiology, and Immunology, Division of Digestive Diseases, University of North Carolina, Chapel Hill, NC, USA

H. Ralph Schumacher Jr Professor of Medicine, Division of Rheumatology, University of Pennsylvania, School of Medicine, Director, Arthritis-Immunology Center, Veterans Affairs Medical Center, Philadelphia, PA, USA

Joachim Sieper Professor, Department of Medicine and Rheumatology, Klinikum Benjamin Franklin, Free University of Berlin, Berlin, Germany

Joel David Taurog Professor of Internal Medicine, Harold C. Simmons Arthritis Research Center, University of Texas Southwestern Medical Center, Dallas, TX, USA

Paavo Toivanen Department of Medical Microbiology, Turku University, Turku, Finland

Jaakko Uksila Department of Medical Microbiology, Turku University, Turku, Finland

Eric M. Veys Professor of Rheumatology, Head of Rheumatology Department, University Hospital, Gent, Belgium

Paul Wordsworth Clinical Reader in Rheumatology, Oxford University; Honarary Consultant Rheumatologist, Nuffield Orthopaedic Centre NHS Trust and Oxford Radcliffe NHS Trust, Oxford, UK

Henning K. Zeidler Professor of Medicine and Rheumatology; Director, Division of Rheumatology, Department of Internal Medicine and Dermatology, Medizinische Hochschule Hannover, Hannover, Germany

Abbreviations

AAU	acute anterior uveitis
ACR	American College of Rheumatology
AIMS	Arthritis Impact Measurement Scale
ANA	antinuclear antibody
ANCA	anti-neutrophil cytoplasmic antibody
ANKENT	ankylosing enthesopathy
APC	antigen-presenting cell
APP	acute-phase protein
ARA	American Rheumatism Association
AS	ankylosing spondylitis
ASIF	Ankylosing Spondylitis International Federation
BAS-G	Bath Ankylosing Spondylitis Global Score
BASDAI	Bath Ankylosing Spondylitis Disease Activity Index
BASFI	Bath Ankylosing Spondylitis Functional Index
BASMI	Bath Ankylosing Spondylitis Metrology Index
BASRI	Bath Ankylosing Spondylitis Radiology Index
CIA	chlamydia-induced arthritis
CK	creatine-kinase
CREG	cross-reacting group
CRP	C-reactive protein
CT	computed tomography
CTL	cytolytic T cells
DIF	direct immunofluorescent (antibody studies)
DIP	distal interphalangeal
DISH	diffuse idiopathic skeletal hyperostosis (aka ankylosing hyperostosis, aka Forestier's disease)
EB	elementary body
EM	electron microscopy
ESR	erythrocyte sedimentation rate
ESSG	European Spondyloarthropathy Study Group
FDA	Food and Drug Administration (USA)
FMLP	formyl–met–leu–phe
GU	genitourinary
HA	hydroxyapatite
HAQ	Health Assessment Questionnaire
hβ2m	human β_2-microglobulin
HIV	human immunodeficiency virus

HLA	human leucocyte antigen (system)
hsp	heat-shock protein
IBD	inflammatory bowel disease
IEM	immunoelectron microscopy
IFN	interferon
IL	interleukin
ISH	*in-situ* hybridization
LCMV	lymphocytic choriomeningitis virus
LGV	lymphogranuloma venereum
LMP	large multifunctional protease
LPS	lipopolysaccharide
MHC	major histocompatibility complex
MOMP	major outer-membrane protein
MPA	murine progressive ankylosis
MRI	magnetic resonance imaging
NASS	National Ankylosing Spondylitis Society (UK)
NSAID	non-steroidal anti-inflammatory drug
PCR	polymerase chain reaction
PDGF	platelet-derived growth factor
PG-PS	peptidoglycan-polysaccharide
PID	pelvic inflammatory disease
PMN	polymorphonuclear (granulocyte)
PsA	psoriatic arthritis
RA	rheumatoid arthritis
RB	reticulate body
Re	rough mutant strain of enterobacteria
ReA	reactive arthritis
RFLP	restriction fragment length polymorphism
RNHRD	Royal National Hospital for Rheumatic Diseases (UK)
SARA	sexually acquired reactive arthritis
SF	synovial fluid
SFBL	self-filling blind loop
SI	sacroiliac (joint)
SpA	spondyloarthropathy
TAP	transporter associated protein
TCR	T-cell receptor
TGF	transforming growth factor
TH1	T-helper cell—type 1 cytokine
TH2	T-helper cell—type 2 cytokine
THR	total hip replacement
TNF	tumour necrosis factor

1 Terminology, introduction, diagnostic criteria, and overview

Andrei Calin

Historical review and terminology

A debate continues as to what name should be given to the spondylarthritides. We find no compelling reason to change from the title of our initial text (Calin 1984) and so continue to favour the use of spondylarthropathies or the spondylarthritides. We accept that François and colleagues (1995) have made some suggestions towards a new glossary for the rheumatic spinal diseases. They base this on pathology and appear to favour the term 'spondylo-arthropathy' originally proposed by Moll and Wright in 1974. However, as pointed out by Braun and Sieper (1996), spondylarthropathy and spondarthritis, and even spondylo-arthropathy, have all been used interchangeably to describe the heterogeneous group of diseases that have a number of features in common. These are summarized in Table 1.1. One reason that François and colleagues gave for avoiding the term 'spondylarthropathy' is that it could be confusing because it refers to any degenerative disease of the spine. We would, however, not accept this, feeling that every rheumatologist accepts spondylarthropathy (or one of the alternative spellings) as relating to a group of conditions with inflammation of both peripheral and axial joints (to a varying degree), together with additional extraarticular features as discussed elsewhere in this text.

Another reason for favouring the term spondylarthropathy (apart from its already being accepted by common usage), is related to the fact that Dougados and colleagues (1991*a*) have

Table 1.1 Individual conditions that overlap to form the spondylarthritides

- Ankylosing spondylitis
- Reiter's syndrome/reactive arthropathy (*Campylobacter, Yersinia, Shigella, Chlamydia* spp.)
- Enteropathic spondylitis (Crohn's disease and ulcerative colitis)
- Psoriatic arthropathy
- Uveitis
- Juvenile ankylosing spondylitis
- Seronegative enthesopathic arthropathy syndrome
- Undifferentiated spondylitis (i.e. subset of patients who have spondylarthropathic features but who fail to meet criteria for ankylosing spondylitis, Reiter's syndrome, or other conditions, e.g. dactylitis, uveitis plus unilateral sacroiliitis)
- Pustulotic arthro-osteitis (considered by the Japanese to be part of spondylarthropathy spectrum (rare in USA and Europe))
- Behçet's disease (argument exists as to whether this should be considered as part of the group)
- ? Remitting seronegative symmetrical synovitis with pitting oedema (RS3PE)

used the term in a European context for the preliminary criteria for classification (the European Spondylarthropathy Study Group Preliminary Criteria for the Classification of Spondylarthropathy). Indeed, the term is frequently used in epidemiological, clinical, imaging, and other investigations (Amor *et al.* 1990; Boyer *et al.* 1993; and Braun *et al.* 1994*a*). In summary, therefore, we accept that Moll and colleagues introduced the concept of 'spondarthritis' in 1974, and developed the field further in 1976 (Wright and Moll 1976) in a text entitled '*Seronegative polyarthritis*'. Later, Wright (1980), in a chapter entitled 'Relationships between ankylosing spondylitis and the other spondarthritides', published in *Ankylosing spondylitis* (1980) edited by Moll pointed out that we had misquoted their term, as spondylarthritis, in our 1978 monograph on the subject (Calin and Fries). We feel that, in spite of the frequent appearance of spondylarthritis, spondylarthropathy, and spondyloarthropathy, the best known and most commonly applied terms are spondylarthropathy, spondylarthritis, or the spondylarthritides, and we therefore will continue to use these names. Regardless of preference, we all agree that the spondylarthropathies include an exciting and intriguing group of disorders that range from asymptomatic sacroiliitis to symptomatic sacroiliitis, widespread multisystem ankylosing spondylitis, enteropathic arthropathies, certain subsets of juvenile-onset arthritis, the reactive arthritides, and other entities. These are sum-

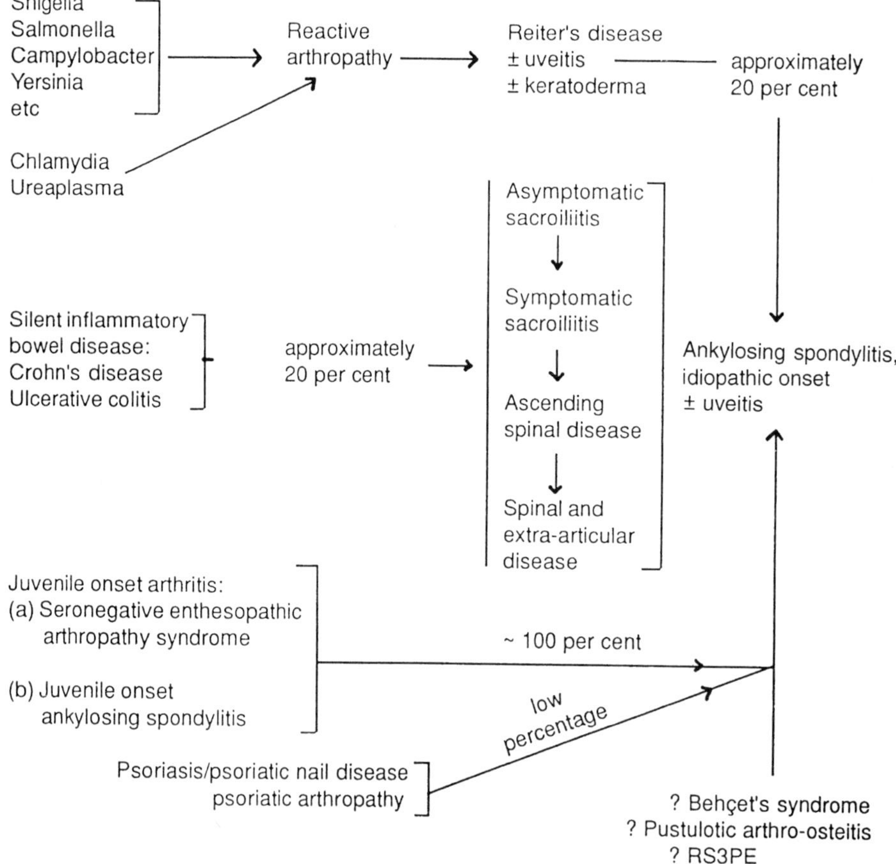

Fig. 1.1 The interrelated conditions making up the spondylarthropathies.

marized in Fig. 1.1. The figure demonstrates how the conditions may overlap with, or develop into, ankylosing spondylitis.

Introduction

As summarized in Table 1.2, the spondylarthritides are characterized by involvement of the sacroiliac joints, by peripheral inflammatory arthropathy, and insertional tendinitis (enthesopathy). (Calin 1989*a*, 1993*a*,*b*).

There are several other important features which include the following.

1. Pathological changes are concentrated at the site of insertion of ligaments or tendons into bone rather than in the synovium. Further pathological changes may also develop in the eye, the aortic valve, lung parenchyma, and skin.
2. There is clinical evidence of overlap between the various seronegative spondylarthritides. Thus, a patient with psoriatic arthropathy may develop uveitis or sacroiliitis and a patient with inflammatory bowel disease may develop ankylosing spondylitis or mouth ulcers.
3. There is a tendency towards familial aggregation, with evidence that these disorders 'breed true' within families (Calin *et al.* 1984).
4. There is an association with HLA-B27, ranging from about 50% (psoriatic and enteropathic spondylitis) to over 95% (primary ankylosing spondylitis). The specific frequency depends on ethnic group and disease type (see Chapter 2).

Diagnostic criteria and classification

Classification or diagnostic criteria for several of the disorders belonging to the spondylarthropathy group have been developed over the last decades. For example, there are the Rome (Kellgren *et al.* 1962), the New York (Bennet and Burch 1968*a*), the van der Linden *et al.* (1984*a*) and other criteria for ankylosing spondylitis. We have long favoured the simple

Table 1.2 Important features of the spondylarthropathy group

- Sacroiliitis, ascending spondylitis
- Peripheral joint disease (juxta- > intra-articular)
- Insertional tendinitis (enthesopathy)
- Insertional capsulitis (enthesopathy)
- Inflammatory eye disease (iritis/uveitis/iridocyclitis)
- Aortitis, valve disease, cardiac conduction defects
- Upper lobe pulmonary fibrosis
- Inflammatory skin disease (balanitis, psoriasis, keratoderma)
- Clinical overlap within the patient
- Clinical overlap within family members
- Tendency towards familial aggregation
- Association with HLA-B27

approach (namely that of symptomatic sacroiliitis; Calin 1989*a*, 1993*a*,*b*). Likewise, criteria exist for Reiter's syndrome (Willkens *et al.* 1981) and for psoriatic arthropathy (Vasey and Espinoza 1984). However, one could consider these criteria sets as being somewhat restricted, there being need to emphasize the existence of a much wider disease spectrum. For example, radiographically detected sacroiliitis in the absence of symptoms would not be included in the existing classification. Moreover, patients with asymmetrical sacroiliitis in addition to, for example, a dactylitis or uveitis would be excluded from classification and yet clearly are part of the spondylarthropathy spectrum. Also, patients with limited or atypical forms of disease would be inappropriately excluded from the typical clinical or epidemiological study. For this reason the European Spondylarthropathy Study Group (ESSG) has proposed a classification criteria for the entire spondylarthropathy group of patients, which now encompass those with clearly defined entities such as Reiter's syndrome or ankylosing spondylitis on the one hand and those with an undifferentiated spondylarthropathy on the other (Dougados *et al.* 1991*a*). In essence, patients with inflammatory spinal pain or asymmetrical synovitis, predominantly of the lower limb, together with at least one of the following—family history positivity, psoriasis, inflammatory bowel disease, enthesopathic lesions, or asymmetrical sacroiliitis, have 'undifferentiated spondylarthropathy' with an acceptable sensitivity and specificity. The proposed classification criteria known as the ESSG criteria for spondylarthropathy, will help broaden our acceptance and understanding of the entire spondylarthropathic disorders (Table 1.3). The ESSG criteria have rapidly gained widespread use. For example, Boyer and colleagues published their assessment of these new criteria for the Inuit, finding them to be appropriate for such study (Boyer *et al.* 1994). In addition, we have followed this same format in clinical pharmacological studies of sulphasalazine in the spondylarthropathy group (Dougados *et al.* 1995*a*).

Parallel to the ESSG criteria, Amor has developed a point-scale that has good sensitivity and specificity in the assessment of patients with spondylarthritis (Table 1.4). The two criteria sets are compared in Table 1.5 (Amor *et al.* 1991). Reactive arthritis and enteropathic arthropathy are readily defined with Amor's criteria. However, it is important to accept that (1) patients may have a limited or atypical form of spondylarthropathy, and (2) that first-degree relatives

Table 1.3 Diagnostic criteria and classification: European Spondylarthropathy Study Group (ESSG) criteria

Inflammatory spinal pain	**or**	Synovitis (asymmetrical or predominantly in the lower limbs*[a])
	and	
	one of more of the following:	
	Positive family history	
	Psoriasis	
	Inflammatory bowel disease	
	Alternate buttock pain	
	Enthesopathy	
	Sacroiliitis*[a]	

[a] Without sacroiliitis: sensitivity, 77%; specificity, 89%. With sacroiliitis: sensitivity, 86%; specificity, 87%.

Table 1.4 Criteria for diagnosing spondylarthropathies (Amor *et al.* 1990)

	Points
A. Clinical symptoms for past history of:	
1. Lumbar or dorsal pain during the night or morning stiffness of the lumbar or dorsal spine	1
2. Asymmetrical oligoarthritis	2
3. Buttock pain—if affecting alternatively the right or the left buttock	1 or 2
4. Sausage-like toe or digit	2
5. Heel pain or other well-defined enthesopathic pain	2
6. Iritis	2
7. Non-gonococcal urethritis or cervicitis accompanying or within 1 month before onset of arthritis	1
8. Acute diarrhoea accompanying or within 1 month before onset of arthritis	1
9. Presence or history or psoriasis and/or balanitis and/or inflammatory bowel ulcerative colitis, Crohn's disease	2
B. Radiological finding	
10. Sacroiliitis (grade ≥ 2 if bilateral, grade ≥ 3 if unilateral)	3
C. Genetic background	
11. Presence of HLA-B27 and/or familial history of ankylosing spondylitis, Reiter's syndrome, uveitis, psoriasis, or chronic enterocolopathies	2
D. Response to treatment	
12. Clear-cut improvement of rheumatic complaints with non-steroidal anti-inflammatory drugs (dramatic improvement or relapse of the pain if NSAIDs discontinued)	2

A patient will be considered as suffering from a spondylarthropathy if the sum of the 12 criteria values is at least 6.

Table 1.5 Comparison of the 12 items criteria (Amor *et al.* 1990) and ESSG criteria

Characteristics	**Set of criteria**	
	Amor	**ESSG**
Sensitivity (%)	91.9	87.1
Specificity (%)	97.9	96.4
Positive predictive value (%)	73.1	60.3
Negative predictive value (%)	99.5	99.2
Likelihood ratio	43.0	24.1
Accuracy (%)	97.5	95.8

of B27-positive probands with classical disease frequently have an inflammatory process that appears to be related in terms of pathology or clinical type to the proband's disease, and yet would not satisfy any of the above criteria. For this reason, several of us have used the term 'undifferentiated spondylarthropathy' (Burns and Calin 1984; Khan and van der Linden 1990*a*) to describe such individuals. With the proposed new classification (Table 1.3) most such individuals would be part of the diagnostic group.

However, it is important to keep the different frameworks in mind, given the different values of each approach. For example, the ESSG criteria are very useful for including all subjects with a spondylarthropathy, but when wishing to study a more homogeneous subgroup of patients, with perhaps different aetiologies, the New York criteria may be best for ankylosing spondylitis, whereas the preliminary ACR criteria (Willkens *et al.* 1981), or our earlier approach (Calin 1984), may be best for Reiter's disease or reactive arthropathy (see Table 1.7).

Overview

Clinical subsets

The interrelated group of conditions constituting the spondylarthropathies have a variety of signs and symptoms (Table 1.8)

Elsewhere in the text, we have focused on chlamydia-induced arthritis, enteric infections, and arthropathy, (from both clinical and bacteriological aspects), the eye and spondylarthritis, the reactive arthritides as an entire group, psoriatic arthropathy, and the link between the bowel and arthritis.

Table 1.6 New York clinical criteria for ankylosing spondylitis (New York 1966)

Diagnosis

- Limitation of motion of the lumbar spine in all three planes—anterior flexion, lateral flexion, and extension
- History or the presence of pain at the dorsolumbar junction or in the lumbar spine
- Limitation of chest expansion to 1 inch (2.5 cm) or less, measured at the level of the fourth intercostal space

Grading—Definite as:

Grade 3–4: bilateral sacroiliitis with at least one clinical criterion

Grade 3–4: unilateral or Grade 2 bilateral sacroiliitis with clinical criterion I (limitation of back movement in all three planes) or with both clinical criteria 2 and 3 (back pain and limitation of chest expansion)

Grading—Probable as:

Grade 3–4: bilateral sacroiliitis with no clinical criteria

Table 1.7 Working definition of Reiter's syndrome

Seronegative asymmetrical arthropathy
(predominantly lower extremity)

Plus one or more of:

Urethritis–cervicitis

Dysentery

Inflammatory eye disease

Mucocutaneous disease

Balanitis

Oral ulceration

Keratodermia

Exclusions: primary AS, PsA, other RD*

* AS, ankylosing spondylitis; PsA, psoriatic arthropathy; RD, rheumatic disease.

Table 1.8 Signs and symptoms within the spondylarthritides

	Ankylosing spondylitis	Reiter's/reactive disease/arthropathy	Psoriatic spondylarthropathy[a]	Enteropathic spondylarthropathy[a]	Juvenile onset spondylarthropathy
Sex	M > F	M = F (enteropathic) M > F (sexually acquired)	M < F	F = M	M > F
Age (years)	16+	20+	Any age	Any age	< 16
Uveitis	+	+	+	+	+
Prostatitis/Urethritis/Cervicitis	—	+	—	—	—
Peripheral joints	+	++	++	+	+
Sacroiliitis (%)	100	20	50	50	80
Plantar spurs (%)	+	++	+	?	+
HLA-B27 (%)	95	⩽ 80	50	50	80
Enthesopathy	+	+	+	+	+
Aortic regurgitation	+	+	+	?	?
Familial aggregation	+	+	+	+	+
Risk for HLA-B27+ positive individual	2–10%	20% of those in contact with trigger	?	?	?

[a] Patients with axial disease.

Table 1.9 Comparison of radiological spinal features between primary ankylosing spondylitis, enteropathic spondylitis, and ankylosing spondylitis associated with Reiter's syndrome or psoriatic arthropathy

	Primary AS[a] and AS[a] associated with IBD[b]	AS associated with RS[c] and Psoriatic arthropathy
Sacroiliac changes	usually symmetrical	often symmetrical
Osteitis pubis	++	+
Facet joint involvement	+++	+
Squaring of vertebrae	++	+
Syndesmophytes	+++	+
Ossification	++	+
Spread	Ascending	Random

[a] Ankylosing spondylitis; [b] inflammatory bowel disease; [c] Reiter's syndrome.

McEwen and colleagues (1971) (Table 1.9) defined radiological differences between primary ankylosing spondylitis, ankylosing spondylitis associated with inflammatory bowel disease, and the spinal arthropathy associated with Reiter's syndrome and psoriasis. The explanation for these intriguing differences remains unknown. Further details regarding the distinct pattern of the clinical subsets are summarized in Table 1.10.

In a large case-controlled study, Edmunds *et al.* (1991) compared primary ankylosing spondylitis with psoriatic and enteropathic disease. Moreover, we have further defined the relationship between disease expression, age at onset, and sex (Kennedy *et al.* 1993*b*). The disorders are categorized according to the specific articular or extra-articular pattern. A specific diagnostic label is given, depending on the associated clinical features (namely urethritis, eye disease, skin involvement) and the way the disease progresses (that is to say remission, relapse). However, as discussed above, clearly defined criteria are frequently absent and one often meets patients who have a spondylarthropathy, but in whom the symptoms and signs are such that one is left with an undifferentiated picture. Family and epidemiological studies confirm this clinical finding. For example, a patient may appear with unilateral sacroiliitis and little else, or chest-wall symptoms due to intercostal muscle insertional tendinitis and, for example, uveitis. Clearly, the specific phenotypic expression is the end-product of a variety of interrelating genetic and environmental factors. Finally, the link between the skin and arthropathy should be stressed (Rosner *et al.* 1993). However, whether hydradenitis suppurativa and acne conglobata-associated arthropathy should be considered as part of the spectrum of spondylarthritis, remains an area of contention. The majority of such cases appear not to be B27-related and only occasionally are the sacroiliac joints involved. However, this is an area where we need to remain open-minded. The Japanese, who see pustulotic arthro-osteitis with some frequency, sometimes consider this to be part of the spondylarthritis picture (Sonozaki *et al.* 1981).

Pathogenesis

Even in the reactive arthropathies where the infective trigger is recognized (for instance, *Yersinia, Shigella, Salmonella, Campylobacter*, and *Chlamydia* spp.) and the genetic background

Table 1.10 Differences between the spondylarthritides

	Ankylosing spondylitis	Reactive arthropathy and Reiter's disease	Psoriatic spondylarthropathy	Enteropathic spondylarthropathy	Juvenile onset ankylosing spondylitis
Onset	Gradual	Sudden	Variable	Peripheral joint: onset predominates	Variable
Urethritis	—	+	—	—	—
Conjunctivitis	—	+++	+	—	—
Skin involvement	—	+	—	—	—
Mucous membranes	—	+	—	(+)	—
Peripheral Joints (%)	25	90	90	50	90
Hips, shoulders	+++	+	++	+/—	++
Spine	+++	+	+	+	Usually late
Symmetry	+	—	—	+	Variable
Self-limiting	No	Yes	Variable	Variable	Uncertain
Remissions, relapses	Variable	Typical	Variable	Typical	Variable

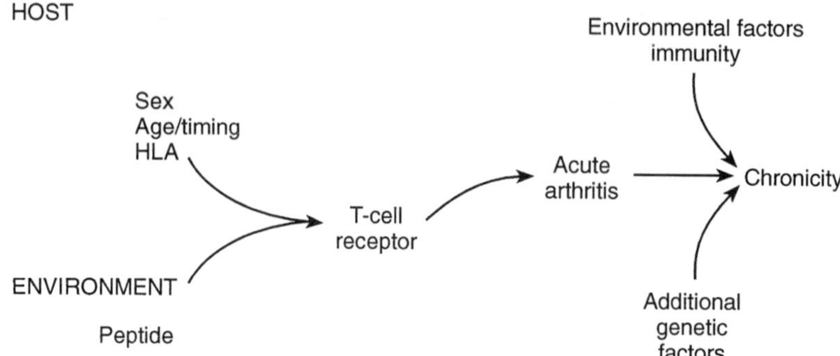

Fig. 1.2 Hypothesized relationship between host, environmental, and other factors in the determination of phenotypic expression.

(HLA-B27) clearly defined, the precise pathogenesis is not well understood. Elsewhere in this book, other authors review the story more fully, but if the hypothesized pathogenesis shown in Fig. 1.2 is approximately correct, we can look forward to elucidation of the following steps.

(1) low-grade inflammatory change in the bowel or genitourinary tract;

(2) the absorption of microorganisms or parts thereof;

(3) interaction of the inciting fragments with antigen-presenting cells or perhaps the presence of persistent viable material;

(4) degradation of the material followed by linking of the putative antigenic peptide with the HLA molecule;

(5) the expression of the combined HLA/peptide complex as a binary product on the cell surface;

(6) and finally, this HLA/antigenic peptide composite interacts with the T-cell receptor determinant, the three forming a tertiary product.

An acute arthropathy results following a relatively poorly defined cascade of events and, perhaps, following further unknown environmental factors and poorly defined genetic characteristics (Figure 1.2), development of the chronic disease state may ensue.

HLA-B27

Over 20 years have passed since we learned of the association between this molecule and the spondylarthritides. At that time, it all seemed very easy. We had an outstandingly good genetic marker, and knew a great deal about the environmental triggers. In theory, at least, we should have been able to complete the jigsaw puzzle within the next few years. If anything, life seems even more complicated now than it did in the 1970s! (Brown *et al.* 1996*a*).

Epidemiology and the spondylarthritides

There are numerous intriguing parts of the puzzle that need to be fitted together:

1. Anecdotal data suggest that reactive arthropathy is more common in the epidemic than the endemic situation.

2. Adults are more at risk than are children (Kaslow 1981), in contradistinction to the situation with acute rheumatic fever.
3. In postdysenteric arthropathy, patients frequently suffer only minimal gastrointestinal symptoms.
4. Reiter's disease can occur postvaccination (salmonella) (Calin *et al.* 1987).
5. Ankylosing spondylitis is seen in both the developing and developed world with an increased age of onset in the latter.
6. Epidemiological studies reveal that ankylosing spondylitis occurs predominantly in the HLA-B27-positive Haida and Pima Indians and the B27-positive relatives of white patients with ankylosing spondylitis, while Reiter's syndrome occurs among the Navaho Indians and Inupiat Eskimo in addition to white family members of B27-positive probands with Reiter's disease. Presumably B27 is itself not sufficient and, as stated, an additional gene (or genes) modifies the phenotypic expression (that is to say, HLA-B27 plus an appropriate environmental trigger together with the ankylosing spondylitis gene(s) results in ankylosing spondylitis, while HLA-B27 plus an environmental trigger and the Reiter's gene(s) leads to Reiter's syndrome (Fig. 1.3).
7. The relationship between sex, phenotypic expression, mode of inheritance, and age at onset in the spondylarthropathies is complicated and intriguing (Kennedy *et al.* 1993).
8. Recent epidemiological studies have focused on the presence of spondylarthritis in Alaskan Eskimos (Boyer *et al.* 1994), the native population of Chukotka in Russia (Alexeeva *et al.* 1994), the Indonesian Chinese and native Indonesians (Nastution *et al.* 1993), and in the population of Togo (Mijiyawa 1993). The varied prevalence rate is of great interest.
9. The risk for the B27-positive individual depends on the nature of that individual. For example, if an individual is related to a B27-positive patient with ankylosing spondylitis the chance of developing that same disease is approximately 1 in 3. B27-positive relatives of healthy B27-positive subjects are at much less risk of developing spondylarthropathy (Calin *et al.* 1983).
10. Interplay between different chromosomes may occur (Brown *et al.*, unpublished data). Chromosome 6 is clearly important with HLA-B27 and BW60 both relevant. In addition, recent interest focuses on the tumour necrosis factor (TNF) and other class III genes

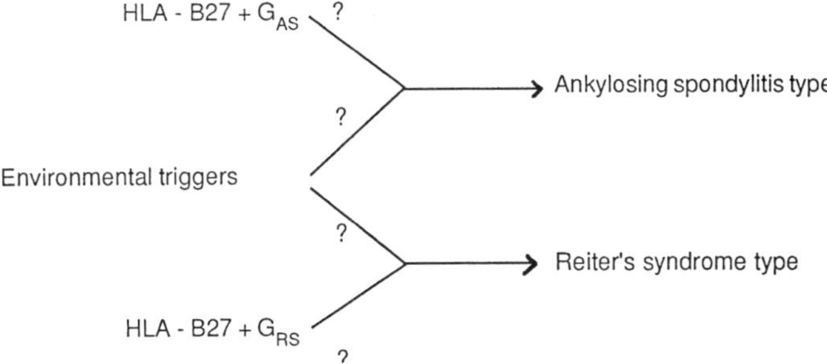

Fig. 1.3 Epidemiology and the spondylarthritides: hypothesis regarding genetic predisposition. G_{AS}, genes determining phenotypic expression of ankylosing type; G_{RS}, genes determining phenotypic expression of Reiter's syndrome type.

(complement) on the same chromosome. Other possible genetic factors relate to the T-cell receptor (TCR) beta gene (encoded by a locus on Chromosome 7) and the TCR alpha gene, α_1 antitrypsin gene and the IgG heavy-chain gene products encoded by loci on chromosome[14]. However, studies using restriction fragment length polymorphisms (RFLP) have failed to confirm the presence of additional genetic material of relevance to disease pathogenesis. For example, no differences have been found between the frequencies of TNF RFLP between patients and controls (Verjans *et al.* 1991).

11. Intracellular proteins are partly degraded by the proteasome, of which the MHC-encoded LMP gene products are subunits. This results in a peptide reaching the endoplasmic reticulum via the transporter associated with peptide (TAP). The TAP genes are also found within the MHC. The nonapeptide then becomes associated with the HLA Class I antigen (B27) and is expressed on the cell surface as a bimolecular product to face the T-cell receptor gene product. The resulting B27/antigen/TCR trimolecular complex causes the release of cytokines and other inflammatory mediators. Application of this system to the spondylarthropathies has recently been the focus for various studies (Burney *et al.* 1994; Lopez-Larrea *et al.* 1996; Maksymowych *et al.* 1994; Rudwaleit *et al.* 1994; Scofield 1996).
12. The observation that psoriatic arthropathy and Reiter's disease thrive in the presence of HIV infection provides support for the hypothesis that CD8-positive T cells play a critical role in these disorders. This is in contrast to the CD4-positive, T-cell maintained arthropathy of rheumatoid arthritis, which sometimes appears to remit in the presence of HIV infection. Ankylosing spondylitis, itself, appears unaffected by the virus, but few data exist.

The changing epidemiology of rheumatic disease (Will *et al.* 1990, 1992).

In rheumatology we recognize that acute rheumatic fever has, at least until recently, become less common, while we perhaps see less acute gout and certainly fewer cases of chronic tophaceous gout. Since the late 1980s, data have become available suggesting that there is also a change in the spondylarthropathies. There are many reasons why the pattern (perceived or real) of a disease may change. Increased interest and recognition by the medical profession and greater concern and pressure from patients may lead to more emphasis being placed on a particular disease. For example, osteoporosis, until recently ignored by rheumatologists, has become a major focus of interest.

Chronic tophaceous gout, once the scourge of medical clinics, is an example of a rheumatic disorder which has become less prevalent, in part due to changing dietary habits, and, in part, because of the introduction of hypouricaemic agents. By contrast, a rise in the prevalence of gout in older females relates to the greater use of diuretics.

Rheumatic fever, at least until recently, had become rare in the more affluent communities. The decline in fatal rheumatic carditis accelerated after 1945, perhaps due to an alteration in the pathogenicity of the streptococcal group A M antigen. Altered streptococcal antigenicity may also be responsible for the recent recognition of a post-streptococcal arthropathy.

Recent studies also suggest that rheumatoid arthritis may be declining in frequency in the developed world—perhaps due to the advent of the contraceptive pill—but is becoming more severe in the developing world. For example, there is a suggestion that, as rural black Africans migrate to an urban environment, rheumatoid arthritis among them increases in frequency and becomes a more destructive disease (Will *et al.* 1990). Hypothetical explanations for this phenomenon may include either exposure to new antigens present in an urban environment, which are uncommon in a less crowded rural setting, or, conversely, a reduction in the antigenic load due to fewer parasitic infestations, which, in turn, could result in less immunosuppression.

Moreover, there is increasing evidence accumulating from developing countries suggesting that the pattern of ankylosing spondylitis may be changing. This relates to both the age of onset of the disease and the pattern of joint involvement. Ankylosing spondylitis develops at an earlier age in countries with poor living conditions, but as these improve the age of onset increases. We have recently suggested that the age of onset of the disease may also be increasing over time in Britain. The influence of potential left- and right-censoring biases on the UK data has been emphasized elsewhere, although the importance of this phenomenon is difficult to quantify (Fries *et al.* 1989). Can the conclusion of an increasing age of onset of ankylosing spondylitis in Britain be substantiated by data from other communities? The putative change may be due to a later age of exposure to the presumed 'infective trigger(s)' or altered pathogenicity of the trigger(s) perhaps due to a modifying factor such as the widespread use of antibiotics.

In France, Amor and colleagues noted that the age of onset of ankylosing spondylitis was influenced by the geographic background of their patients. They observed that 25% of patients from North Africa develop disease before 15 years of age, whereas only 10% of patients in France did so. Moreover, 47 second-generation North Africans with ankylosing spondylitis born and living in France (but whose parents were born in North Africa) were identified from a survey conducted by the French Society of Rheumatology in 1983. None of these 'Beur', as they are known, developed disease before the age of 15 years. Other studies have also noted a lower frequency of juvenile-onset ankylosing spondylitis (less than 16 years of age) in White-Caucasian populations as compared to subjects in the developing world. In spite of the inevitable ascertainment biases, there is now a series of studies consistently demonstrating a greater frequency of patients with a lower age of disease onset from developing countries.

We have recently taken an entirely separate epidemiological route and studied the changing pattern of new patient referrals to the London Hospital (Will *et al.* 1992). Of interest, over the last 30 years patients with non-specific mechanical back pain have progressively presented at a younger age, whereas new patients with ankylosing spondylitis have presented later. We feel that these data, together with the Bath and the French data of Amor add further support for the changing pattern.

Family studies of sibling pairs with ankylosing spondylitis also suggest that the time of onset in each sib is similar, while the age at onset is discordant, suggesting exposure to the trigger at about the same time. This emphasizes the importance of the environment trigger in determining the time of onset of disease in sibling pairs who have a similar genetic predisposition (Calin and Elswood 1989*a*).

The age of disease onset also influences the need for total hip replacement (THR). Calin and Elswood (1989*b*) have shown that 16% of a juvenile cohort (10–15 years of age), 10% of an early onset (18–20 years), and 1% of a late-onset cohort (30–40 years) underwent THR. Amor *et al.*, (1987*b*) also observed that the frequency of THR in a spondylitic population correlates well with the mean age of disease onset. A study of THRs performed in patients from four French hospitals between 1977 and 1983 was undertaken. Of a total of 71 patients, 22 (31%) who had THRs were born in North Africa compared with only 7.9% of non-surgical spondylitic patients treated in French hospitals during this same period. The explanation for more severe hip-joint involvement in a juvenile cohort is unknown, but the developing hip joint may be at greater risk of damage. Conversely, a more marked inflammatory response may result in greater joint destruction in juveniles compared with patients who develop the disease at an older age.

A changing pattern in inflammatory bowel disease is now also recognized; in many studies the incidence of Crohn's disease, which became progressively more common until the mid 1970s, has now begun to decline. The intriguing interrelationship between the bowel and ankylosing spondylitis is, of course, well known (see later chapters).

In conclusion, chronic rheumatic disease should not be considered immutable processes. A changing pattern of disease is to be expected given the interaction of genes and the environment: ankylosing spondylitis, and perhaps the other spondylarthropathies, should now be considered as another example of a rheumatic disorder whose characteristics may be altering as a result of a changing environment. We might expect to see less need for THR as a consequence of the increasing age of onset in patients in the West, and also, perhaps, in developing countries, as the environment changes. Physicians will need to be increasingly aware that patients may present with symptoms of disease in their third decade or later. The epidemiological pattern among the other spondylarthropathies is less well defined.

Treatment

The management of the various components of spondylarthropathy are discussed in the chapters that follow. However, there are some general points that should be stressed. Drug therapy is often disappointing. For example, for ankylosing spondylitis itself, the major thrust of treatment relates to an exercise programme. In contrast to the situation in rheumatoid disease where rest is good for the joints, the patient with ankylosing spondylitis deteriorates with rest and improves with exercise. For those with reactive arthritis, the role of antibiotics has been considered, but even the proponents of this approach would agree that the outcome is only marginally improved (Bardin *et al.* 1992; Cuéllar and Espinoza 1996; Lauhio *et al.* 1991, 1992; Leirisalo-Repo 1993; Toivanen and Toivanen 1996; Toivanen *et al.* 1993). One difficulty relates to the interpretation of the effect, if any, of an antibiotic. Does this relate to the antimicrobial action or, for example, the anticollagenolytic potential of the drug? There are theoretical reasons why sulphasalazine should be efficacious in the spondylarthropathies given the relationship between bowel inflammation and arthropathy. However, again, improvement is marginal and, in large part, beneficial only for peripheral joints rather than axial disease (Dougados 1995*a*; Job-Duslandre and Menkes 1993; Kirwan *et al.* 1993; Youssef *et al.* 1992).

The sacroiliac joints

These are central to the disease process. Why they should be the focus of pathology remains unknown. An excellent review addressing this issue has been written by Braun and Sieper (1996).

Natural history and prognosis

Outcome in spondylarthropathy is notoriously difficult to define. Since our early studies in the 1970s when we showed that Reiter's syndrome typically is not a self-limiting disorder (Calin and Fries 1976; Fox *et al.* 1979), there have been numerous studies showing that the outcome can be relentlessly progressive for many patients. In ankylosing spondylitis, the natural history is varied, although most believe that an intensive exercise programme has an excellent effect on limiting disease progression. No longer is it held that the disease 'burns out' for the majority of patients (Kennedy *et al.* 1993*a*). Pierre *et al.* (1995) have attempted to define predictive factors for the long-term outcome of the spondylarthropathies and have suggested that those individuals with hip involvement, an erythrocyte sedimentation rate over 30, a poor response to non-steroidal anti-inflammatory drugs, a decreased Schober's test, dactylitis, oligoarthropathy, and a young age of onset have the worse prognosis. Although this study was not a formal prospective investigation, few would disagree that these phenomena relate to a poorer outcome.

As discussed in Chapter 16 and elsewhere, we do, at last, have good outcome measurements for ankylosing spondylitis. These also need to be developed for the other spondylarthropathies in order to define the natural history, prognosis, and effects of treatment more precisely.

Finally, the influence of gender in arthritis and its relationship to cartilage damage cannot be ignored (Cutolo, 1997).

Conclusion

During the next few years, hopefully we will understand why and how HLA-B27, other genes, the bowel, sex and environmental triggers interact, resulting in the development of spondylarthropathy in its many guises. Once we understand this intricate interrelated network we will know how to manage and perhaps cure our patients.

2 A worldwide overview: the epidemiology of HLA-B27 and associated spondyloarthritides

Muhammad Asim Khan

The spectrum of the spondyloarthropathies

The discovery of a remarkable association between HLA-B27 and ankylosing spondylitis (AS) and related disorders a quarter of a century ago helped to revitalize interest in the clinical features, pathogenesis, and genetic epidemiology of these disorders, and also broadened our understanding of their clinical spectrum (Khan and van der Linden 1990*b*, 1990*c*). The concept of spondyloarthropathies no longer necessarily implies the presence of sacroiliitis or spondylitis, but rather a spectrum that may start with features such as enthesitis, dactylitis, or oligoarthritis on the one hand, and sacroiliitis and spondylitis on the other, that may also be accompanied by certain extra-articular features, including acute anterior uveitis or mucocutaneous lesions. The strength of the disease association with HLA-B27 varies markedly both among the various spondyloarthropathies and also among racial and ethnic populations (Gran and Husby 1993; Khan 1985, 1987, 1995, 1996*a,b,* 1997*a,b,c*; Khan and van der Linden 1990*b,c*; Tiwari and Terasaki 1985).

In clinical practice, it is not always possible to differentiate clearly between the various forms of spondyloarthropathies, especially in the early stages of disease, but this ambiguity usually has little impact on treatment decisions. Moreover, features typical of the spondyloarthropathies may occur as isolated findings or in a variety of different combinations (reviewed in Zeidler *et al.* 1992; Olivieri *et al.* 1997). For example, there are now well-defined B27-associated clinical syndromes such as isolated seronegative oligoarthritis, polyarthritis, or dactylitis (sausage digits), and heel pain caused by plantar fasciitis and/or calcaneal periostitis. The onset of undifferentiated spondyloarthropathy both in children and in individuals over 45 years of age has been documented. The frequency of undifferentiated spondyloarthropathy may be higher than that of AS or reactive arthritis in some developing parts of the world. In recognition of this phenomenon, Amor *et al.* (1995*b*) and the European Spondylarthropathy Study Group (Dougados *et al.* 1991*a*) formulated classification criteria that are complementary to each other, and encompass, to a large extent, the currently recognized wide disease spectrum under the single rubric of spondyloarthropathy.

There are marked differences in the prevalence of these diseases among many of the world's racial and ethnic groups, as well as that of HLA-B27 and its 11 subtypes. The author has recently reviewed all these aspects elsewhere (Khan 1995, 1996*a,b,* 1997*b*), and they are summarized in Tables 2.1 to 2.8 in this chapter.

The prevalence of HLA-B27 and the spondyloarthropathies

HLA-B27 is present throughout Eurasia, but it is virtually absent among the genetically unmixed native populations of South America, Australia, and among equatorial and southern

Table 2.1 HLA-B27 antigen (phenotype) frequency in native American Populations

Linguistic groups		B27 phenotype frequency[a] (%)
Eskimo-Aleut:	Inupiaq Eskimo	25
	Inuit Eskimo	25
	Inuit Eskimo (Greenland)	30
	Yupik Eskimo	40
	(Siberian Eskimo)	40
Na-Dene:	Tlingit	20
	Dogrib	30
	Navajo	35
	Haida	50
Amerind:		
North American:		
	Bella Coola	26
	Yakima	21
	Pima	18
	Cree	14
	Zuni	13
	Chippewa	11
	Papago	9
	Hopi	9
	Havasupai	7
	Mexicans Mestizo	3–6
Central American:		4–20
South American:		0

[a] The numbers are rounded off for simplicity in this and the subsequent tables.

African Bantus and Sans (Bushmen). In striking contrast, it has a very high prevalence among the native peoples of the circumpolar arctic and subarctic regions of Eurasia and North America, and in some regions of Melanesia. Tables 2.1 to 2.5 list the phenotype frequencies of HLA-B27 in these population subgroups.

The prevalences of AS and related spondyloarthropathies (SpA), in general, seem to correlate directly with that of HLA-B27 in the general population (Table 2.6). The highest prevalences of both B27 and AS have been observed among the Haida Indians living on the Queen Charlotte Islands of the Canadian province of British Columbia. They show a 50% prevalence of B27 (Table 2.1), and definitive AS has been reported to occur in 4% of the adult male Haida population (Gofton 1980). Yupik and Inupiaq (Inupiat) Eskimos of Alaska show a 40% and a 25% prevalence of B27, respectively, and they show a 0.4% prevalence of AS in the adult general population. The overall prevalence of all forms of SpA, including AS, is 2.5% in this population. Both undifferentiated SpA and reactive arthritis (ReA) are more common than AS, and the disease prevalence is quite similar in men and women. A high prevalence of SpA, especially ReA (including Reiter's syndrome), has also been observed in Inuit Eskimos of Canada and Greenland, and among other North American natives (reviewed in Bardin and Lathrop 1992, and Khan 1996*b*). A retrospective analysis of the prevalence of rheumatic diseases among a tribe of

Table 2.2 HLA-B27 antigen (phenotype) frequency among North and Central Asiatic linguistic population groups

Linguistic groups		B27 phenotype frequency (%)
Chukchic:	Siberian Chukchis	19–34
Uralic:	Ural mountain natives	8–15
	Samis (Lapps)	24
Altaic:		
Siberians:	Yakuts	17–19
	Tofs	13
	Buryats	3–6
	Tuvinians	1
	Todjans	2
Japanese		1
Ainu		4
Koreans		3–8
Mongolians		3–9
Uygurs		5
Kazakhs		8
Turkic		3–7
Uzbeks		3
Sino-Tibetan:		
Chinese (Mainland)		2–6
Chinese (Overseas)		4–9
Tibetans		12

Table 2.3 HLA-B27 prevalence in caucasoid population groups

Groups	B27 phenotype frequency (%)
Ugro-Finnish	12–16
Northern Scandinavians	10–16
Slavic populations	7–14
Western Europeans	6–9
Southern Europeans	2–6
Sardinians	5
Basques	9–14
Gypsies (Spain)	16–18
Arabs[a], Jews, Armenians, and Iranians	3–5
Pakistanis	6–8
Indians (Asian)	2–6

[a] Prevalence of B27 may be much lower (closer to 1%) in United Arab Emirates, Kuwait, and adjacent parts of Saudi Arabia, and among Lebanese Maronite Christian Arabs.

Table 2.4 HLA-B27 prevalence in other population groups

Groups	B27 phenotype frequency (%)
Southeast Asians:	
Vietnamese	9
Thais	5–12
Khmer	5
Taiwanese Aborigenes	6
Filipinos	5–8
Malaysians	5–10
Indonesians	5–12
Micronesians:	
Nauru	2
Guam	5
Melanesians:	
Papua New Guineans[a]	12–26
Vanuatuans	23
New Caledonians	18–22
Ouveans	11
Fijians	4–6
Polynesians:	
Hawaians	2
Samoans	2–3
Marquesas Islanders	3
Maoris	0–3
Tokelau and Society Islanders	0
Rapanui (Easter Islanders)	0
Australian Aborigines:	0

[a] An isolated community (Pawaia) in Papua New Guinea showed a B27 prevalence of 52%.

2300 Nuu-Chah-Nulth native Indians of Vancouver Island, located only 150 miles (241 km) south of Queen Charlotte Island (inhabited by Haida Indians) on the western Canadian coast, had noted the absence of definite AS (Atkins *et al.* 1988). These authors did not study the prevalence of B27 in this native Indian population. Psoriasis and psoriatic arthritis are very rare among the Eskimos and other native Americans.

The native Chukchis of Siberia show a 19–34% prevalence of B27 (Table 2.2), while the Siberian Eskimos, like their North American counterparts, show a 40% prevalence of B27. (Table 2.1). There is a correspondingly high prevalence of spondyloarthropathies in their general population. Recent collaborative epidemiological studies (Table 2.6) of four indigenous population groups—in Siberia (the Chukchi and Eskimo) and in Alaska (the Inupiaq and Yupik Eskimo)—show an overall prevalence that varies between 2 and 3.4%. The prevalence of all types of spondyloarthropathies was 4.2% among the B27-positive individuals in the four groups combined, while that of AS alone was 1.6%. The natives of northern Scandinavia (Lappland) known as Samis (or Lapps) have a 24% prevalence of B27, and the prevalence of AS in their general population is 1.8%. It has also been estimated that 6.8% of B27-positive Samis suffer from AS (reviewed in Khan 1995, 1996*b*).

Table 2.5 HLA-B27 prevalence in African population groups

Groups	B27 phenotype frequency (%)
North Africans:	
Arabs	3–5
Berbers	2
Ethiopians	1.4
West Africans:	
Gambia and Senegal	2–4
Gambia (Fula ethnic group)	6
Mali	10
Equatorial and Southern Africans:	
Pygmies	7–10
San (Bushmen)	0
Bantu	
Nigerians	0
Zimbabweans	0
South African Xhosas	0–0.3
Zaireans	0–0.7

Table 2.6 Recent prevalence studies of AS and related spondyloarthropathies (SpA)

	B27 frequency	Prevalence of AS (%)		Prevalence of SpA (including AS) (%)	
Populations	(%)	General population	B27(+) population	General population	B27(+) population
Eskimos (Alaska)	40	0.4		2.5	
Eskimos (Alaska and Siberia) + Chukchi	25–40		1.6	2–3.4	4.2
Samis (Lapland)	24	1.8	6.8		
Northern Norway	14	1.4	6.7		
Mordovia	16	0.5			
Holland	8	0.2	2		
Germany	9	0.86	6.4	1.9	13.6

The B27 prevalence in Hungary, Finland, and Estonia ranges between 12 and 16%. The populations of these countries are genetically related to the Ugro-Finnish people of the Autonomous Mordova Republic in Russia, who show an approximately 16% prevalence of B27 and a 0.5% prevalence of AS. The prevalence of B27 is between 10 and 16% among northern Norwegians and northern Swedes, and that of AS is up to 1.4%. This contrasts with a

B27 prevalence of 8% and that of AS of 0.2% (200 cases per 100 000) among western European and United States Caucasoid populations (reviewed in Khan 1995, Khan and van der Linden 1990*b*). The data, indicate that among unrelated B27-positive Caucasoid adults, anywhere between 1 and 7% may suffer from AS, with appreciable regional differences (Braun *et al.* 1997). On the other hand, the risk for AS in B27-positive first-degree relatives of AS patients is much greater than among the B27-positive population at large; anywhere between 11 and 29% of B27-positive first-degree relatives of AS patients develop the disease, compared with only 1.3–1.9% of the general population of B27-positive adults in the same study (Khan and van der Linden, 1990*b*, van der Linden *et al.* 1984*b*).

Thus, the prevalence of AS ranges between 0.2% to 0.86% for the adult Caucasoid populations of western European extraction. The prevalence increases to more than 2% among the B27-positive individuals in the general population, and to a range of 10% to 30% among the B27-positive first-degree relatives of B27-positive AS patients.

Clinically diagnosable AS may be three times more common in men than in women in the general population, but the prevalence rates of sacroiliitis may not differ. Although axial disease is more severe in males, the overall pattern seems to be similar in both sexes. The overall annual incidence (age and gender adjusted) of AS is 7.3 per 100,000 population in Rochester, Minnesota (Carbone *et al.*, 1992).

Studies of B27-positive twins have shown a 67% pairwise concordance rate for AS among monozygotic twins and only 23% among dizygotic (see Chapter 12). Susceptibility to AS in B27-positive individuals may be further increased by a factor of three when HLA-B60, (which is a split of B40), is also present (Robinson *et al.* 1989). An individual inheriting both HLA-B27 and B44 has a higher risk for concurrent Crohn's disease and AS. The co-occurance of HLA-B27 and HLA-DR8 has been described among Japanese patients with both AS and acute iritis (Islam *et al.* 1995). Moreover, polymorphism in the HLA-linked LMP2 gene (proteasome) has been reported to be associated with acute iritis and peripheral arthritis in AS (Maksymowych *et al.* 1995*a*). Thus genetic factors, in addition to HLA-B27, influence susceptibility as well as phenotypic expression of AS, and this subject is reviewed in Chapter 12. HLA-B27 homozygous individuals seem to be no more susceptible to developing AS, or to having more severe disease, than HLA-B27 heterozygotes, but further studies are needed.

Spondyloarthropathies should be regarded as a group of phenotypically similar, but multifactorial diseases, with heterogeneity of the genetic predisposing factors, while the putative environmental (possibly bacterial) triggers have their own heterogeneity. Disease heterogeneity is best exemplified by the differences between B27-positive vs. B27-negative disease. If AS is defined as low-back pain in the presence of early radiographic sacroiliitis and one looks at individuals with only these two features, then there are no differences between B27-positive and B27-negative patients. But if one looks at the more classical AS with limitation of motion of the lumbar spine, one finds that more typical spinal radiographic features, such as bamboo spine, seem to occur primarily in B27-positive patients. Generally speaking, B27-negative AS is somewhat later in its onset, significantly less frequently complicated by acute anterior uveitis, and more frequently accompanied by psoriasis, ulcerative colitis, and Crohn's disease, and less often shows familial aggregation (Khan and van der Linden 1990*b*). In fact, only rare instances have been observed among people of Northern European extraction with two or more first-degree relatives affected with B27-negative primary AS in the absence of psoriasis or chronic inflammatory bowel disease in the family. There is an over-representation among B27-negative AS patients of other HLA-B alleles, including the B7 cross-reacting group (CREG) of HLA antigens (HLA-B7, B22, B40, and Bw42), Bw62, Bw35 CREG, the Bw38 split of HLA-Bw16, and the psoriasis-associated HLA alleles B13, B17, B37, and B39 (Cedoz *et al.* 1995, Khan 1983, Kidd *et al.* 1995, Yamaguchi *et al.* 1995). A recent British study (Brown *et al.* 1996*a*) has noted an excess of B60 (a split of B40) among B27-negative patients, and confirmed a previous report of a three fold increased risk of AS among those who co-inherit B27 and B60, as compared with those who only inherit B27 (Robinson *et al.* 1989).

Factors other than HLA-B alleles are also involved (see review by Brown and Wordsworth, 1997*b*). Both B27 and AS are absent among the Australian aborigines of unmixed ancestry. However, in Papua New Guinea B27 is quite prevalent (Table 2.4) but AS is very uncommon, even though B27-associated oligoarthritis is frequently observed (Richens and McGill 1995). HLA-B27 is not uncommon in West African countries (Table 2.5) but AS is rare (Brown *et al.* 1996*b*).

In sub-Saharan equatorial and southern Africa, B27 is virtually absent among the Bantu and San populations of unmixed ancestry, and AS and related spondyloarthropathies are reported to be very rare among them. B27 is present among pygmies (Table 2.5), but it is not known whether they suffer from spondyloarthropathies. In Bantu populations, B27 has been found in only 2 of 19 unrelated patients with AS and in none of 10 patients with Reiter's syndrome (reviewed in Khan 1995, 1996*b*).

The prevalence of B27 among African-Americans varies between 2 and 3%, most likely resulting from genetic admixture with Americans of European descent (Whites), 8% of whom possess B27, and native Americans. A study of 176 Caribbean Blacks (98 Jamaican and 78 Colombian) showed an absence of B27. There is a comparatively lower prevalence of AS among American Blacks than among Whites, and the association of AS with B27 has also been found to be weaker among Blacks (close to 50%) than among Whites (more than 90%) (reviewed in Khan 1995, 1996*b*; Khan and Kellner, 1992).

Juvenile spondyloarthropathy

Four recent studies (reviewed by Malleson and Petty, 1997) have demonstrated that SpA form a large proportion of childhood arthropathies. A study based on data collected from all provinces in Canada estimates the incidence rate for juvenile SpA (excluding juvenile psoriatic arthritis) at 1.44 per 100 000 children at risk per year, and 0.3 for juvenile psoriatic arthritis (Malleson *et al.* 1996); the male to female ratio for juvenile SpA was 1.9 to 1. However there is a marked variance in the reported annual incidence rates of juvenile SpA among various regions and ethnic or racial groups in the world, varying from a low of 0.1 per 100 000 in Finland to a high of 69 per 100 000 among Inuit Eskimos of Canada (Oen and Cheang, 1996; Kaipiainen-Seppanen and Savolainen, 1996). The high incidence of juvenile SpA among Inuit Eskimos is of interest in light of a very high (25%) prevalence of HLA-B27 in their general population (Table 2.1).

Reactive arthritis

The occurence of ReA (including Reiter's syndrome) varies with the prevalence of B27 and that of the triggering bacterial infections (reviewed in Khan, 1992, Silman and Hochberg, 1993; Toivanen and Toivanen, 1997). It occurs in about 1–4% of individuals following chlamydial urogenital infection or enteritis due to Gram-negative bacteria. Recent reports indicate that the incidence of ReA after salmonella enteritis is almost 7%, and whereas the initial episode of arthritis is relatively weakly associated with HLA-B27 (in some studies, not more than 33% of these patients may possess this gene), it is more likely to become chronic and demonstrate acute anterior uveitis and other extra-articular features among those who possess HLA-B27

(Mattila *et al.* 1994; Thomson *et al.* 1995). The incidence of ReA after some epidemics of bacterial enteritis among B27-positive individuals in the general population can be as high as 20%. The current understanding of the role of bacteria in B27-associated ReA has been recently reviewed by Taurog (1995) and Hughes and Keat (1994), and is discussed in detail in Chapters 5, 6 and 11 of this book.

The annual incidence of ReA, especially chlamydia-induced ReA, has declined in Europe and the USA since 1985. In a 3-year study (between 1988 and 1990) in Oslo, Norway, the annual minimal *incidence* of chlamydia-induced ReA (confirmed by positive genitouretheral culture of *Chlamydia spp.*) was 4.6 per 100 000 population aged 18 to 60 years, and the triggering genitourinary infection was asymptomatic in 36% of the patients; while the annual incidence of postenteritic ReA was 5 per 100 000, and the triggering enteric infection was asymptomatic in 26% (Kvien *et al.* 1994). Postvenereal chlamydial ReA is very frequent in Inuit Eskimos (reviewed by Bardin and Lathrop, 1992), a population with 25 to 30% prevalence of HLA-B27 (Table 2.1).

A recent study of the *prevalence* of ReA in Germany (Braun *et al.* 1997) has demonstrated that 0.7% (700 per 100 000) of the HLA-B27 positive population of Berlin suffers from this disease, and also calculated that the prevalence in the general population is 0.01% (10 per 100 000). According to prior studies, the prevalence of ReA among males in the United States has varied from 0.03% in Rochester, Minnesota to 0.3 to 0.5% among homosexuals. Navajos living in Keams Canyon, with a 35% prevalence of HLA-B27 (Table 2.1), have a 0.3% prevalence of ReA that is mostly triggered by Shigella enteritis, and an annual incidence of 0.133%.

Enteropathic arthritis

Up to 20% of patients with ulcerative colitis or Crohn's disease develop arthritis and up to 25% of them have axial disease. Subclinical inflammatory gut lesions have been observed in many spondyloarthropathy patients; the lesions are histologically acute in 25% and chronic in 30%. Follow-up studies indicate that 15–25% of those with chronic lesions develop clinically obvious Crohn's disease. These Crohn-like gut lesions are not associated with the presence of B27, and support the existence of a B27-independent pathogenic link between gut inflammation and spondyloarthropathy (Mielants *et al.* 1995*a*) (see Chapters 9 and 11).

Psoriatic arthritis

The prevalence of this disorder in various population groups differs markedly, reflecting differences in the prevalence of psoriasis. The disease is very uncommon among Africans, native American Indians, and Eskimos of unmixed ancestry, and is also relatively less common among Orientals. Psoriasis affects more than 1% of the population of the USA, and is most common among people of northern European extraction. Recent studies, primarily from Europe, suggest that 20–36% of patients with psoriasis may show some features of psoriatic arthritis, and that the existing criteria for this disease are inadequate and need to be improved (Hanly *et al.* 1988, Salvarani *et al.* 1995, Veale *et al.* 1994). The annual incidence rate of joint inflammation in patients with psoriasis is estimated at 6 to 7 per 100,000 in two recent studies (Kaipianen-Seppanen 1996; Shbeeb *et al.* 1995). The observed prevalence of psoriatic arthritis in the HLA-B27-positive population of Berlin, Germany, is 1.4%, and the prevalence in the general population has been calculated to be 0.29% (Braun *et al.* 1997). HLA-B27, B39, and DQw3 are risk factors for severe progressive psoriatic arthritis (Gladman and Farewell 1995).

Table 2.7 HLA-B27 subtypes in world populations

Populations	HLA-B27 subtypes
North American Natives	HLA-B*2705
Siberian Chukchis	HLA-B*2705
Siberian Eskimo	HLA-B*2705
	HLA-B*2702 (rare)
Euro-Caucasoids	HLA-B*2705
	HLA-B*2702
	HLA-B*2701 (rare)
	HLA-B*2708 (rare)
	HLA-B*2709 (rare)
	HLA-B*2710 (rare)
Semitic and Eastern Mediterranean	HLA-B*2702
	HLA-B*2705
	HLA-B*2704 (rare)
	HLA-B*2707 (rare)
Indians (Asians)	HLA-B*2705
	HLA-B*2704
	HLA-B*2707 (rare)
	HLA-B*2702 (rare)
Chinese	HLA-B*2704
	HLA-B*2705
	HLA-B*2706 (rare)
	HLA-B*2707 (rare)
Japanese	HLA-B*2704
	HLA-B*2705
	HLA-B*2711 (rare)
Koreans	HLA-B*2705
Polynesians	HLA-B*2705
	HLA-B*2704
Thais	HLA-B*2704
	HLA-B*2706
	HLA-B*2705 (rare)
	HLA-B*2707 (rare)
Indonesians	HLA-B*2706
	HLA-B*2704
	HLA-B*2705
	HLA-B*2707 (rare)
West Africans	HLA-B*2705
	HLA-B*2703
African Americans	HLA-B*2705
	HLA-B*2703 (rare)

HIV infection ans spondyloarthropathies

Occurrence of arthritis and psoriasis in association with HIV infection has added a new dimension to the prevalence of reactive arthritis (including Reiter's syndrome) and psoriatic arthritis in various parts of the world. For example, spondyloarthropathies and psoriasis were virtually absent among the native African population of Zimbabwe prior to the present outbreak of HIV infection among them. The occurrence of psoriasis and arthritis now raises the suspicion of underlying HIV infection in this and many other populations with high prevalence rates of HIV infection (Stein and Davis 1996).

In a recent retrospective study from Togo (Mijiyawa 1993), a small African country on the west coast, 8 out of 31 (26%) spondyloarthropathy patients seen in rheumatological consultation between October 1989 and January 1992 were infected with HIV, whereas the local HIV prevalence rate in blood donors was 4%. This suggests that the prevalence of spondyloarthropathy in Black Africans is likely to increase in the future because of HIV infection. These 8 patients had no sacroiliitis and they mostly suffered from oligoarthritis, spinal pain, diarrhoea, and weight loss. Of the remaining 23 patients, 9 had AS with bilateral sacroiliitis and 14 had reactive arthritis without sacroiliitis. B27 typing was not performed in any of the 31 patients.

The link between HIV infection and increasing prevalence of SpA has been more clearly demonstrated in a recent study from Lusaka, Zambia (Njobvu *et al.* 1997). This study defined the relative frequency of rheumatic diseases in 507 consecutive patients attending an arthritis clinic at University Teaching Hospital between April 1994 and December 1995. There were 244 patients with SpA (ReA 119, undifferentiated SpA 113, psoriatic arthritis 11, ankylosing spondylitis 1), 21 with RA, 21 with gout, 122 with undifferentiated arthritis, and 99 with other miscellaneous diagnoses. The HIV seroprevalence in Lusaka is approximately 30%, but it is approximately 50% among adults attending medical outpatient clinics, 94% in patients with SpA, 64% in undifferentiated arthritis, 23% in gout, and 0% in RA.

Thus there has been a dramatic change in the epidemiology of SpA in sub-Saharan Africa from a relative rarity before the HIV epidemic to its current overwhelming prevalence. This is all the more remarkable given the almost complete absence of HLA-B27 in Bantu populations (Table 2.5), and the fact that the HIV-associated SpA in Eurocaucasoid populations, on the other hand, retains a strong association with HLA-B27.

The subtypes of HLA-B27

Table 2.7 lists the HLA-B27 subtypes observed in various world populations. The occurence of AS or related SpA has been observed in individuals possessing any of the subtypes except B*2708, B*2709, and B*2711 (Khan 1997*b*, Brown and Wordsworth 1997*b*, Reveille *et al.* 1996, Feltkamp *et al.* 1996, Gonzalez-Roces *et al.* 1997). B*2708 is a rare subtype observed in Caucasoid populations (Hildebrand *et al.* 1994); in a recent British study it was present in none of 172 B27-positive AS patients and in only 2 of 154 B27-positive healthy controls (Brown *et al.* 1996). B*2709 has been observed among Italians, primarily among those living on the Island of Sardinia; it is of interest that among B27-positive Sardinians, B*2709 was present in 25% of controls but in no patient with AS (del Porto *et al.* 1994). B*2710 has been identified in an American Caucasian family with spondylitis (Peter Stastny, Personal communication). B*2711 has only been detected in a healthy Japanese individual (Hasegawa *et al.* 1996, 1997).

Three recent studies have demonstrated a lack of association of HLA-B*2706 with AS and related SpA in Thailand (Lozez-Larrea *et al.* 1995), Singapore (Ren *et al.* 1997), and Indonesia (Nasution *et al.* 1997). Such studies are going to lead to a more precise understanding of the disease association for the different subtypes of HLA-B27, and any influence of these subtypes on the phenotypic expression of the disease. This will help provide a clearer insight into the molecular mechanism of disease (reviewed by Parham, 1996, and see Chapter 12).

3 Ankylosing spondylitis: clinical aspects

Muhammad Asim Khan

Ankylosing spondylitis (AS) is a chronic systemic inflammatory rheumatic disorder of the axial skeleton, that is to say the sacroiliac (SI) joints and the spine; the presence of sacroiliitis is its hallmark. Hip and shoulder joints, and less commonly peripheral joints or certain extra-articular structures, may also be involved. Its aetiology is as yet not fully understood, but there is a strong genetic predisposition in association with the histocompatibility antigen HLA-B27. The disease sometimes occurs in association with reactive arthritis (including Reiter's syndrome), psoriasis, ulcerative colitis, or Crohn's disease. In such cases it is called secondary AS. Most cases, however, show no evidence of these associated diseases and are classified as primary or uncomplicated AS (Khan 1993, 1997*a*).

Typically, the earliest and most consistent findings are seen in the SI joints. The other axial sites characteristically affected include discovertebral, apophyseal, costovertebral, and costo-transverse joints of the spine, and the paravertebral ligamentous structures. A striking feature is the high frequency of inflammation at entheses, which are the sites of musculotendinous and ligamentous attachments to bones, and this enthesitis is particularly prominent in the axial skeleton. The inflammation affects the synovium, articular cartilage, and subchondral bones of the involved joints, and can also involve juxta-articular ligamentous structures. The site of enthesitis is infiltrated by plasma cells, lymphocytes, and polymorphonuclear cells, and there can also be oedema and infiltration of the adjacent bone-marrow space. The inflammatory process frequently results in gradual fibrous and bony ankylosis (Ball 1971; Khan 1990, 1992; Resnick and Niwayama 1995).

The symptoms usually begin in late adolescence or early adulthood (the average age of onset is 25 years); onset after the age of 45 is very uncommon. The disease is three times more common in men than in women, and the clinical and radiographic features of the disease probably evolve more slowly in women (Khan and van der Linden, 1990*b*). In industrialized countries, only a small subset of patients have juvenile onset (before the age of 16 years), but in many developing countries this form of the disease is quite common (Burgos-Vargas and Vasquez-Millado 1995; Malleson and Petty 1997).

Clinical features

The major clinical features of AS can be divided into skeletal and extraskeletal manifestations.

Skeletal manifestations

Back pain and stiffness

Chronic low back pain and stiffness are the most common and characteristic initial presenting complaints in adult-onset AS. The backache is usually of insidious onset, dull in character, difficult to localize, and felt deep in the gluteal area or the sacroiliac region. It can be unilateral or intermittent at first, but within a few months becomes persistent and bilateral. Pain and stiffness in the lumbar area, rather than the more typical buttock-ache, may be the initial symptom in some patients. The backache and stiffness tend to worsen after prolonged periods of inactivity, and at night or early morning. At times, the pain may awaken the patient from sleep, and some may have difficulty sleeping well or find it necessary to wake up at night to exercise or move about for a few minutes before returning to bed. The back stiffness tends to be eased by movement or other mild activity, and by a hot shower or exercise. In some patients fatigue can be a major complaint in addition to pain and stiffness.

Back complaints are the first clinical manifestations in approximately 75% of patients with adult-onset AS. Occasionally, back pain may be absent or too mild to impel the patient to seek medical care. Some patients may complain only of back stiffness, fleeting muscle aches, or musculotendinous tender spots. These symptoms become worse on exposure to cold or dampness, and such patients are often misdiagnosed as having rheumatism or fibrositis. Pain in the buttocks or superior posterior thigh can be misdiagnosed as lumbago or sciatica, despite a normal neurological examination. Some patients in the early stages of the disease may have mild constitutional symptoms, for example anorexia, malaise, weight loss, and even mild fever.

Enthesitis

Extra-articular or juxta-articular bony tenderness due to enthesitis can be a major or presenting complaint in some patients, and persistent or recurrent bouts of enthesitis and/or peripheral arthritis may precede the onset of definite axial disease by many years, especially among those with juvenile-onset AS (Burgos-Vargas and Vasquez-Mellado 1995; Olivieri *et al.* 1997, Malleson and Petty 1997).

Hip and shoulder joint involvement

Sometimes the first symptoms may result from the involvement of root or girdle joints (the hips and the shoulders). Hip involvement, with resultant limitation of motion or flexion contracture, can be a presenting manifestation. Accurate assessment of the hip joints is crucial because their involvement can result in severe physical limitation or disability, and they are involved at some stage of the disease in one-third of the patients, and perhaps even in a majority of those with juvenile-onset AS. The hip joint involvement is usually bilateral and potentially more crippling than involvement of any other joint of the extremities. If hip involvement has not occurred during the first 10 years of the disease it is unlikely to occur later. However, loss of extension at the hip joints and even some degree of flexion contracture tends to be present in most patients with the advanced stage of AS. Involvement of the shoulder girdle (glenohumeral, acromioclavicular, or sternoclavicular joints) is less common and often leads to only a minor disability, mostly resulting from some loss of thoracoscapular movement.

Peripheral joint involvement

Involvement of peripheral joints other than hips and shoulders is infrequent in primary AS. When present it is usually asymmetrical, mild and transient, rarely persistent or erosive, and tends to resolve without any residual joint deformity in most patients. Peripheral joint involvement can sometimes occur after the axial disease has become inactive. Intermittent knee hydroarthrosis is occasionally the presenting manifestation of juvenile-onset AS. Temporomandibular joint pain and local tenderness may occur in more than 10% of patients, sometimes resulting in a decreased range of motion of this joint (Ramos-Remus *et al.* 1997). A few male patients over 50 years of age with an undifferentiated spondyloarthropathy syndrome have recently been described. This arthropathy may sometimes resemble somewhat the syndrome of remitting seronegative symmetrical synovitis with pitting oedema. At onset of the disease, the patients may show little or no clinical involvement of the axial skeleton, but many of them later develop bilateral sacroiliitis or even go on to develop AS (Olivieri *et al.* 1995).

Spinal involvement

Chest pain may result from inflammation of the thoracic spine (including the costovertebral joints), enthesitis at costosternal areas, and inflammation of manubriosternal or sternoclavicular joints. The pain may be accentuated on coughing or sneezing, and at times may even mimic symptoms of atypical angina or pericarditis. Some patients notice an inability to fully expand the chest on inspiration.

Most patients with AS breathe primarily with the diaphragm because involvement of the costovertebral and costotransverse joints results in restriction of chest expansion. Limited chest expansion in an individual with an insidious onset of chronic low-back pain and without a chest disease such as emphysema or scoliosis should strongly raise the possibility of AS.

There is often some limitation of motion of the lumbar spine, most easily recognized on hyperextension, axial rotation, or lateral flexion. Neck involvement with resultant pain and stiffness may occur, generally after some years, but it sometimes occurs in relatively early stages of the disease. The early loss of spinal mobility can result from pain and muscle spasm rather than bony ankylosis, and therefore marked improvement in spinal mobility can occur after treatment with non-steroidal anti-inflammatory drugs (NSAIDs) and proper physical therapy. There is often tenderness in the midline over the vertebral spinous processes due to enthesitis at those sites. Important additional early, but often overlooked, physical findings that can result from enthesitis include tenderness over the anterior chest wall at costochondral or manubriosternal junctions, or over anterosuperior iliac spines, iliac crest, pubic symphysis, ischial tuberosities, greater femoral trochanters, tibial tubercles, or calcanea.

Spinal ankylosis develops at a variable rate and pattern; occasionally the disease may remain confined to one part of the spine. Typically, after many years of disease progression, the patient loses normal posture because of flattening of the lumbar spine and accentuation of the thoracic kyphosis. The anterior chest wall becomes flattened, the abdomen becomes protuberant, and the breathing becomes increasingly diaphragmatic. Finally, involvement of the cervical spine may result in progressive limitation of neck motion, and a forward stoop of the neck. At this advanced stage the diagnosis is readily apparent because of the characteristic posture and gait, and the back pain and stiffness tend to regress, although some degree of inflammatory pain is usually present. These typical deformities usually evolve after 10 or more years of the disease. In the rare extreme case, the hips and shoulders may become ankylosed and the spine may fuse in a flexed position.

The rigid, ankylosed, osteoporotic spine can break like a long bone and is unduly susceptible to fractures. The fracture line is usually transverse. Fractures occur after even a relatively minor trauma, including events that may not be noticed or remembered by the patient. The most common site is the cervical spine, usually at the C5–6 or C6–7 levels (Murray and Persellin 1981; Khan *et al.* 1993). Cervical fracture dislocation, with resultant quadriplegia, is a very serious complication with a high mortality. The possibility of spinal fracture must be considered in any patient with advanced AS who complains of new or altered neck or back pain, particularly after even a mild trauma. An undiagnosed or improperly treated fracture results in spondylodiscitis and pseudoarthrosis.

Extraskeletal manifestations

Acute anterior uveitis (also called acute iritis or iridocyclitis), the most common extraskeletal involvement in patients with AS, occurs in up to 30% of patients, and is more common in HLA-B27 positive than negative patients. Occasionally, it may be the presenting symptom which draws attention to the diagnosis of AS or related spondyloarthropathy (Rosenbaum 1992) (see Chapter 10). The uveitis is virtually always unilateral, but frequently recurrent, and when recurrent it can affect the contralateral eye. The symptoms usually begin acutely and include pain, increased lacrimation, photophobia, and blurred vision. There is circumcorneal congestion, a small oedematous iris, and a copious exudate in the anterior chamber of the eye, which can be seen on slit-lamp examination. An individual attack of uveitis usually subsides within 2–3 months, and usually with no sequelae. Residual visual impairment is rare, and tends to occur in cases in which treatment is inadequate or delayed.

Clinically silent (asymptomatic) enteric mucosal inflammatory lesions in the terminal ileum and colon have been detected by endoscopy in many patients with AS, and it is quite likely that they have some role in the pathogenesis of AS (Mielants *et al.* 1995*a*). The presence of such gut lesions in patients with spondyloarthropathy who do not meet criteria for AS or symptomatic inflammatory bowel disease (IBD) increases the risk of subsequent development of AS and/or IBD (see Chapters 9 and 14).

Cardiac involvement can occur in some patients, usually those with severe and long-standing AS with peripheral joint involvement (Aranson *et al.* 1996; Bergfeldt *et al.* 1988; O'Neill and Bresnihan 1992, Sun *et al.* 1992). Dilatation of the aortic ring and aortic valve incompetence can result from aortitis of the ascending aorta. Cardiac conduction abnormalities can result from involvement of the bundle of His and/or atrioventricular node, and very rarely it may even involve the anterior leaflet of the mitral valve to cause mitral valve incompetence. Complete heart block causing Stokes–Adams attacks may supervene in some patients, necessitating implantation of cardiac pacemakers.

Rigidity of the chest wall does not usually result in ventilatory insufficiency because of compensatory increased diaphragmatic contribution. A rare pleuropulmonary complication of AS is a slowly progressive apical pulmonary fibrosis of the upper lobes of the lungs (Rosenow *et al.* 1977). It appears, on average, two decades after the onset of AS, and is usually bilateral, appearing as linear or patchy opacities on chest radiographs, eventually becoming cystic. Recent studies using high-resolution computed tomography suggest that this complication may be more common than previously realized, and there may also be a possible association between interstitial lung disease and AS (Canvin *et al.* 1995, Casserly *et al.* 1997). The fibrobullous disease is usually asymptomatic and diagnosed as an incidental radiographic finding. However, the cavities may become colonized by fungi or bacteria, and infection with *Aspergillus* species may result in the formation of a mycetoma. Such patients may complain of cough, increasing dyspnoea, and occasionally haemoptysis.

Neurological involvement may occur in some patients with AS and is most often related to fracture dislocation of the spine, atlantoaxial subluxation, or cauda equina syndrome. Spontaneous anterior atlantoaxial subluxation is a well-recognized complication of AS, presenting as occipital pain with or without signs of spinal cord compression. It occurs in about 2% of patients, mostly in those with peripheral joint involvement and advanced axial disease, although in rare cases it may be an early manifestation. A slowly progressive cauda equina syndrome is a rare but significant complication of long-standing AS (Tullous *et al.* 1990). A few AS patients with multiple sclerosis have been reported but any association between the two diseases has not been established (reviewed by Whitman and Khan 1989). Convincing evidence for the involvement of skeletal muscles in AS is lacking. The marked muscle wasting seen in some patients with advanced disease probably results from disuse, although some ultrastructural changes in muscle and a raised level of serum creatine kinase have occasionally been observed.

Amyloidosis (secondary type) is nowadays a very rare complication of AS, especially in the USA (Escalante *et al.* 1995). A recent study from Spain (Gratacos *et al.* 1997) has documented that amyloid deposits in abdominal fat are not a rare finding in AS, but most of these patients do not develop clinical amyloidosis after a followup of several years. However, amyloidosis should be considered in the differential diagnosis of proteinuria with or without progressive azotaemia in a patient with AS or a related spondyloarthropathy. Quite a few cases of IgA nephropathy and six cases of IgA multiple myeloma have been reported in AS patients, and this is of interest because of the frequently observed elevation of serum IgA in AS (Bruneau *et al.* 1986, O'Neill *et al.* 1997). The presence of renal abnormalities on electron microscopy and immunofluorescent studies, as well as proteinuria, impairment of renal function, and renal papillary necrosis induced by analgesics and NSAIDs have also been noted in AS patients (Vilar *et al.* 1997). There may also be a modestly increased incidence of chronic prostatitis among patients with AS.

Investigations

Laboratory tests

An elevated erythrocyte sedimentation rate (ESR) is present in up to 75% of patients with AS, but it may show a lack of correlation with clinical disease activity. A normal ESR has been noted in some patients with clinically active AS in the presence of elevated levels of serum C-reactive protein (CRP). Possibly, ESR and CRP relate more to the peripheral than to the axial arthropathy of AS. Mild to moderate elevations of the serum concentration of IgA are frequently observed in AS, and its level correlates with acute phase reactants (Mackiewicz *et al.* 1989). Serum complement levels are normal or elevated. Some investigators have detected circulating immune complexes, while others have not confirmed these findings. There is no association with rheumatoid factor or antinuclear antibodies. The synovial fluid in AS patients does not show markedly distinctive features compared with other inflammatory arthropathies. Mild elevation of cerebrospinal fluid protein has been noted in some patients, perhaps as a result of a mild arachnoiditis. Modest elevations of serum alkaline phosphatase (primarily derived from bone) are seen in some patients, but are unrelated to disease duration or activity, and mild, normocytic-normochromic anaemia is present in 15% of patients. Persistent but mild elevation of serum creatine kinase (CK) of muscle origin (confirmed by isoenzyme testing) in the presence of normal levels of serum aldolase has been reported in 15% of patients with AS or related spondyloarthropathies. This CK elevation does not correlate with disease activity, therapy, ESR, or the presence or absence of HLA-B27. Moreover, these patients do not develop muscle weakness and the elevated CK requires no treatment. There is no evidence of any circulating endotoxin (Mäki-Ikola *et al.* 1997). The clinical assessment of disease activity in patients with AS is difficult, especially in uncomplicated disease confined to the SI joints and spine. This subject is discussed in detail in two recently published reviews (van der Linden and van der Heijde 1995; Calin 1995). (See also Chapter 16).

Radiography

The characteristic radiographic changes of AS are seen in the axial skeleton, especially in the SI, discovertebral, apophyseal, costovertebral, and costotransverse joints (Khan 1990, Resnick and Niwayama 1995). These changes evolve slowly over many years. The earliest, most consistent, and most characteristic findings are seen in the SI joints. Various methods have been used to examine the SI joints radiographically; none is ideal because of the complex configuration and individual variations of these joints. A standard anteroposterior view suffices in most situations (Fig. 3.1), but if it does not provide adequate demonstration of the changes in these joints because of undulating articular surfaces, one may require angulation of the X-ray tube (Ferguson's view) (Fig. 3.2). There is rarely a need for oblique views of the individual SI joints.

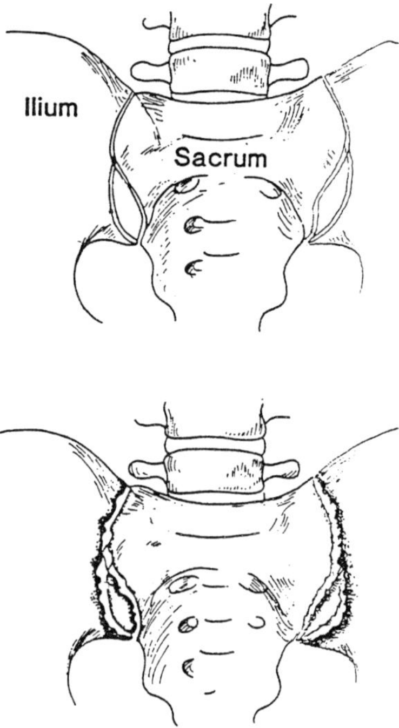

Fig. 3.1 A schematic drawing illustrating bilateral sacroiliitis (lower half of the figure) as seen on a conventional anteroposterior view of the pelvis, and compared with normal findings (upper half of the figure). The sacroiliac joint looks like a pear hanging by a stalk due to the obliquity of the lower half of the articulating surface on this view.

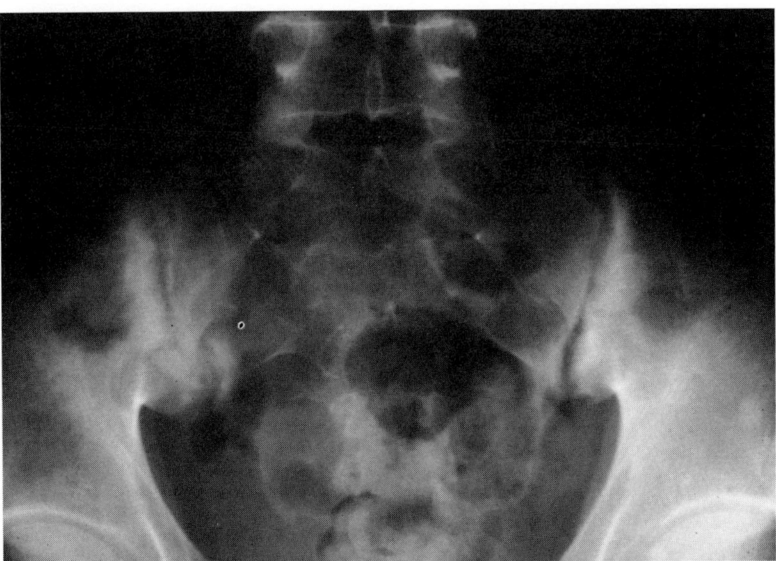

Fig. 3.2 X-ray of sacroiliac joints, Ferguson's view.

The radiographic findings of sacroiliitis are usually symmetrical, and consist of blurring of the subchondral bone plate, followed by erosions and sclerosis of the adjacent bone. They are typically seen first on the iliac side, and tend to be more prominent on that side. These subchondral bone erosions can resemble postage-stamp serrations, and can progress to lead to pseudowidening of the SI joint space. With time there is gradual fibrosis, calcification, interosseous bridging, and ossification. Erosions become less obvious, but the subchondral bony sclerosis persists, or becomes more prominent. Ultimately, there may be complete bony ankylosis of the SI joints after several years, with resolution of bony sclerosis. In occasional patients, SI joints remain normal on plain films for many years (Mau *et al.* 1988).

The inflammatory lesions in the vertebral column affect the superficial layers of the annulus fibrosus at their attachment to corners of vertebral bodies, the apophyseal joints, and intervertebral ligaments. There is reactive bone sclerosis, seen radiographically as highlighting of the corners of vertebral bodies, and subsequent erosive bone resorption. This can lead to squaring of the vertebral bodies, followed by a gradual ossification of the superficial layers of

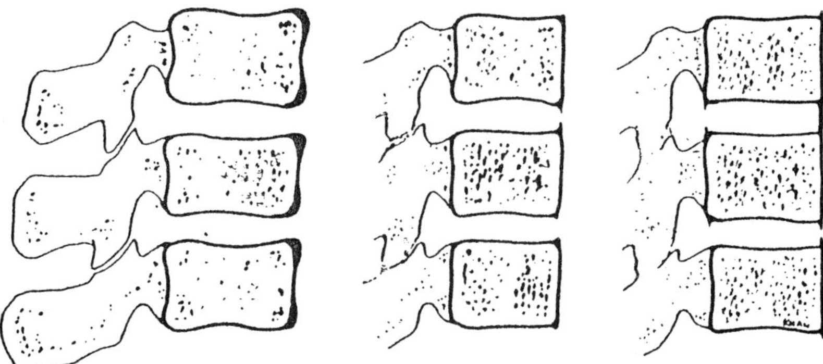

Fig. 3.3 A schematic drawing illustrating progressive changes (from left to right) of ankylosing spondylitis affecting the lumbar spine as visualized on a lateral view. There is a gradual development of syndesmophytes of the marginal type (with eventual bony bridging), fusion of apophyseal joints, and spinal osteoporosis.

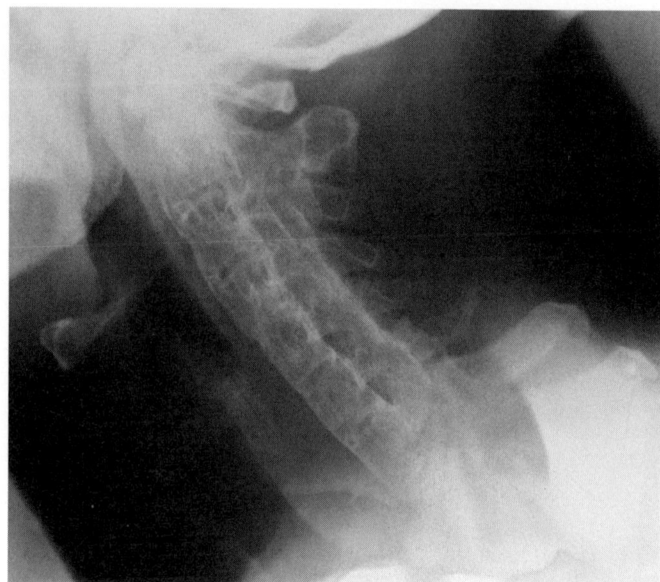

Fig. 3.4 X-ray of cervical spine, lateral view, showing complete fusion. There is also anterior stooping of the neck.

the annulus fibrosus and eventual bridging between vertebrae. These vertical bony bridges are called syndesmophytes (Fig. 3.3). There are often concomitant inflammatory changes and resultant ankylosis in the apophyseal joints, and ossification of some of the spinal ligaments. These processes can ultimately result in virtually complete fusion of the vertebral column in many patients with severe AS of long duration (Fig. 3.4). Spinal osteoporosis is frequently observed in patients with severe long-standing AS. This has been thought to result from ankylosis and lack of mobility. However, the presence of a marked reduction in bone mineral density of the lumbar spine and femoral neck has been reported in a group of young patients with early AS (Will *et al.* 1989), and thus exposure to inflammatory cytokines or some other aspect of the inflammatory process may be involved.

Involvement of the hip joints can lead to symmetrical concentric joint-space narrowing, irregularity of the subchondral bone plate with subchondral sclerosis, osteophyte formation at the outer margins of the articular surfaces of the acetabulum and the femoral head, and ultimately in some cases bony ankylosis. Shoulder girdle involvement can result in concentric joint-space narrowing and, rarely, osseous ankylosis of the glenohumeral joint. Erosions on the superolateral aspect of the humeral head, erosive abnormalities or osseous ankylosis of the acromioclavicular joint, and osseous proliferation (enthesophytes) at the acromial attachment of the acromioclavicular ligament (bearded acromion) are also part of shoulder involvement in AS. There is absence of periarticular or widespread osteopenia in the involved hip or shoulder girdles. Bony erosions and osteitis (whiskering) at sites of osseous attachment of tendons and ligaments are frequently observed. These radiographic findings result from enthesopathic lesions, and are seen particularly at the ischial tuberosities, iliac crest, calcanei, femoral trochanters, and spinous processes of the vertebrae (Resnick and Niwayama 1995).

Radionuclide quantitative scintigraphy, computed tomography (CT), and magnetic resonance imaging (MRI) have been used for evaluating patients with early disease in whom standard radiography of the SI joints may show normal or equivocal changes (Battafarano

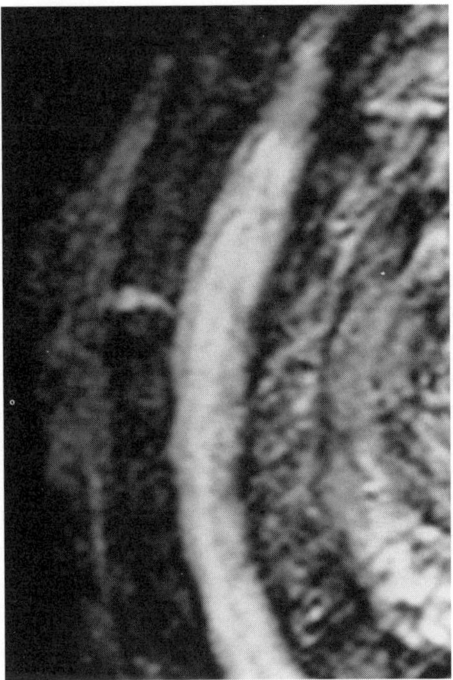

Fig. 3.5 MRI of cervical spine, lateral view, showing transverse fracture of lower cervical spine.

et al. 1993; Ryan and Fogelman 1995). Quantitative scintigraphy has generally been found to be too sensitive and too non-specific to be of much clinical value, while CT is more sensitive and equally specific in the recognition of sacroiliitis when compared with conventional radiography (Khan 1990, Khan and Kushner, 1984). However, CT should only be used for those few patients whose conventional radiographs give normal or equivocal results, and in whom the presence of AS is strongly suspected but cannot be firmly established on clinical grounds alone. MRI in such a clinical situation also produces excellent, although costly, computer-generated imaging, and has the added advantages of a lack of ionizing radiation and the ability to detect early lesions of the articular cartilage and oedema of the adjacent bone marrow. MRI is also very useful in spinal fractures in AS (Fig. 3.5), and for visualizing arachnoid diverticuli in cauda equina syndrome (Tullous *et al.* 1990, Ginsburg *et al.* 1997).

HLA-B27 typing

The clinical use of HLA-B27 typing as an aid to the diagnosis of AS has been discussed elsewhere in detail by the author (Khan 1997*a*, Khan and Khan 1982). HLA-B27 shows a strong association with AS, but the strength of this association and its prevalence in the general population differs appreciably among various ethnic and racial groups (Khan 1995, 1997*b*). The HLA-B27 test has no place as a routine, diagnostic, confirmatory, or screening test for AS in patients presenting with back pain. A large majority of patients with AS can be readily diagnosed clinically on the basis of history, physical examination, and radiographic findings, and they do not need to be tested for HLA-B27. In general, the usefulness of a test depends on the clinical setting in which it is performed. A test that is very valuable in a particular clinical setting might be useless if performed on a random population. The predictive value of a test depends on the pretest estimate that the disease is present in that particular clinical setting. The pretest estimation of the likelihood of the disease presence has to be sought prior to and independent of the test, in order to properly discern the probability that the disease is present once the test result is known. As a rule, in those patients in whom history and physical examination suggest AS, but whose radiographic findings are equivocal, the HLA-B27 test may allow the presumptive diagnosis of AS to be accepted or rejected with greater certainty. In patients with back pain in whom AS is suggested by neither history nor physical examination, HLA-B27 testing is inappropriate; a positive result would still not permit the diagnosis of AS to be made.

Although HLA-B27 typing can define the population at a higher risk for AS and related spondyloarthropathies, it is of very limited practical value for that purpose because no effective means of prevention are currently available. Moreover, most B27-positive persons never develop AS or related diseases. It does not help to distinguish between AS and other spondyloarthropathies, because all these diseases are associated with HLA-B27 (although the strength of the association varies). Differentiation between these diseases is based primarily on clinical grounds. The test is not a useful indicator of the prognosis of AS, although familial aggregation and acute iritis are more common in patients possessing HLA-B27. There are 11 different subtypes of HLA-B27 (B*2701 to B*2711) and the ones that are most prevalent (B*2705, B*2704, B*2702) are equally disease-associated (Feltkamp *et al.* 1996; Khan 1996*a*, 1997*b*). Proper epidemiological studies need to be done to investigate whether there is any preferential association or lack of association with any of the subtypes among the various population groups. Current data indicate that B*2709 among Sardinian Italians and B*2706 in Thailand, Singapore and Indonesia do not show an association with AS and related SpA (see Chapters 2, 12, and 18).

Differential diagnosis

The clinical diagnosis of AS depends primarily on history and physical examination, and is confirmed by radiographic examination (Khan 1992, Khan 1997*a*, Khan and Kushner, 1984). The clinical and radiographic findings can sometimes be minimal in the early stages of the disease. Therefore, a detailed clinical history and a thorough physical examination, particularly of the SI joints and the spine, are critical in making an early diagnosis. Clinical involvement of the SI joints may be evident from palpation or physical stressing of these joints with resultant tenderness or pain. Direct pressure over the SI joint frequently, but not always, elicits pain. Sometimes SI pain may be elicited by pressure over the anterior superior iliac spines, and by compressing the two iliac bones of the pelvis towards each other, or forcing them away from each other, while the patient is lying supine, as has been illustrated by the author elsewhere (Khan 1984; 1997*a*). The pain can also be elicited by maximal flexion of one hip and hyperextension of the other. Maximal flexion, abduction, and external rotation of the hip joints, or compression of the pelvis with the patient lying on the side, or pressing the sacrum forcefully forward when the patient is lying prone can also cause pain if the SI joints are inflamed. If two or more of these manoeuvres elicit pain in the region of the SI joints in a patient with symptoms of inflammatory back pain, the likelihood of the presence of sacroiliitis will be quite strong. These signs may be absent in some patients despite sacroiliitis because the SI joints have strong ligaments that limit motion, and the signs disappear completely in the late stages of the disease, when inflammation is replaced by fibrosis and bony ankylosis.

Chronic back pain and stiffness are the most common presenting symptoms in patients with AS, although a variety of other presentations may antedate back symptoms in many patients. Back pain, however, is very prevalent in the general population, and AS is by no means the most common cause (Khan and Wilber 1997). In non-inflammatory spondylogenic causes of back pain, the symptoms are generally aggravated by activity and relieved by rest, there is no limitation of chest expansion, lateral flexion of the lumbar spine is usually within normal limits, and the ESR is frequently normal. Radiography of the pelvis can be helpful in differentiating AS from other causes of back pain because the likelihood of AS is markedly increased by the presence of bilateral sacroiliitis. However, early sacroiliitis is difficult to identify with certainty by plain radiography, as indicated above. Moreover, sacroiliitis is not unique to AS among the spondyloarthropathies.

In comparing the radiographic features of primary and secondary forms of AS, patients with AS in association with ulcerative colitis and Crohn's disease tend to show radiographic changes identical to those seen in primary AS. Spondylitis that accompanies psoriasis or follows reactive arthritis usually shows subtle differences from primary AS. For example, in primary AS, syndesmophytes usually form in an ascending fashion, initially forming in the lower thoracic and the adjacent lumbar spine and then appearing in the upper thoracic and, ultimately, the cervical spine (Fig. 3.4). In contrast, patients with spondylitis in association with reactive arthritis and psoriasis tend to develop asymmetric, bulky, non-marginal syndesmophytes. In the end, of course, differentiation of these diseases is based much more on the accompanying clinical features rather than on radiographic differences.

At times, other diseases can be confused radiologically with AS, particularly degenerative joint disease and ankylosing hyperostosis. In degenerative joint disease of the spine, changes are seen in discovertebral junctions and apophyseal joints, with adjacent osteophytes. The SI joints are usually normal or show only mild degenerative changes; the erosions and subchondral sclerosis typical of sacroiliitis are absent. In some elderly patients severe degenerative changes of the SI joint, such as joint-space narrowing, subchondral bone sclerosis, and bridging osteophytes in the lower part of the joints may erroneously suggest sacroiliitis.

Ankylosing hyperostosis, also called Forestier's disease or diffuse idiopathic skeletal hyperostosis (DISH), is a condition usually seen in elderly individuals and is characterized by hyperostosis affecting the anterior longitudinal ligament and bony attachments of tendons and ligaments (Khan 1990). It may be radiographically confused with AS. There is no association between HLA-B27 and DISH. Occasionally, in some patients with DISH, severe degenerative and hyperostotic changes of the SI joints, such as joint-space narrowing, subchondral bone sclerosis, and capsular ossifications give a radiographic appearance superficially resembling that of sacroiliitis on anteroposterior view of the pelvis. Chronic treatment with retinoids (synthetic derivatives of vitamin A) for skin disease such as acne and psoriasis can sometimes lead to bone abnormalities mimicking spondyloarthropathies or DISH. The syndesmophytes in those AS patients who have concomitant degenerative disc disease at the time syndesmophytes are forming may also lead to some diagnostic confusion.

Miscellaneous conditions that might be confused with AS because of SI joint involvement or a syndesmophyte-like spinal appearance include fluorosis, chondrocalcinosis, ochronosis, Paget's disease, tuberculous spondylitis, Scheuermann's disease, congenital kyphoscoliosis, and chronic brucellosis. Primary and secondary hyperparathyroidism can lead to irregularity of the SI joint surfaces, particularly on the iliac side, as a result of subchondral resorption and adjacent bony sclerosis; however, narrowing and ankylosis of the joint space do not occur. SI joint changes superficially resembling sacroiliitis, and even complete fusion of these joints, can be observed in paraplegics and quadriplegics. These changes probably do not result from an inflammatory process but may be a consequence of immobility and appear to be related to the duration and level of spinal paralysis. Malignancies should also be considered in the differential diagnosis of back pain, in both young and old individuals. Other causes of back pain include pelvic inflammatory disease, septic (pyogenic) sacroiliitis or discitis, axial osteomalacia or osteoporosis, and sacral insufficiency fractures.

Osteitis condensans ilii, a disorder seen primarily in young multiparous women and quite often asymptomatic, is characterized by radiographic evidence of a triangular area of dense sclerosis in the iliac bones of the pelvis adjacent to the lower half of the SI joints. The SI joints themselves are normal. It is a self-limiting condition that shows no association with HLA-B27, and there is no evidence to indicate that it is a form of AS.

Osteoarticular manifestations of a collection of unusual skin conditions (including acne conglobata, acne fulminans, hidradentitis suppurativa, palmoplantar pustulosis), sternocostoclavicular hyperostosis, and chronic recurrent multifocal osteomyelitis may be nosologically related to (psoriatic) spondyloarthropathy. These manifestations include seronegative asymmetrical oligoarthritis, sacroiliitis, syndesmophytes, enthesopathies, anterior chest-wall involvement, and a possible weak association with HLA-B27. Kahn and his colleagues in France have suggested the eponym: synovitis–acne–pustulosis–hyperostosis–osteomyelitis (SAPHO) syndrome for this entity (Reviewed in Kahn and Khan 1994).

The distinction of AS from rheumatoid arthritis (RA) is usually not difficult. Patients with RA usually have polyarthritis which is symmetrical in distribution and affects small and large joints of the extremities; involvement of the SI, apophyseal, and costovertebral joints is very rare. In AS, on the other hand, any involvement of peripheral joints (other than hip and shoulder joints) is oligoarticular and asymmetrical, affecting more often the larger joints of lower extremities; serological tests for rheumatoid factor are negative; and subcutaneous nodules are absent. Rare instances of concurrent AS and RA have been described.

Disease course

The course of AS is highly variable, but the outcome is generally favourable because the disease is often relatively mild or self-limiting, and responds well to treatment with NSAIDs (Khan and Kushner, 1984; Carette *et al.* 1983). Only rarely does AS show persistent disease activity that results in early and severe disability. Earlier studies suggesting a generally unremitting course of AS primarily consisted of patients with severe disease studied in hospitals or clinics. Good functional capacity and the ability to work are maintained in most patients, even in cases of protracted disease, especially if the patient can avoid carrying heavy loads, prolonged standing, and excessive bending, jarring, and twisting. Those patients with hip-joint involvement or complete ankylosis of the cervical spine with kyphosis are more likely to be disabled. The results of total hip arthroplasty in recent years are very gratifying in preventing partial or total disability in many such patients. Although it is difficult to predict the ultimate prognosis for an individual patient, some factors that influence the overall prognosis include severity in early disease, development of extra-articular complications, stage of disease at the time of diagnosis and initiation of appropriate treatment, quality of management, and the degree of patient compliance with suggested therapy. Clinically diagnosable AS may be three times more common in men than in women in the general population, although the prevalence of sacroiliitis may not differ. The clinical features of AS may not differ between the sexes with regard to spinal symptoms, chest expansion, peripheral arthritis, and extra-articular features, except that males show more pronounced radiological changes and demonstrate radiographically detectable sacroiliitis earlier than females. Although axial disease is more severe in males, the overall pattern seems to be similar in both sexes. Recent evidence indicates that smoking is associated with a poor long term outcome (Averns *et al.* 1996).

An excess mortality of AS patients was observed in the past, and this was ascribed primarily to complications of radiotherapy and amyloidosis. Excess mortality has also been observed among non-irradiated patients seen at treatment centers, but only after more than 20 years subsequent to the diagnosis of AS (Callahan and Pincus 1995; Khan *et al.* 1981). In these studies, the patients had disease severe enough both to impel them to seek specialized care and to be correctly diagnosed at a time when AS was felt to be a rare disease. A population-based study, which included milder cases not seen at referral centres, showed no effect of AS on lifespan (Carter *et al.* 1979). It is quite likely that the survival of those patients with mild disease, who form the majority of patients with AS, is comparable to the general population. However, spinal fracture, surgery, cardiovascular involvement, associated medical conditions—including ulcerative colitis and Crohn's disease—and complications of treatment with NSAIDs, may contribute to premature mortality in some patients.

Management

There is currently no preventive measure or cure for AS, but most patients can be well managed and long-term prognosis has improved in recent years. An early diagnosis, a compliant patient, and a competent physician can substantially influence the outcome for the better (Amor *et al.* 1995*a*, Khan 1993*a*; 1997*a*, Toivanen and Khan 1994). Aspirin seldom provides an adequate therapeutic anti-inflammatory effect. NSAIDs should be used regularly in full therapeutic anti-inflammatory dose during the active phase of the disease. Compliance with this regimen requires deliberate patient education, since otherwise the drugs are likely to be used occasionally and for their analgesic effect only. The responses to NSAIDs vary among patients, as do the side-effects, and it is worthwhile searching out the best alternative NSAID for each patient. Although phenylbutazone (Butazolidin) is probably the most effective NSAID for AS patients, it is not used in the USA because of its potentially greater risk of bone-marrow toxicity, while in the UK it can only be prescribed by rheumatologists in hospital practice and for those patients with severe disease who have not responded adequately to other NSAIDs. The NSAIDs that are most commonly used in the USA include indomethacin, naproxen, diclofenac, or sulindac. There are additional NSAIDs that may be equally effective in AS, but they are not currently approved by the Food and Drug Administration (FDA) for such use.

When the disease is not being adequately controlled by NSAIDs, or for those intolerant to such drugs, sulphasalazine may be effective in some AS patients, particularly those with peripheral arthritis, but it has no appreciable influence on the persistence of axial disease and peripheral enthesopathy (Lehtinen *et al.* 1995). Because of its efficacy in inflammatory bowel disease and psoriasis, it would appear to be especially useful for AS associated with those diseases. With regard to agents used in other rheumatic diseases, D-penicillamine is ineffective, and antimalarial drugs and gold have not been well studied in AS, but appear to have no role. A few patients with severe AS with peripheral joint involvement unresponsive to NSAIDs and sulphasalazine have responded to oral methotrexate therapy (Creemers *et al.* 1994*b*; Creemers *et al.* 1995, Amor *et al.* 1995*b*). Oral corticosteroids have no therapeutic value in the long-term management of the musculoskeletal aspects of AS because of their serious side-effects, and they do not halt disease progression.

Recalcitrant enthesitis and persistent synovitis may respond quite well to a local corticosteroid injection, and the therapeutic contribution of steroid injections into the sacroiliac joints is being evaluated (Braun *et al.* 1996; Cunnane *et al.* 1996). There seems to be a consensus that spinal radiotherapy has no role in the modern management of patients with AS because of the high risk of leukaemia and aplastic anaemia. None the less, there are occasional uncontrolled reports of the efficacy of low-dose external beam radiotherapy on persistent peripheral enthesitis and synovitis resistant to standard treatments (Popert *et al.* 1996). Splints, braces, and corsets are generally not helpful and are not advised. There is no special diet and there is no evidence that any specific food has something to do with the initiation or exacerbation of AS, unconfirmed claims to the contrary (for example, Ebringer and Wilson 1996) notwithstanding. Pregnancy does not usually affect the symptoms of AS, and fertility, the course of pregnancy, and childbirth have been reported to be normal (Gran and Husby 1990).

Regular exercises are of fundamental importance in preventing or minimizing deformity (Gall 1994). Spinal extension exercises and deep-breathing exercises should be done routinely once or twice daily, and smoking should be avoided. The patient should keep the spine as straight as possible, walk erect, avoid prolonged stooped posture, and sleep on a firm mattress with as thin a pillow as possible. Formal physiotherapy is especially of value in teaching the patient the proper posture, appropriate exercises, and recreational sports, and in making sure that the exercise programme is maintained. Group exercise sessions that include hydrotherapy are very helpful. Regular swimming is considered to be one of the best exercises for AS patients.

Acute anterior uveitis, discussed in detail in Chapter 10, can usually be managed with dilatation of the pupil and use of corticosteroid eye drops, and rarely requires periocular or systemic corticosteroids (Careless and Inman 1995). Interestingly, during a recent double-blind, placebo-controlled, 6-month study of sulphasalazine in the treatment of spondyloarthropathies, acute anterior uveitis was less frequent among those taking this medicine than those on placebo (Dougados *et al.* 1995*a*).

Total hip arthroplasty gives very good results, and prevents partial or total disability from severe hip disease. Vertebral wedge osteotomy may be needed for correction of severe kyphosis in some patients, although it carries a relatively high risk of paraplegia. Cardiac complications may require aortic valve replacement or pacemaker implantation. Infected apical pulmonary fibrosis is not easy to manage; surgical resection may rarely be required.

Many patients may have difficulty driving an automobile because of their impaired neck mobility, and special wide-view mirrors can be very helpful. Similarly, special prism glasses can help improve the field of view of patients who are so kyphotic that they cannot look ahead while walking. There are many patient support groups that enlist enthusiastic patient co-operation, provide information about the disease, and advice about life and health insurance, jobs, the working environment, wide-view mirrors, and other useful items (See Chapter 17).

4 Reactive arthritis and Reiter's syndrome—the clinical spectrum

Andrei Calin

Introduction

Reactive arthropathy and Reiter's syndrome are two terms that are used more or less interchangeably. The latter defines a triad or more of features, while the former relates to the inflammatory joint process and relationship to infection. In theory, reactive arthropathy may be defined as an inflammatory arthropathy distant in time and place from the original inciting infection, which is usually in the bowel or genitourinary tract. More recently, we have come to suspect that respiratory organisms can also precipitate disease and, of more importance, we accept that the synovial joint is not free of bacterial insult. As discussed elsewhere, there is growing evidence that fragments of organisms and antigenic determinants are found within the joint cavity or synovial tissues. The importance of this phenomenon and the relationship to potential antibiotic therapy remains unclear but of paramount interest and importance.

During the 1970s and 1980s, the significance of Reiter's syndrome transcended its incidence, prevalence, and intriguing natural history. The focus on the disease related, in part, to the striking relationship between a specific infective trigger (shigella, salmonella, and other organisms), and the specific genetic background (HLA-B27) together with a clearly defined acute or chronic natural history. There are few areas in medicine where these three aspects come together so precisely.

For the purpose of this discussion, we will use reactive arthritis as an umbrella term for those with the arthropathy alone, or the extra-articular stigmata that make up the spectrum of Reiter's disease.

Historical background

A review of the literature (Calin 1984) takes us from the Old Testament book of Leviticus (Chapter 15, vs. 2) to 1997. No doubt exciting developments will occur during the coming years. Leviticus described an individual with a urethral discharge, but there is no clinical follow-up as to whether he developed eye disease, skin involvement, or indeed arthropathy. Stoll, in 1776, was the first to describe the triad of urethritis and conjunctivitis following dysentery, while Sir Benjamin Brodie, in 1818, found the same to be true following venereal infection. The story was next taken up in 1916 by Reiter on the Balkan front, and the French physicians, Fiessenger and Leroy, on the Somme, who described 'spirochaetosis arthritica' on the one hand, and 'conjunctival–urethral–synovial syndrome' on the other. Given the more recent evidence of the Lyme borrelia causing both an infective and reactive arthropathy, it is intriguing to speculate whether Reiter's description of the 'hitherto unrecognised spirochaetal arthritis' may indeed have been Lyme disease, rather than what we now recognize as Reiter's disease itself! (Toivanen and Toivanen 1995 *a,b*).

Two major epidemics of reactive arthritis have played a major role in our understanding of the disease process. The first was described by Paronen in 1948 and the second by Noer in 1966. Both resulted in follow-up publications which throw light on the natural history of the disorder. Specifically, Paronen described an epidemic in Finland of *Shigella flexneri*, during which 344 subjects developed Reiter's syndrome. In the second, Noer reported on nine cases of Reiter's disease, that developed among 602 crew members with shigella dysentery. None of those who remained free of the original infection developed arthropathy. The original Paronen epidemic of 1944 was reviewed 20 years later (Sairanen *et al.* 1969). At follow-up, 100 of the original 344 were available for study (no doubt including a bias towards those with more severe disease). Of these, 80 still had active disease and the group included 32 with ankylosing spondylitis, 18 with a recurrent acute arthropathy, and 30 with chronic joint disease. In addition, seven had recurrent uveitis and two aortic regurgitation. Some 40 (over 10% of the original) were unemployable because of persistent active disease. In turn, we followed up Noer's original study (Noer 1966) and found that four of the five traceable patients had active and severe disease 13 years after the original epidemic. All four had persistent joint problems, two had deteriorating vision, and two had ankylosing spondylitis.

Elsewhere, we studied 131 consecutive endemic patients at a University and Community Medical Centre, and at a mean follow-up of 5.6 years, found that 122 (93%) were still available for follow-up (Fox *et al.* 1979). Polyarthropathy persisted in 83% of cases, urethritis and/or cervicitis in 42%, back pain and heel pain in about 50%, eye disease in 33%, and balanitis with mouth ulcers in 25%. Over 25% were either unemployable or forced to change occupation. A chronic course was also described in a followup study (Leirisalo-Repo *et al.* 1982), in which 68% of 160 patients with Reiter's syndrome had chronic joint symptoms and 16% had chronic destructive peripheral arthritis. A much more favorable outcome was described in a recent community-based study from Norway (Glennas *et al.* 1994), in which almost all patients with reactive arthritis recovered.

In summary, therefore, reactive arthropathy/Reiter's syndrome is a major chronic rheumatic disease, and although many such individuals will have a self-limiting disorder, the prognosis is varied and can be relentlessly progressive.

Definition

Reiter's syndrome may be defined in many different ways. For example, one could rely, as originally suggested, on the classical triad of urethritis, arthritis, and conjunctivitis/iritis. Alternatively, a working diagnosis has been suggested as summarized in Table 4.1. (Calin a 1984). A working party provided preliminary criteria under the auspices of the American Rheumatism Association (ARA) (Willkens *et al.* 1981); an episode of arthritis within four weeks of a bowel or sexually acquired infection, but this suggestion has never been widely followed. In addition, the European approach of the Spondylarthropathy Study Group (ESSG) is given in Chapter 1, Table 3, while Amor (1991) provides a different framework (Table 4, Chapter 1).

In summary, an individual with a seronegative asymmetrical arthropathy which is predominantly of the lower extremity, plus one or more of urethritis or cervicitis, dysentery,

Table 4.1 Working definition of Reiter's syndrome

Seronegative asymmetrical arthropathy (predominantly lower extremity)
Plus one or more of
Urethritis–cervicitis
Dysentery
Inflammatory eye disease
Mucocutaneous disease
Balanitis
Oral ulceration
Keratodermia
Exclusions: Primary AS PsA, other RD[a]

[a] AS, ankylosing spondylitis; PsA, psoriatic arthropathy; RD, rheumatic disease.

inflammatory eye disease, or mucocutaneous problem has Reiter's disease. This definition is simple and readily applicable and would certainly satisfy the definition for reactive arthritis. Inevitably there are exceptions. For example, an individual may develop gonococcal urethritis followed by an inflammatory or mechanical arthropathy of unrelated aetiology. Nevertheless, in the subcommittee's experience the sensitivity and specificity of the criteria were over 85%. Needless to say, difficulties arise with women, in whom urethritis or cervicitis can be missed.

Other terms such as sexually acquired reactive arthropathy and incomplete Reiter's syndrome have been popularized, but the former suffers from an implicit criticism of social activity, while the latter suggests that there exists a 'complete Reiter's picture'. As we become bacteriologically more sophisticated, specific labels will be used such as post-chlamydial arthropathy, post-salmonella arthritis, and other labels depending on the defining genus. Another concern regarding the concept of 'sexually acquired reactive arthropathy' relates to the fact that individuals with shigella, salmonella, or other bowel infections can develop an arthropathy associated with a urethritis, the latter being clearly unrelated to sexual activity, but rather an 'allergic' event.

Various *formes frustes* of Reiter's syndrome are recognized, such as persistent balanitis or calcaneodynia, in the absence of other stigmata.

Incidence and prevalence

The incidence and prevalence of Reiter's syndrome/reactive arthritis are difficult to assess for the following reasons:

1. There is no diagnostic test that defines all cases.
2. The arthropathy tends to affect young adults, members of a mobile community, who are often difficult to follow.
3. The early genitourinary features of the disease may be suppressed or forgotten, and the patient carries a diagnostic label of undifferentiated arthropathy, or other non-specific entity.

4. The enteric features may have been minimal or ignored.
5. Many individuals with an inflammatory reactive arthropathy have neither urethral nor bowel symptoms, and only sophisticated laboratory tests can suggest a recent sexually acquired or bowel infection.
6. Several diagnostically significant features of the disease are clinically minimal or inapparent. For example, mouth ulcers, balanitis, and urethritis or cervicitis may all be overshadowed by the more severe arthritic component.
7. Non-specific, but clinically significant, features may be overlooked such as eye or skin signs. For example, the latter may be misdiagnosed as fungal disease or psoriasis rather than the keratodermia of Reiter's syndrome.
8. Urethritis, which is often difficult to recognize in the male, is frequently impossible to establish with certainty in the female.
9. Cervicitis, likewise, is non-specific, and often asymptomatic. It may not be identified as a relevant feature in a woman, presenting with, for example, a swollen ankle.
10. In chronic cases, those with a persistent arthropathy are often misdiagnosed as having a seronegative rheumatoid arthritis, given that the chronicity of reactive arthritis is not generally well established.
11. Because of the overlap between the various members of the spondylarthritides, some patients, considered to have ankylosing spondylitis as a primary event with secondary peripheral arthropathy, may in fact have started with the arthritis of a reactive nature or Reiter's disease itself, which in turn has developed into ankylosing spondylitis.
12. Even in individuals with the classical triad of urethritis, arthritis, and iritis, the eye or urethral symptoms may have preceded the arthropathy by days or weeks, or the eye problem may occur at a later stage. Thus, those expecting the classical triad to be contemporaneous in nature may be disappointed.
13. Because Reiter's syndrome is a multisystem disorder, care is often fragmented and the patient may be followed independently by the ophthalmologist, orthopaedic surgeon, rheumatologist, genitourinary physician, orthodontist, or other subspecialist.

Nevertheless, it is often claimed that one of the most common forms of inflammatory arthropathy in a young man is indeed reactive arthritis/Reiter's syndrome. The same may well be true in a woman.

Csonka (1958, 1960) stated that Reiter's syndrome develops in about 1% of subjects with non-specific urethritis, and many of the more recent epidemiological studies have confirmed that reactive arthritis develops in 1–3% of individuals with infective diarrhoea. Thus, some 20% of those with HLA-B27 appear to be at risk of developing arthropathy following contact with the inciting organism (Kaslow *et al.* 1979). Why the other 80% are protected remains unknown. Clearly, HLA-B27 itself is not sufficient, (at least 20–30% being HLA-B27 negative), and other factors, most likely genetic, are decisive (Kaslow *et al.* 1981).

Geographic distribution

In large part, reactive arthropathy has a worldwide distribution, roughly following the prevalence of HLA-B27 (Khan 1995). Presumably, depending on genetic and other factors, certain individuals will develop a reactive arthropathy after an inciting infection, whereas others will have the full-blown picture of Reiter's disease on the one hand, or perhaps ankylosing spondylitis on the other. In certain areas of sub-Saharan Africa, reactive arthropathy has become much more prevalent with the advent of widespread HIV infection and is unrelated to B27 (Njobvu *et al.*, 1997; Davis and Stein 1991) (see chapter 2). The prevalence is also particularly high in certain circumpolar populations such as the Inuit Eskimo (Erdesz *et al.* 1994). Whether this relates to the genetic make-up alone, or a higher prevalence of sexually acquired or other infection, or both, is unclear. By contrast, reactive arthropathy and spondylarthropathy are exceptionally rare in West Africa, except in conjunction with HIV infection (Brown *et al.* 1996*b*; Mijiyawa 1993).

Sex distribution

Given the difficulty in defining the syndrome in women, the sex distribution remains difficult to determine. In the past, it was said that 20 males were affected for every female, but we now know that sex distribution is much nearer unity. In our report of 131 patients, 15% were women (Fox *et al.*, 1979), but it may well be that postdysenteric Reiter's syndrome/reactive arthritis has an equal sex distribution and that for many women with oligoarticular inflammatory disease, the diagnosis is simply missed. That sexually acquired reactive arthritis is more common in men than women may relate to the simple fact that non-specific urethritis itself occurs more frequently in men.

Age distribution

Urethritis is difficult to recognize in children and there are few documented cases of Reiter's syndrome in this age group. However, it is clear that in the epidemic setting of dysentery, with many family members affected, children only rarely are affected (Kaslow *et al.* 1981). The reason for this is unclear.

The peak age at onset is probably in the third decade, but no age group is exempt and onset of disease in the sixth decade or later does occur. Children with the so-called seronegative enthesopathic arthropathy syndrome with features that occur both in Reiter's syndrome and adult spondylarthritis do exist, but on the whole these evolve into ankylosing spondylitis rather than recurrent Reiter's disease.

Aetiology

Environmental considerations

Although reactive arthropathy has been considered to occur in two forms—the epidemic or postenteric on the one hand, and the endemic or postvenereal on the other, this artificial grouping may be untenable since some patients do not fall so readily into one or other of these categories. For example, there are individuals who develop a reactive arthropathy that relates to one of the classical triggers but in whom neither bowel nor genitourinary symptoms have occurred. Moreover, the distinction between urethritis as a precipitating factor and urethritis as an integral manifestation of the postdysenteric syndrome remains unclear. It is certain that urethritis, itself, can be a reactive rather than infective phenomenon (Paronen 1948). What determines the chronicity of reactive arthritis is also uncertain. Whether additional infective triggers are required to maintain the ongoing disease activity is unknown, although there are certainly documented cases where reinfection has precipitated a flare of disease. For the rest, the immune response is presumably self-generating. The list of aetiological agents associated with reactive arthritis is given in Chapter 11.

Epidemic Reiter's syndrome

There have been several clearly defined epidemics of postenteric reactive arthritis. Paronen's patients were known to have *Shigella flexneri* dysentery, but the specific shigella serotype was not defined. We recognize (Kaslow *et al.* 1981) that *Shigella flexneri* serotype 1b and 2a are both arthritogenic, but in spite of only the very occasional case report of *Shigella sonnei* causing arthritis the organism appears to be virtually trouble-free in terms of a succeeding arthritis. For example, in our controlled follow-up study of an epidemic of *Shigella sonnei* in Puerto Rico, no cases of Reiter's syndrome occurred (Kaslow *et al.* 1979). As discussed elsewhere, salmonella, yersinia, campylobacter, and other organisms have all been associated with reactive arthritis.

Postsexually acquired reactive arthritis

Chlamydia is certainly the most common aetiological factor, although ureaplasma has also been incriminated.

Genetic considerations

Since 1973, when Brewerton and colleagues first defined the association between HLA-B27 and Reiter's syndrome, there have been numerous studies addressing this phenomenon. The first included patients with 'non-specific' urethritis and thus no definitive organism. We looked at patients with epidemic Reiter's syndrome following Noer's original outbreak and confirmed that shigella-induced arthropathy was also B27-associated, thus defining a specific link between a recognized infective trigger and a well-defined genetic background (Calin and Fries 1976). This was also confirmed in a followup study of the 1944 epidemic in Finland (Sairanen and Tiilikainen 1975).

It has long been recognized that the Haida Native Americans, for example, with a high prevalence of HLA-B27, predominantly develop ankylosing spondylitis as do the Pima Indians, whereas other ethnic groups such as the Inuit Eskimos or Navaho Indians appear to be more likely to develop a reactive arthropathy/Reiter's syndrome type of picture. This difference presumably relates to additional gene or genes, defining the specific phenotypic expression, although environmental factors may be of at least equal importance in these particular populations.

Likewise, in Caucasian families, it appears that reactive arthropathy appears to 'run in some families', while ankylosing spondylitis does so in others, again arguing for the phenotypic expression being under genetic control (Calin *et al.* 1984).

Clinical features

Almost every system in the body can be affected by Reiter's syndrome. The prevalence of the various features is difficult to ascertain precisely since different authors have used different

Table 4.2 Reiter's syndrome characteristics at diagnosis (n = 131)

	%
Arthritis:	
Mono	4
Poly	96
Urethritis/Cervicitis	90
Diarrhoea	18
Eye disease	63
Back pain	72
Heel pain	56
Tendinitis	52
Mucocutaneous–oral	27
Balanitis	46
Nails	6
Keratodermia	22

From Fox *et al.* 1979

definitions for the condition—some only making the diagnosis when the full triad of features was present. In our study of 131 patients (Fox *et al.* 1979) 4% had a monoarthropathy and 96% polyarthritis, with 90% having urethritis or cervicitis, 18% diarrhoea, 63% inflammatory eye disease, 72% back pain, 56% heel pain, 52% tendinitis, 27% mucocutaneous changes in the mouth, 46% with balanitis, 6% nail changes, and 22% keratodermia (Table 4.2) (also see Leirisalo *et al.* 1982; Leirisalo-Repo *et al.* 1987, 1988; and Glennas *et al.* 1994).

Every patient presenting with a mono- or an oligoarticular arthropathy, especially if the lower limb joints are involved, must be questioned about possible urethritis, balanitis, eye disease, and mouth ulcers. A previous history of bowel change, even in the absence of obvious diarrhoea, must be sought, and likewise any possibility of a sexually acquired infection. The urethritis is frequently minimal from the patient's point of view. Some stinging on passing urine, or a small discharge may have been noticed by the patient, but perhaps only after being alerted by direct questioning may such a finding become obvious. Balanitis is rarely evident unless the prepuce is retracted, and stomatitis is usually asymptomatic and only apparent on close inspection. A minimally inflamed eye is easily forgotten or passed off as a reaction to irritating fumes. The various skin lesions typified by keratodermia blenorrhagica may not be seen until later in the course of the disease, and may be then considered as a non-specific fungal infection or due to psoriasis. The two most important features—that of diarrhoea or urethritis—are frequently missed, the latter because of the patient's natural diffidence in disclosing such an event, and the former because symptoms are so often minimal.

The typical latent period between the infective process and the rheumatological syndrome is 1–3 weeks, but studies of chlamydia-induced reactive arthritis have shown that much longer intervals are not uncommon (see Chapter 6). Conjunctivitis or uveitis may be seen, followed perhaps by tendinitis, arthralgias, or frank arthritis. As discussed above, the urethritis that can follow an episode of diarrhoea should be considered a reactive rather than an infective phenomenon. Although less common, diarrhoea and endoscopically evident mucosal abnormalities can also occur in those who clearly have sexually acquired reactive arthritis—see Chapter 9.

Arthritis

Until the late 1970s, the arthritis of Reiter's disease was often considered to be acute, short-lived, and transient. Indeed, the fortunate patient does have such a self-limiting process. Frequently, however, patients are seen with a persistent or recurrent rather than transient arthropathy. Arthralgia, monoarthritis, polyarthritis, tendinitis, tenosynovitis, fasciitis, and spinal symptoms occur. Weight-bearing joints, particularly the knees and ankles, are most frequently involved. The arthritis may be florid, with large effusions, and knee involvement has been known to result in popliteal rupture early in the course of the disease, before the capsule thickens. The 'sausage' digit or dactylitis represents a typical lesion, the extrasynovial swelling associated with dactylitis characterizes the enthesopathic nature of the disease process. Patients frequently complain primarily of ankle or heel pain. Why Reiter's syndrome preferentially involves the Achilles tendon, plantar fascia, and ankle and subtalar joints remains unknown.

Ligament, tendon, and fascial problems

Achilles tendinitis, planter fasciitis, chest-wall pain, and other problems including back pain, frequently occur in Reiter's disease. One can assume that symptoms relate to an insertional tendinitis, or enthesopathic change, as described by Ball (1971) and later by Bywaters (1984). Indeed, intercostal muscle insertional tendinitis can present with a pleuritic-type of chest pain and such individuals may be inappropriately investigated for intrathoracic disease.

Urogenital lesions

Urethritis may present a minor or severe problem. Acute haemorrhagic cystitis has been recognized, and there are suggestions that at least the urethral component can respond to long-term antibiotic therapy. There are few data relating to the possible association with prostatitis and epididymitis.

Ocular lesions (see Chapter 10)

Conjunctivitis is recognized as part of the classical triad of Reiter's syndrome. However, patients may have pure conjunctivitis, a conjunctival reaction to uveitis, iritis alone, or a mixture. The symptoms may be mild (minimal redness and/or discharge) and escape notice, or a major component (severe photophobia, eye pain) of the disorder. It is recognized that approximately one-third to one-half of patients presenting to an ophthalmologist with acute uveitis have an underlying rheumatological disorder. The eye disease may become the most significant problem, causing serious debility (that is to say a panophthalmitis with deteriorating vision or even blindness).

Mucocutaneous manifestations (see Calin 1979)

Why the skin should be involved in Reiter's syndrome is unknown. Keratodermia blennorrhagica has been recognized for 100 years, and occurs predominantly on the soles of the feet, the toes, palms of the hand, and the glans penis, together with the shaft. Discrete lesions may, in fact, be found anywhere on the limbs or scrotum, trunk, and scalp. Very rarely, whole-body involvement occurs with exfoliation. Macroscopically, the skin lesions begin as discrete vesicles that become opaque as their walls thicken. Hyperkeratotic nodules result. There may be an erythematous base around the lesion, with little evidence of local inflammation. The vesicles may coalesce, resulting in a hyperkeratotic crust that lasts for days, weeks, or longer. They can then disappear without trace, but frequently recur.

Microscopically, the lesions cannot be distinguished from those of psoriasis. The characteristic changes include hyper- and parakeratosis with elongation of the rete pegs. Spongiform pustules are found in the upper Malpighian layer with varying degrees of polymorphonuclear leucocyte infiltration. Well-defined microabscesses occur.

There is no specific treatment for these skin lesions, although anecdotal reports suggest that methotrexate or azathioprine can have a favourable effect on the lesions. Mouth ulcers are intriguing in view of their asymptomatic nature. They can appear on the palate, tongue, buccal mucosa, and lips. They start as shallow ulcers, sometimes with an irregular erythematous base. Therapy is not required.

Circinate balanitis occurs as a painless superficial erosion on the glans penis—the lesions coalescing to form a circinate pattern. The coronal margin of the prepuce and adjacent glans are most frequently affected. In circumcised individuals, the lesions develop a hard crust in contrast to uncircumcised patients, where the lesions remain moist and may develop secondary infection. Balanitis can predate other manifestations of Reiter's syndrome and can be considered as a *forme fruste* of Reiter's disease—particularly in B27-positive individuals (Lassus 1975).

Nail involvement may be seen in association with keratodermia, or it may occur as a separate entity. Subungual corny material accumulates and may lift the nail plate, which becomes yellow and thickened. The brittle nail may shed. Inflammatory areas in the skin adjacent to the subungual hyperkeratotic material may mimic paronychiae.

Late sequelae of disease

The natural history of reactive arthritis ranges from a self-limiting minor arthropathy lasting for a few days to long-term catastrophic disease with spinal rigidity, loss of vision, heart involvement, and death. Naturally, there are numerous steps in between. Some individuals with an episode of arthropathy have asymptomatic asymmetrical sacroiliitis, whereas another individual may have an hitherto unrecognized degree of aortic regurgitation. Fusion of joints, particular in the ankle and foot, is not uncommon.

Spinal disease

Some 20% of individuals with B27-positive Reiter's disease develop unilateral or bilateral sacroiliitiis and even the full-blown picture of ankylosing spondylitis. There are relatively few long-term follow-up studies of those presenting simply with a monoarthropathy, but a small percentage of such individuals will progress to develop spinal symptoms, or may be found to have sacroilitis at the start of their illness. Those with long-standing recurrent disease have a higher prevalence of spinal involvement. Whether the spinal disease should be considered a complication of Reiter's syndrome or a manifestation of HLA-B27 disease remains unclear. The fact that the spinal disease is said to occur more frequently in those with severe Reiter's syndrome, and that the involvement may be asymmetrical (McEwen *et al.* 1971) would suggest that the process is related to the Reiter's disease itself, rather than to the underlying genetic background. Moreover, one can see ankylosing spondylitis develop in the patient with chronic Reiter's syndrome at an age of onset that is older than that usually seen in primary ankylosing spondylitis. This is analagous to the situation where patients with inflammatory bowel disease may develop sacroiliitis and spondylitis only after the fifth or sixth decade. Whether a B27-positive individual who develops Reiter's syndrome is more likely to develop sacroiliitis and ankylosing spondylitis than an otherwise healthy B27-positive subject, is not certain, but this would appear to be the case. The typical features of the back pain in such individuals include gradual onset of predominantly early morning stiffness, discomfort after prolonged periods of rest, and improvement with exercise. There may be decreased spinal mobility and these symptoms and signs can occur before radiological change.

Late eye disease

Progressive iridocyclitis with other problems (eg panophthalmitis) can occur in Reiter's disease. Blindness may result.

Cardiovascular disease

Involvement of the heart is well recognized. Electrocardiographic changes include prolongation of the PR interval, complete heart block, S–T segment changes, and abnormal Q waves. The patient may develop palpitations, transient murmurs, pericardial rub, and aortic regurgitation. This last complication is clinically and histologically identical to that seen in ankylosing spondylitis. Clinically inapparent heart changes may also be seen with the use of more sophisticated equipment (Tucker *et al.* 1982; Good 1974; Paulus *et al.* 1972).

Central nervous system involvement

The presence of neurological complications is in the region of 1%. These include peripheral neuropathy, transient hemiplegia, cranial nerve lesions, and other non-specific changes (Oates and Hancock 1959; Good 1974).

Pulmonary complications

Pleurisy and pulmonary infiltrates have been described. Since patients with Reiter's syndrome may have insertional tendinitis of the intercostal muscles and ligaments, a pleuritic-like chest-wall pain may occur. Likewise, the costochondral joints can be involved.

Miscellaneous complications

In rare instances, purpura, thrombophlebitis, amyloidosis, and other entities have been described. The majority of patients have fatigue, malaise, and weight loss, while some have fever suggesting an infective aetiology (Wright and Moll 1976*a*).

Radiological evaluation

There are no characteristic radiological changes found early in the active arthritis of Reiter's syndrome. However, given the genetic background of the individual, sacroiliitis may be apparent often without the patient's knowledge. With progression of disease, juxta-articular osteoporosis, narrowing of the joint spaces, and erosive changes may occur. Periosteal reaction is seen particularly around the pelvis, metatarsals, tarsal bones, phalanges, and elsewhere. New bone formation is also found at the insertion of the plantar fascia. The plantar spurs are fluffy with a poorly defined margin, in contrast to the clearly demarcated edge of the mechanical spurs.

In time, the asymmetrical sacroiliitis may become symmetrical with spread up the spine, involving the apophyseal joints. Ankylosis can result. There are more likely to be skip lesions present in reactive arthritis and in psoriatic arthropathy, in contrast to the situation in primary ankylosing spondylitis where the progressive radiological change is seen from the lower to the upper spine (Calin 1996, Guerra and Resnick 1984). Naturally, more expensive forms of imaging, such as CT and MRI, will reveal more widespread evidence of disease. For example, plain radiography may miss the subtle changes of sacroiliitis seen on MRI or CT.

Laboratory evaluation

The erythrocyte sedimentation rate can vary from normality to 130—there appearing to be little correlation between the laboratory mediators of inflammation and the disease process. Mild anaemia may be present, and immune complexes have been described in some two-thirds of patients (Rosenbaum *et al.* 1981). Synovial fluid analysis is rarely contributory to the differential diagnosis, since the white cell count may range from 500 to 50 000 cells/mm^3. Indeed, the synovial fluid can appear cloudy and purulent, but culture reveals no viable organism.

HLA-B27

As discussed throughout this text, B27 is of major interest in terms of disease pathogenesis. However, routine typing for the B27 antigen is usually unnecessary and inappropriate. Up to 80% of individuals with reactive arthritis are B27 positive, and therefore at least 20% do not carry this antigen, and so the diagnosis must often depend on clinical acumen rather than the presence of this genetic marker.

Pathology

Synovial biopsy changes are non-specific and show inflammatory cells with oedema, vascular congestion, and infiltration with neutrophils, lymphocytes, and plasma cells. There may be proliferation of synoviocytes and fibroblasts. These changes are quite similar to those seen in rheumatoid arthritis, apart from the absence of germinal centres (Bywaters 1984).

Many of the clinical features of Reiter's syndrome can be explained by the enthesopathic nature of the disease. Whereas inflammation of the synovium is central to the disease process of rheumatoid arthritis, inflammation at the site of ligament and capsule insertion is the focus for disease activity in Reiter's Syndrome. Typical examples of this enthesopathic process include insertional tendinitis of the Achilles tendon, dactylitis with juxtra-articular inflammation, and radiological evidence of periostitis, peri-insertional osteoporotic change, erosions, and plantar spurs.

Table 4.3 Reiter's syndrome (RS) and gonococcal arthropathy (GcA) compared

	RS	vs	GcA[a]
Polyarthritis	+[a]		+
Tenosynovitis	+		+
Conjunctivitis[a]	+		+
Urethritis	+		+
Skin lesions	+		+
Fever	+		+
Uveitis[a]	+		—
Urethritis	+		+
Gc culture			
Urethra	?+		+
Joint	—		+
Skin	—		+
Synovial fluid	variable		variable
White blood cell count			
HLA-B27	≤ 80%		7%
History of previous arthritis	+		—
Family history of arthritis	+		—
Back pain	+		—
Migratory arthralgias	—		+
Joint distribution[b]	L > U		U = L
Achilles tendinitis	+		+
Calcaneal symptoms plantar fasciitis	+		—
Massive recurrent knee effusion (> 100 ml)	+		—
Oral lesions	+		—
Balanitis	+		—
Palmar–plantar macules	+		—
Keratodermia blenorrhagica	+		—
Response to antibiotics appropriate for GC	—		+

[a] Conjunctivitis may occur in GcA, particularly in the homosexual community.
[b] L, lower; U, upper

Differential diagnosis

When Reiter's syndrome presents with a triad or tetrad of features, there should be no problem in reaching a correct diagnosis. However, if only a single joint is involved, then the differential diagnosis must include infective arthropathy, crystal disease, and other disorders. The most common cause of an oligoarticular inflammatory arthropathy in a young male is Reiter's syndrome, and although gonococcal disease provides a diagnostic dilemma, this is more prevalent in women. The similarities and differences between the two disorders are summarized in Table 4.3. Since both of the conditions can be sexually acquired, a coincidental positive culture for the gonococcus may be found in Reiter's syndrome. As discussed above, B27 typing is frequently unhelpful, and should not be used to confirm or refute a diagnosis.

Psoriatic arthropathy and Reiter's syndrome have many features in common, and these are summarized in Table 4.4.

Table 4.4 Comparison between Reiter's syndrome and psoriatic arthropathy

	Reiter's syndrome	Psoriatic arthropathy
Peripheral joint disease	+	+
Axial disease	25%	25%
Eye disease	+	+
Skin disease	+	+
Nail involvement	+	+
HLA-B27	⩽ 80%	20–50%
Sex	10 M:1 F	3 F:2 M
Age (years)	20–30	Any age
Onset	Acute	Insidious
HLA	B27	B27, B13, Bw17, Bw38, Cw6
Skin lesions	Plantar, palmar, penile	Widespread
Relationship of arthritis to severity of skin lesions	None	Good
Mouth ulcers	Yes	No
Urethritis	Yes	No
Joint predilection	Lower limb	Upper limb
Distal interphalangeal joints	Rare	Frequent

Table 4.5 Similarities between ankylosing spondylitis (AS) and Reiter's syndrome (RS)

	AS	RS
Sex	M > F	M > F
Age (years)	15 & up	15 & up
Uveitis	++	++
Prostatitis	Common	Common
Peripheral joints	Lower limb often	Lower limb often
Sacroiliitis	Always	Often
Plantar spurs	? Common	Common
Rheumatoid factor	—	—
HLA-B27	+	+
Enthesopathy	+	+
Aortic regurgitation	+	+
Indomethacin–phenylbutazone therapy	+++	+++
Risk for HLA-B27 individual	⩽ 10%[a]	?20%

[a] Depending upon family history.

Table 4.6 Differences between ankylosing spondylitis (AS) and Reiter's syndrome (RS)

	AS	RS
Onset	Gradual	Sudden
Urethritis	—	+++
Conjunctivitis	—	+
Uveitis	+	++
Skin involvement	—	+
Mucous membranes	—	+
Peripheral joints	25%	90%
Hips, shoulders	+++	+
Spine	+++	+
Symmetry	+	—
Self-limiting	—	+
Remissions, relapses	—	+

Relationship of Reiter's syndrome to ankylosing spondylitis

The patient with progressive spinal disease may be followed for many years with a diagnosis of 'ankylosing spondylitis', forgetting that the episode began with urethritis and conjunctivitis several decades earlier. Whether one considers the situation as that of ankylosing spondylitis being a manifestation of severe Reiter's disease, or coincidental to the same background, is a question for debate, but as discussed above, there are several characteristic features of the spinal disease in those who began with reactive arthritis. The two conditions are compared in Tables 4.5 and 4.6. One intriguing difference is that HLA-B27 is present in over 95% of those with primary ankylosing spondylitis, but perhaps in only 70 or 80% of those with reactive arthritis. The patient with reactive arthritis and HLA-B27 is more likely to develop spinal changes than those without.

HIV and reactive arthritis (Quinn 1996)

The relationship between HIV infection and rheumatic/autoimmune syndromes remains controversial (Naides 1995) and is clearly dependent on geographic location. Indeed, Solinger and Hess (1993) have even questioned whether the association is real. By contrast, Blanche and colleagues (1993) identified 36 patients with acute arthritis at a referral hospital in Kigali, Rwanda, and found 72% to be HIV positive, compared with a background seroprevalence of 21%. Certainly, septic arthropathy is seen in HIV-positive individuals, but it would also appear that reactive arthropathy, and more particularly Reiter's disease and psoriatic arthropathy are perhaps more prevalent and/or more severe in those who are HIV positive, particularly where there is a full-blown picture of AIDS.

In terms of treatment, anti-inflammatory drugs can help the HIV-associated arthropathy, and some have suggested that sulphasalazine has a role in HIV-associated Reiter's disease (Disla *et al.* 1994). Methotrexate usually must be avoided in any patient with reactive arthritis who is HIV positive, given the potential disastrous effect on the underlying infection and immunosuppression.

Of interest, a change in the incidence of Reiter's syndrome has been noted during the last few years, both anecdotally and more formally in a study of a military population in Greece (Iliopoulos *et al.* 1995). The suggestion is that as the campaigns about the risk of HIV infection are intensified, an influence on sexual behaviour results, and so the use of condoms may protect both against HIV infection and chlamydia or other arthritogenic agents. In the Greek study, four cases of Reiter's syndrome were seen during a 4-year period following the introduction of the anti-AIDS campaign, while in a previous 4 year period, 27 patients presented with Reiter's syndrome.

Natural history and prognosis

Earlier texts stated that 'joint symptoms are characteristically acute, short-lived and transient' (Wright 1978). This may well give both patient and physician a false expectation. In fact, the prognosis of reactive arthritis is notoriously difficult to assess. Long-term follow-up studies are relatively few and suffer from the inherent problem that they are usually performed in academic centres where patients with more severe disease are followed. Nevertheless, for the fortunate individual, reactive arthritis may indeed be self-limiting. However, as stated above, the experience of the Paronen and Noer patients in the two classical follow-up studies suggested that where long-term investigations are performed, the outcome is much less benign than originally supposed (Fox *et al.* 1979, Sairanen *et al.* 1969).

In Csonka's (1958) follow-up study of 185 patients with sexually acquired disease, after a period ranging from 2 to 15 years, he found 62% had active disease, and suggested a recurrence rate of 15% per patient per year. Elsewhere Good (1974) followed 34 patients for 2 years and found that 24 had persistent disease at the end of this period, including 13 with sacroiliitis. More recently, the study of Glennas *et al.* (1994) suggests a more benign course and prognosis, perhaps influenced by earlier recognition and treatment.

In summary, Reiter's syndrome may be a major chronic rheumatic disease for the unfortunate individual, while at the other end of the spectrum the problem may be self-limiting.

Management

There is no cure for reactive arthropathy/Reiter's syndrome, and few rheumatic disorders are more frustrating to treat. The major difficulties in managing the condition are summarized in Table 4.7. Explanation and education play a major role in disease management. Reiter's syndrome can be a bewildering and disturbing event for the patient and family alike. There may be feelings of guilt and anxiety about sexual matters, and even in the absence of sexually acquired disease, persistent balanitis is a difficult component to manage in terms of the patient and sexual partner. Anecdotally, a condom may well protect the patient from a postvenereal exacerbation of disease. As discussed, the one advantage of the HIV/AIDS epidemic is that society is more attentive to the concept of 'safer sex', and there is evidence for a decrease in sexually acquired disease over the past decade (Iliopoulous 1995). Of course, those with post-dysenteric disease are unaffected by modification of sexual activity.

Table 4.7 The major difficulties and errors in the management of Reiter's syndrome

Difficulties	Errors
Inability to define prognosis	Failure to reach diagnosis
Multisystem disease with 'unusual' problems	Inability to provide patient with insight
Tendency toward 'physician shopping'	Danger of thrusting feelings of guilt on patient
Lack of 'expected' response to therapy	Recourse to corticosteroid therapy
Toxicity of available drugs	Too many NSAIDs[a] administered without appropriate plan
Frustrated patients and physicians	
Fragmented care (orthopaedic vs. rheumatological vs. primary care)	Loss of contact with patient due to patient's loss of confidence

[a] Non-steroidal anti-inflammatory drugs.

In counselling patients, it is useful to provide an 'allergic analogy'. Some individuals have a tendency to develop asthma or hay fever on exposure to known or unknown allergens, whereas others have a genetically determined susceptibility to develop Reiter's syndrome following contact with an unrecognized (or recognized) precipitating event. This allergic approach provides the patient with some insight into the recurrent nature of the condition, and aids discussion about prognosis.

Symptomatic management of the acute episode includes the use of analgesics, NSAIDs, and physical therapy.

Antibiotic therapy is of major interest. Although viable bacteria have not been cultured from the synovial space, antigenic debris may be present. A series of long-term follow-up studies have shown only moderate response to therapy. There is a consensus that post-chlamydial arthropathy responds best, whereas yersinia and other bowel-related reactive arthritidies are less likely to improve (Bardin *et al.* 1992; Lauhio *et al.* 1991, 1992; Leirisalo-Repo 1993, 1995; Toivanen *et al.* 1993). However, even with the post-chlamydial disease, long-term antibiotic therapy over 3 months is required, and the results, although encouraging, are not very impressive (see Chapter 6). In general, the earlier the therapy, the better the response—as suggested by Zhang and colleagues' data (1996) with yersinia-induced arthropathy in an experimental model. A debate continues as to whether any benefit relates to the antimicrobial effect of the agent, or, as seems more likely, an anticollagenolytic activity.

Indomethacin has often been considered the drug of choice in terms of non-steroidal anti-inflammatory drugs, but for patients who fail to respond adequately to this drug, or one of the other NSAIDs, methotrexate or azathioprine have a role to play. The latter has been studied in a single, formal, placebo-controlled study (Calin 1986). Specifically with azathioprine, 1–2 mg/kg bodyweight was shown to be useful in controlling disease within 4–8 weeks. Thereafter, the drug can be tapered and withdrawn. Sulphasalazine would appear to be of modest benefit only (Dougados *et al.* 1995; Clegg *et al.* 1996). Systemic corticosteroids should be avoided, but intra-articular or subperiosteal injection therapy is often efficacious where synovitis or dactylitis predominate. For those subjects with severe, persistent, or recurrent iritis, conjoint management with an ophthalmologist is appropriate. For some, an intraocular steroid is required.

The role of irradiation therapy remains unclear and anecdotal. In ankylosing spondylitis, meaningful long-term efficacy seems improbable (Calin and Elswood, 1989), whereas in reactive arthropathy, no formal study has been carried out. The possibility that the odd patient with persistent ankle arthropathy, unresponsive to an intralesional steroid, will respond to local irradiation should be considered, but definitive data are unavailable.

The major goals in the management of Reiter's syndrome are summarized in Table 4.8.

Table 4.8 Major goals in the management of Reiter's syndrome

1.	Explanation and insight
2.	Family counselling
3.	Indomethacin
4.	Other NSAIDs
5.	Exercise programme as able, preferably swimming
6.	Attention to spine, if involved
7.	Occasional use of local steroid injections
8.	Early eye care for inflammatory eye disease
9.	Avoidance of fragmented care
10.	Azathioprine and methotrexate
11.	Physical modalities as needed (foot care, etc.)
12.	Selected referrals for complications (ophthalmology, cardiovascular, etc)
13.	Antibiotics in sexually acquired disease
14.	Occasional use of methotrexate, azathioprine, or sulphasalazine

5 Enteric infections and arthritis: clinical aspects

Marjatta Leirisalo-Repo

Enteric infections associated with sterile joint inflammation include infections with Gram-negative bacteria such as yersinia (especially *Y. enterocolitica*, less frequently *Y. pseudotuberculosis*), salmonella, shigella, and campylobacter (Aho *et al.* 1985). There are also sporadic reports on the association of joint symptoms with *Clostridium difficile* (Putterman and Rubinow 1993). On the other hand, bacteria belonging to the normal gut flora (such as *Escherichia coli* or *Klebsiella* spp.) are not associated with reactive arthritis.

The clinical spectrum of enteric infections with Gram-negative bacteria varies from mild gastrointestinal upset to extraintestinal complications, such as erythema nodosum or other skin manifestations, aberration in the function of kidneys and liver, (occasionally associated with septic infection), and reactive arthritis. The spectrum of the manifestations of infection is partially determined by age, gender, and genetic background of the patient.

Two factors, environmental (infectious) and genetic (HLA-B27) are usually required for the development of acute reactive arthritis. The arthritis is usually preceded by gastrointestinal (enteroarthritis) or urogenital (uroarthritis) infections. In about 60% of the patients, evidence of previous infection can be detected either by serology or by cultures from urogenital or stool samples (Keat 1983). In other cases, the role of infection is less distinct. There is increasing evidence for the role of the gut in the maintenance of joint symptoms in patients with spondylarthropathies even without the history of preceding enteritis (Leirisalo-Repo *et al.* 1994; Mielants *et al.* 1993); analogous to those patients with inflammatory bowel disease, in whom an increased load of Gram-negative pathogens via an inflamed and therefore 'leaky' gut mucosa is probably contributing to the development of peripheral and axial arthritis (Leirisalo-Repo and Repo 1992).

Epidemiology of enteric infections

Reports of yersinia infections as well as reactive complications associated with the infection have come mostly from Scandinavia (Aho *et al.* 1985), while salmonella infections are reported worldwide with increasing interest especially in the food industry (Baird-Parker 1990). The strains of shigella vary within countries, with industrialized countries mostly having sporadic infections with *Shigella sonnei*. In the developing countries, *Shigella flexneri* and *Shigella dysenteriae* are more prevalent and often endemic (Guerrant *et al.* 1990).

The prevalence of infections capable of triggering reactive arthritis in different populations is unknown. Although the proportion of subjects with raised antibody titres against Gram-negative bacteria depends greatly on the serological methods applied, some estimates of the prevalence of such infections can be made, based on the presence of antibodies in healthy populations. Yersinia antibodies have varied between 1 and 4% in surveys of general populations and healthy blood donors (Ahvonen *et al.* 1969; Granfors *et al.* 1983; Hazelton *et al.* 1985; Winblad 1970). In Denmark, the prevalence of positive serology for yersinia was shown to increase from 1.0% in 1967 to 7.7% in 1978 (Agner *et al.* 1981). The proportion of subjects with elevated levels of antibodies has been reported to vary between different countries: low-level positive antibodies for *Salmonella enteritidis* were detected more frequently in normal blood donors from England (26%) than from Finland (8%), while antibodies against *S. infantis* were observed in half of the subjects studied concurrently in both countries (Mäki-Ikola *et al.* 1993). On the basis of serological studies, recent yersinia infection has been suggested to play a role in 19% of patients with acute inflammatory arthritis (Tamburrino *et al.* 1993) and in 9–18% of patients with inflammatory joint disease of less than 6 months' duration (Granfors *et al.* 1983; Mäki-Ikola *et al.* 1991). Salmonella (7%) and campylobacter (6%) were less frequently associated with inflammatory joint diseases (Mäki-Ikola *et al.* 1991).

Epidemiology of reactive arthritis triggered by enteric infections

The annual incidence of acute reactive arthritis has been estimated to be 4/10 000 inhabitants in Finland (Isomäki *et al.* 1979) and 1/10 000 inhabitants in Norway (Kvien *et al.* 1994). Patients with this condition comprise about 10% of those seen in early synovitis clinics (Amor 1983; Hülsemann and Zeidler 1995; Isomäki *et al.* 1979). Most cases of reactive arthritis arise sporadically, but single-source epidemics provide considerable insight into the process (Table 5.1). The prevalence of reactive joint complications varies greatly among these studies (from 1 to 21%). The age of the susceptible cohort, infective load, and genetic background all probably contribute to the differences, but the contribution played by different bacterial species cannot be ruled out. This is most frequently discussed in the context of shigella infections. The reported outbreaks with reactive arthritic complications have been caused by *Shigella flexneri* (Paronen 1948; Simon *et al.* 1981), while *Shigella sonnei* infection has been only rarely associated with reactive arthritis (Lauhio *et al.* 1988). Children seem to develop reactive arthritis less frequently than adult subjects. Also, the joint complications seem to be more frequent in Scandinavia and in Finland, where the populations have higher frequency of HLA-B27 (12–16%) than is the case in other Caucasian populations (4–7%) or in the Japanese (< 1%).

According to the few reports in which the aetiological spectrum of reactive arthritis has been investigated, the proportions of different triggering infections seems to be changing. In a series of patients with chronic Reiter's disease, 16% had a history of diarrhoea at the onset of arthritis (Fox *et al.* 1979). In the 1970s, *Chlamydia trachomatis* was shown to be the most frequent cause of Reiter's disease, that is reactive arthritis with extra-articular features (Bengtsson *et al.* 1983; Kousa *et al.* 1978), and as frequent as yersinia in the aetiology of unselected patients with reactive arthritis (Hülsemann and Zeidler 1995; Valtonen *et al.* 1985), whereas salmonella was either not observed at all (Bengtsson *et al.* 1983) or was only occasionally identified as a triggering factor (Leirisalo *et al.* 1982; Valtonen *et al.* 1985). In contrast, chlamydia and enterobacteria have been described as playing an equally frequent aetiological role in a recent community-based epidemiological study from Norway (Kvien

Table 5.1 Clinical symptoms (%) of patients during major outbreaks of gastroenteritis with respect to age, population studied, and infective agent

Country	Infection	Source	Number of patients	Diarrhoea	Fever	Joint symptoms	
						Pain	Arthritis
Japan							
Children[(1)]	*Y. e.* 3*	?	183	60	76	0	0
Children[(1)]	*Y. e.* 3*	?	544	64	50	0	0
Children[(2)]	*Y. e.* 3*	?	198	36	61	0	0
USA							
Community[(3)]	*Y. e.*	Water	129	71	36	0	0
Children[(4)]	*Y. e.* 8*	Chocolate milk	38	47	97	0	0
Community[(5)]	*Y. e.* 13*, 18*	Milk	172	83	93	15	0
Canada							
Adults[(6)]	*S. heidelberg* and *S. hadar*	Potato salad	83	88	?	?	7
Adults[(7)]	*S. typhimurium*	Food	473	?	?	7	5
Adults[(8)]	*S. typhimurium*	Food	919	100	?	40	1–14
England							
Community[(9)]	Campylobacter	Milk	130	68	?	?	1
Finland							
Community[(10)]	*Y. e.* 3*	?	26	69	85	4	8
Community[(11)]	*Y. ps.* III	?	19	21	58	32	21
Adults[(12)]	*Y. e.* 3* or 9*	?	117	?	?	0	0
Children[(13)]	Salmonella	Sprouts	155	91	?	18	3
Adults[(13)]	Salmonella	Sprouts	91		?		13
Sweden							
Adults[(14)]	*S. enteritidis*	Food	113	96	?	26	15
Community[(15)]	*S. typhimurium*	?	330	?	?	?	4

Abbreviations: Y. e., *Yersinia enterocolitica*; Y. ps., *Yersinia pseudotuberculosis*; S., *Salmonella*.

* serotype. [(1)] Asakawa *et al.* 1973; [(2)] Zen-Yoji *et al.* 1973; [(3)] Eden *et al.* 1977; [(4)] Black *et al.* 1978; [(5)] Tacket *et al.* 1984; [(6)] Thomson *et al.* 1992; [(7)] Inman *et al.* 1988; [(8)] Samuel *et al.* 1995; [(9)] Eastmond *et al.* 1983; [(10)] Tuori and Valtonen 1983; [(11)] Tertti *et al.* 1984; [(12)] Lindholm and Visakorpi 1991; [(13)] Mattila *et al.* 1994; [(14)] Locht *et al.* 1993; [(15)] Håkansson *et al.* 1975.

et al. 1994). Moreover, there are reports on the decrease of chlamydia-triggered reactive arthritis, whereas no such trend has been observed for enteroarthritis (Iliopoulos *et al.* 1995). On the contrary, salmonella seems to be an increasingly important factor in enteroarthritis (Krüger and Schattenkirchner 1983; Kvien *et al.* 1994; Mäki-Ikola and Granfors 1992*a*).

Clinical picture of reactive enteroarthritis

Reactive arthritis shows similar features when triggered by enteric or urogenital infections (Keat 1983). The preceding infection can be asymptomatic in a proportion of patients. For unknown reasons, the preceding infection in yersinia arthritis is often mild or asymptomatic (Toivanen *et al.* 1985), whereas in patients with salmonella arthritis the preceding infection is more severe (Inman *et al.* 1988) than in patients with uncomplicated gut infection. There is usually an interval of 1–2 weeks between the preceding infection and the first joint symptoms, which then proceed within a short time to a full picture of mono- or oligoarthritis. Joints of the lower extremities are almost always affected, but joints of the upper extremities are also affected in about half of the patients. Even then, the clinical picture is easily distinguishable from early rheumatoid arthritis, the patients with reactive arthritis having an asymmetrical pattern of arthritis with a predilection to large joints. The patients also have other characteristic extra-articular features of spondylarthropathy (Table 5.2). Recently, more interest has been focused on the frequent presence of enthesopathy in such patients (Lehtinen *et al.* 1994; Thomson *et al.* 1994). Extra-articular symptoms occur in about 15–30% of the patients. These features are much like those observed in uroarthritis, although full-blown Reiter's syndrome (arthritis, urethritis, and conjunctivitis) is less frequently observed in enteroarthritis except when triggered by *Shigella flexneri* (Table 5.2) (Keat 1983; Leirisalo *et al.* 1982). The clinical picture does not vary greatly between patients with different enteric infections, with few exceptions. Erythema nodosum is most commonly observed during yersinia infection (Keat 1983).

Radiological examination of the joints during acute reactive arthritis shows either no changes or mild transient osteoporosis. Compared with chronic Reiter's syndrome, periosteal or erosive changes are only occasionally observed in acute enteroarthritis, whereas radiological sacroiliitis is detected in 3–20% of patients during acute enteroarthritis (Table 5.2), most of the patients having the first attack of reactive arthritis.

Natural course of reactive arthritis

The median duration of acute reactive arthritis is about 3–5 months, but a few patients continue to have prolonged arthritis for more than one year (Table 5.2). Enthesopathy seems to persist even after the joint inflammation has disappeared and laboratory markers of inflammation have returned to normal (Glennås *et al.* 1994; Lehtinen *et al.* 1995). The long-term prognosis is best known for yersinia and shigella arthritis (Table 5.3). Mild peripheral arthralgia or enthesopathy is frequent in patients with previous reactive arthritis. Also, one-third have occasional attacks of low-back pain. During follow-up of 10–20 years, recurrent attacks of acute reactive arthritis seldom occur in patients with previous yersinia arthritis, but are more frequent in patients with previous salmonella or shigella arthritis (Table 5.3). About

Table 5.2 Clinical features of reactive arthritis triggered by enteric infections

	Triggering infection Yersinia[1]	Salmonella[2]	Shigella[3]	Campylobacter[4]	Clostridium difficile[5]
Number of patients	322	306	364	29	17
Sex (M/F)	1:1.1	1.2 : 1	2.2 : 1[6]	1.4 : 1	0.5 : 1
Age, years, mean (range)	32 (4–76)	34 (2–69)	46 (27–57)[7]	35 (18–76)	42 (23–61)
Number of joints					
mean (range)	6.5 (1–22)	6.0 (0–22)	4 (2–11)	3 (1–10)	NA
Low-back pain (%)	30 (16–45)	37 (18–67)	3 (2–50)	24	NA
X-ray sacroiliitis (%)	19 (11–20)	11[8]	NA	NA	NA
Urethritis (%)	15 (4–23)	14[8]	69 (50–89)	NA	NA
Conjunctivitis (%)	6 (6–7)	13 (6–18)	72 (17–78)	NA	NA
Iritis (%)	7 (6–17)	3[8]	4 (3–17)	NA	NA
Skin lesions (%)	5 (4–7)	2 (2–6)	17[8]	NA	NA
Duration of arthritis, months					
mean (range)	3 (1–13)	5 (0.5–24)	NA	NA	NA
Chronic course					
(> 12 months) (%)	4 (1–24)	19 (0–30)	1	0	NA
HLA-B27 + (%)	71 (56–72)	77 (0–94)	83 (83–85)	59	57

Data derived from the following references: [1] Leirisalo *et al.* 1982; Tertti *et al.* 1984; Thomas *et al.* 1975; Dequeker *et al.* 1980; Winblad 1975; Marsal *et al.* 1981; Leino and Kalliomäki 1974; Herrlinger and Asmussen 1992; Leirisalo-Repo *et al.* 1987; Borg *et al.* 1992; Yli-Kerttula *et al.* 1995; [2] Mäki-Ikola and Granfors 1992*b*; Locht *et al.* 1993; Thomson *et al.* 1992; Thomson *et al.* 1994; Mattila *et al.* 1994; Hannu and Leirisalo-Repo 1988; Aho *et al.* 1975; [3] Simon *et al.* 1981; Paronen 1948; Sieper *et al.* 1993; Noer 1966; [4] Peterson 1994; [5] Putterman and Rubinow 1993 [6] Paronen *et al.* (1948) excluded; [7] 6 patients (Simon *et al.* 1981); [8] average from the review by Mäki-Ikola and Granfors (1992)

NA = not available

15–30% of the patients develop chronic arthritis or sacroiliitis (Leirisalo-Repo and Suoranta 1988) or ankylosing spondylitis (Sairanen *et al.* 1969). It is still uncertain whether reactive arthritis contributes to the development of sacroiliitis or ankylosing spondylitis, or whether sacroiliac changes would have occurred anyway in a subject with a genetic tendency to spondyloarthropathy even in the absence of intervening reactive arthritis. As discussed previously, some of the patients with the first known attack of arthritis already had radiological sacroiliitis (Leirisalo *et al.* 1982). Also, a recent report from Finland describes a 1.7% frequency of ankylosing spondylitis in patients who had had yersinia gastroenteritis but no reactive arthritis 13 years previously (Lindholm and Visakorpi 1991). This figure is slightly, but not markedly, higher than the frequency of AS of 0.4–1.0% estimated in a Finnish population study (Julkunen and Korpi 1984). In addition to different triggering infections, the patient cohort, number of patients, and follow-up time vary in the studies referred to in Table 5.3, all of which confound comparisons of the specific infections in the long-term prognosis.

Factors contributing to the development of chronic spondyloarthropathy are incompletely known, but persistent infection and/or a chronic inflammatory focus in the gut are reasonable candidates. Yersinia structures have been shown to persist in the intestinal submucosa (Hoogkamp-Korstanje 1987) and in lymph nodes in patients with chronic yersinia arthritis (Hoogkamp-Korstanje *et al.* 1988; 1992).

HLA-B27 and enteroarthritis

There is a close association between reactive arthritis and genetic background, as evidenced by a high association with HLA-B27. HLA-B27 is by no means mandatory for the development of reactive arthritis, and examination of cohorts from several salmonella epidemics has indicated frequencies of B27 lower than in reports on patients treated in rheumatological centres (Table 5.2). The presence of HLA-B27 seems to contribute to the severity and extra-articular complications during acute yersinia arthritis (Leirisalo *et al.* 1982). Erythema nodosum is, however, usually observed in B27-negative patients. During 10 years' follow-up, yersinia arthritis patients with HLA-B27 also have a higher risk of developing sacroiliitis compared with patients without the genetic marker (Leirisalo-Repo and Suoranta 1988). However, this distinction has not been observed in investigations with shorter follow-up times (Dequeker *et al.* 1980; Glennås *et al.* 1994; Thomson *et al.* 1995).

Treatment of reactive arthritis

Treatment of this condition encompasses a number of distinct aspects, including treatment of joint inflammation, treatment of the triggering infection, and prevention of recurrent attacks of arthritis.

Treatment of acute joint inflammation

Because the knees and ankles are often involved, overuse of the inflamed joints is best avoided by bed rest or the use of crutches. In the case of knee synovitis, atrophy of the vastus medialis of the quadriceps muscle will occur within a few weeks if preventive measures, such as isometric excercises, are not started.

Table 5.3 Prognosis of reactive arthritis triggered by enteric infections with respect to follow-up time

	Triggering infection Yersinia[1]		**Salmonella**[2]		**Shigella**[3]		**Campylobacter**[4]
Follow-up time, years	4–5	10	1.5–2	5	2	20	5
Number of patients	58	111	17	27	6	100	7
Recovered (%)	19	45	5/6*	33	1/6*	20	7/7*
Arthralgia (%)	32	20	0/6*	NA	3/6*	NA	0/7*
Recurrent arthritis (%)	3	6	8/17*	37	3/6*	18	1/7*
Chronic arthritis (%)	8	2	NA	52	2/6	18	0/7*
Ankylosing spondylitis (%)	7	15	NA	NA	NA	14	0/7*
Radiological sacroiliitis (%)	7	20	NA	NA	NA	32	0/7*

Data derived from the following references: [1] Kalliomäki and Leino 1979; Marsal *et al.* 1981; Herrlinger and Asmussen 1992; Yli-Kerttula *et al.* 1995; Leirisalo-Repo and Suoranta 1988. [2] Mäki-Ikola and Granfors 1992*b*; Thomson *et al.* 1992, 1994, 1995. [3] Simon *et al.* 1981; Sairanen *et al.* 1969. [4] Bremell *et al.* 1991

* absolute numbers; NA: not available

The use of non-steroidal anti-inflammatory drugs, often in high dose, together with the local application of cold and local corticosteroid injections into joints and entheses are usually of major benefit. Systemic use of corticosteroids is indicated in unusual cases, such as a patient who is bedridden from severe polyarthritis or one with atrioventricular conduction disturbances.

Treatment of infection

Often the triggering microbe can no longer be isolated by the time the patient presents with arthritis (Hannu and Leirisalo-Repo 1988; Leirisalo *et al.* 1982). None the less, the question of antibiotic therapy arises both with respect to the treatment of infection and the treatment of arthritis. For chlamydia infection, the use of antibiotic therapy for the patient and the partner is mandatory with respect to the infection itself. For gut infections, uncomplicated enteritis is usually of short duration and does not need treating with antibiotics. Moreover, there is no evidence that standard (namely 2-week) antibiotic treatment of acute enteric infection either prevents reactive arthritis or alters its course (reviewed in Leirisalo-Repo 1993).

Prolonged chemotherapy in acute reactive arthritis

A 3-month, placebo-controlled, prospective study of patients with acute reactive arthritis showed a modest positive effect on the duration of acute arthritis in patients with *Chlamydia trachomatis* triggered arthritis when treated with lymecycline (a tetracycline) compared with those treated with placebo (Lauhio *et al.* 1991). Such a difference in favour of chemotherapy was not observed in patients with enteroarthritis.

The deviating-response antimicrobial chemotherapy depending on whether the infection was due to *C. trachomatis* or gastroenteritis is hard to explain. A difference in the sensitivity of the bacteria to tetracycline is one explanation. However, most enteric pathogens are sensitive to tetracyclines *in vitro*. If whole bacteria persist in the host, they would probably have been eradicated by the long-term course of tetracyclines. There is a possibility that the pathogenesis of chlamydia-triggered reactive arthritis and that triggered by enteric pathogens are different. So far, evidence for the persistence of whole (viable?) bacteria (chlamydial DNA and RNA) in the inflamed joints has been presented only with respect to *C. trachomatis*. In contrast to chlamydia, only stable bacterial degradation products such as lipopolysaccharide and outer-membrane proteins have been detected in patients with enteroarthritis (see Leirisalo-Repo 1993).

Treatment of chronic reactive arthritis

In the case of a prolonged or chronic reactive arthritis, general measures aim to alleviate the patient's symptoms. Regular excercise and the use of non-steroidal anti-inflammatory drugs help in patients with inflammatory low-back pain. Non-steroidal anti-inflammatory drugs also help in the case of peripheral arthritis. Sulphasalazine, which is effective in attenuating the inflammatory flare-ups of patients with ankylosing spondylitis, especially in cases of peripheral arthritis, has been used with some success in patients with chronic spondyloarthropathies (Dougados *et al.* 1995*a*; Clegg *et al.* 1996; Mielants *et al.* 1986). Sulphasalazine may exert its beneficial effect in spondylarthropathies either by diminishing the mucosal inflammation or by acting directly on the arthritic joint. It could also be antibacterial and could modify the gut flora. Auranofin, aurothiomalate, azathioprine, and methotrexate have all been used in the treatment of chronic reactive arthritides. Large-scale controlled studies are, however, lacking.

In an open uncontrolled study, Hoogkamp-Korstanje *et al.* (1992) observed a decrease in IgA class anti-yersinia antibodies with the simultaneous disappearance of yersinia antigenic structures in intestinal biopsies in patients with spondylarthropathy who were treated with antibiotics. However, a placebo-controlled study on patients with chronic reactive arthritis, in most cases triggered by yersinia, treated with a 3-month course of ciprofloxacin, showed a varying effect of active treatment of some joint symptoms, while no consistent pattern was observed in the specific antibody levels (Toivanen *et al.* 1993).

Early treatment of infection in the prevention of arthritis

There is a delay of a few days to 1–2 weeks between the triggering enteric infection and the onset of arthritis. In theory, early eradication of bacteria would possibly diminish the antigen load and/or limit the dissemination of the infection, thereby modulating the development of joint symptoms. Contrary to the promising effect of early antimicrobial chemotherapy of acute non-gonococcal urethritis in the prevention of recurrent Reiter's disease (Bardin *et al.* 1992), there are no prospective studies in patients with enteritis to answer the question whether the early treatment of enteritis would prevent the development of reactive arthritis. The indirect evidence available at the moment is against such a preventive effect (Locht *et al.* 1993; Mattila *et al.* 1994).

Conclusions

The spectrum of reactive enteroarthritis varies between mild monoarthritis and severe polyarthritis. Most patients do recover within a few months, but in a minority the joint symptoms persist for more than one year. During long-term follow-up studies, recurrent arthritis can occur, and many patients have waxing and waning symptoms in joints, low-back pain, and enthesitis. The development of chronic progressive arthritis varies in different series of patients. Radiological sacroiliitis, and even ankylosing spondylitis, occurs in 20–30% of patients within 10–20 years. The treatment of acute reactive arthritis consists of general measures such as non-steroidal anti-inflammatory drugs, local corticosteroid injections, and rest, with exercise aimed at retaining good muscle strength. Contrary to the evidence favouring antibiotic treatment in the case of reactive arthritis triggered by *Chlamydia trachomatis*, the evidence in favour of a short or prolonged course of antibiotic treatment for the patient with enteroarthritis is still lacking.

6 Chlamydia-induced arthritis

Henning K. Zeidler and H. Ralph Schumacher, Jr

Introduction

An aetiological connection between urogenital infections with *Chlamydia trachomatis* and arthritis has long been presumed, but chlamydial antigen in synovium and synovial fluid was only recently identified in patients with Reiter's syndrome, sexually acquired reactive arthritis, and undifferentiated seronegative oligoarthritis (Ishikawa *et al.* 1986; Keat *et al.* 1987; Schumacher *et al.* 1988; Taylor-Robinson *et al.* 1988). Meanwhile, an increasing number of investigations have confirmed the presence of chlamydial antigens, nucleic acid, and chlamydia-like particles in arthritic joints, which has led to the present view of an intra-articular inapparent infection with viable, non-culturable or difficult to culture Chlamydia (Bas *et al.* 1995; Beutler *et al.* 1994; Hammer *et al.* 1992; Mascia *et al.* 1992, Rahman *et al.* 1992*a*; Taylor-Robinson *et al.* 1992).

The triad of inflammation in the genital tract, eye, and joint has traditionally been regarded as Reiter's syndrome and this term is still widely used both as a nosological entity and as a diagnosis. However, the development of Reiter's symptoms has been observed following a variety of genitourinary and enteric infections with different organisms such as *Chlamydia*, *Ureaplasma*, *Yersinia*, *Salmonella*, and *Shigella* (Horowitz *et al.* 1994; Keat 1983; Svenungson 1994). Moreover, the classical triad of Reiter's syndrome is rather rare compared with the more frequent manifestations of seronegative oligoarthritis, enthesopathy, or sacroiliitis in context with the above infections. Today, the term Reiter's syndrome can therefore only be used to describe a clinical subgroup of patients in the microbiologically defined and non-defined spectrum of reactive arthritis and spondylarthritides. The same argument can be applied to the more recent term SARA, which has mostly been used to describe arthritis associated with urogenital infections due to chlamydia, but it has also been discussed in the context of infections with *Ureaplasma urealyticum, Mycoplasma genitalis* and, most recently, human immunodeficiency virus (HIV) (Cole *et al.* 1985; Forster *et al.* 1988; Keat *et al.* 1978). Moreover, the term seronegative spondylarthritides much better covers the whole spectrum of musculoskeletal and extra-articular lesions associated with the different causative organisms and the high frequency of HLA-B27 in this interrelated group of disorders. The term 'chlamydia-induced arthritis' (CIA), instead of Reiter's syndrome and sexually acquired reactive arthritis (SARA), was therefore chosen to describe the rheumatological manifestations following urogenital chlamydial infections with *C. trachomatis* serotypes D to K (Wollenhaupt *et al.* 1989*a*; Zeidler 1992; Zeidler and Wollenhaupt 1991). CIA refers to a non-purulent arthritis which develops in predisposed patients following a primary extra-articular infection with *C. trachomatis*. However, other *Chlamydia* species, especially the recently described *C. pneumoniae,* may also precipitate arthritis (Beaudreuil *et al.* 1995; Braun *et al.* 1994*d*; Gérard *et al.* 1995*b*; Gran *et al.* 1993; Saario and Toivanen 1993). Therefore one should enlarge the definition of CIA to all *Chlamydia* species and the relevant subgroups of *C. trachomatis*.

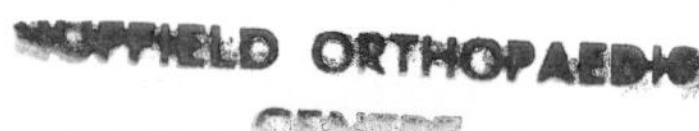

Only a small proportion of all chlamydia-infected persons develop CIA. Studies of SARA suggest that approximately 1–3% of patients with chlamydial urethritis go on to develop arthritis (Keat *et al.* 1980). A community-based study of patients with recent onset synovitis, primarily seen by general practitioners, estimated the annual minimum incidence of CIA to be 4.6/100 000 individuals between 18 and 60 years of age (Kvien *et al.* 1994). The frequency of CIA in patients with undiagnosed arthritis attending an early synovitis clinic of a university out-patient service was approximately 20% (Wollenhaupt *et al.* 1995) and at a similar clinic at the National Institutes of Health, about 30% (unpublished study in progress). In the clinical setting, nearly 50% of all reactive arthritides may be diagnosed as having CIA (Amor *et al.* 1983; Hülsemann *et al.* 1989; Kvien *et al.* 1994; Zeidler *et al.* 1987).

The following overview will concentrate on the infectious, morphological, and clinical features of CIA. Other aspects of the clinical status of reactive arthritis will be discussed in Chapter 4. The triggering mechanisms and T-cell responses in spondylarthritides are reviewed more generally in Chapter 13, as well as an integrative hypothesis for the pathogenesis of the spondylarthritides put forward in Chapter 15.

Classification, biology and morphology of *chlamydia* spp.

Although once thought to be viruses, the *Chlamydiae* have now been recognized as Gram-negative bacteria. The order Chlamydiales consists of one family, the Chlamydiaceae, which in turn contains one genus, *Chlamydia*. The genus *Chlamydia* comprises three species: *C. psittaci*, *C. pneumoniae* (formerly TWAR agent), and *C. trachomatis*. Three subgroups of *C. trachomatis* can be distinguished on the basis of clinical manifestations, and 15 serotypes have been defined immunologically according to the antigenic specificity of the chlamydia-specific major outer-membrane proteins (MOMP) (Table 6.1 and Pearlman and McNeeley

Table 6.1 Characteristics and properties of the three *Chlamydia* species (Modified from Grayston 1989, 1992)

	C. psittaci	*C. trachomatis*	*C. pneumoniae*
Natural hosts	Birds, lower mammals	Human	Human
Major human diseases	Pneumonia	Trachoma, sexually transmitted disease	Pneumonia, bronchitis
Number of serovars	Unknown	18	1 (TWAR)
Morphology			
of EB	Round	Round	Pear-shaped
of inclusion	Variable, dense	Oval, vacuolar	Oval, dense
MOMP contains species-specific antigens	Yes	Yes	No
Plasmid	Usually	Yes	No
Glycogen inclusion	No	Yes	No

1992). The major diseases caused by *C. trachomatis* are trachoma and genital infections. Endemic trachoma is usually produced by infection with *C. trachomatis* serotypes A, B, or C, whereas sexually transmissable chlamydial infections are caused by *C. trachomatis* serotypes D to K and are responsible for sexually acquired CIA. Lymphogranuloma venereum is associated with *C. trachomatis* serotypes L1, L2, or L3. The other two species, *C. pneumoniae* and *C. psittaci*, cause respiratory infections.

Chlamydia spp. are very similar to other Gram-negative bacteria in that they possess both an inner and an outer membrane. Between 50 and 60% of all protein in the outer membrane consists of MOMP, which determines the antigenic specificity of the different serovars of *C. trachomatis* (Pearlman and McNeeley 1992; Ward 1995). Another important constituent of the outer membrane is the genus-specific chlamydial lipopolysaccharide (LPS), which shares significant structural and antigenic similarity to the Re LPS of various enterobacteria (Re is a rough mutant strain of enterobacteria). Special attention has recently been attached to the chlamydial heat-shock proteins (hsp) 12 kDa, 60 kDa, and 75 kDa which show considerable amino-acid homology with their human and microbial counterparts. Expression of chlamydial hsp 60 and hsp 70 in persistently infected cells has been implicated in playing a significant role in the pathogenesis of chronic chlamydial diseases (Lehtinen and Paavonen 1994).

Biologically, because of a metabolic defect, *Chlamydia* spp. are obligate intracellular parasites. These organisms lack the enzymes required for net ATP production and depend on ATP obtained from the host cell. Nevertheless, in adapting to an intracellular lifestyle, *Chlamydia* spp. retained considerable biosynthetic capacity, including elements of glycolysis, respiration, and pentose biosynthesis. Although they possess all the cell machinery for prokaryotic DNA, RNA, and protein synthesis, the organisms are dependent on their host cells for many precursors such as nucleotides and amino acids. In addition, *Chlamydia* spp. are in continuous competition with host cells for vitamins, nutrients, and co-factors.

Chlamydia spp. have developed a unique developmental cycle during which they pass through two clearly distinct functional and morphological forms: the infectious, extracellular elementary body (EB) and the obligate intracellular reticulate body (RB) (Fig. 6.1) (Ward 1988). The small (300–400 nm), dense EB has a rigid cell wall conferred by extensive disulphide cross-linking of the major outer-membrane protein (MOMP) and two cysteine-rich proteins: the 60-kDa envelope protein and the 12-kDa outer-membrane lipoprotein. The structural integrity of EBs confers resistance to environmental factors during transit from cell to cell as well from host to host. In contrast, the RBs are less rigid, highly labile forms that do not survive outside the host cell. The RB is the larger (800–1000 nm), metabolically active form of the organism, synthesizing DNA, RNA, and proteins.

The recent establishment of TWAR as a new species of chlamydia was based primarily on the lack of homology of its DNA with either *C. trachomatis* or *C. psittaci*, and the unique morphology of the EB (Grayston 1992, Pearlman and McNeeley 1992). The EB of *C. pneumoniae* is pear-shaped and has a large periplasmic space. In addition, small electron-dense bodies ('minibodies') of undetermined function were seen in the periplasmic space of the EB. The MOMP of *C. pneumoniae* is less immunogenic and antigenically more complex than those of the other two species (Grayston 1992).

Infection of the host cell and the chlamydial growth cycle is initiated when the EB attaches to specific host-cell receptors, possibly sialic acid residues. Cells that lack this receptor are apparently immune to infection. Subsequently, the EB is actively ingested by endocytosis and sequestered within a host-derived phagosome (Fig. 6.1). Inhibition of fusion with host lyso-

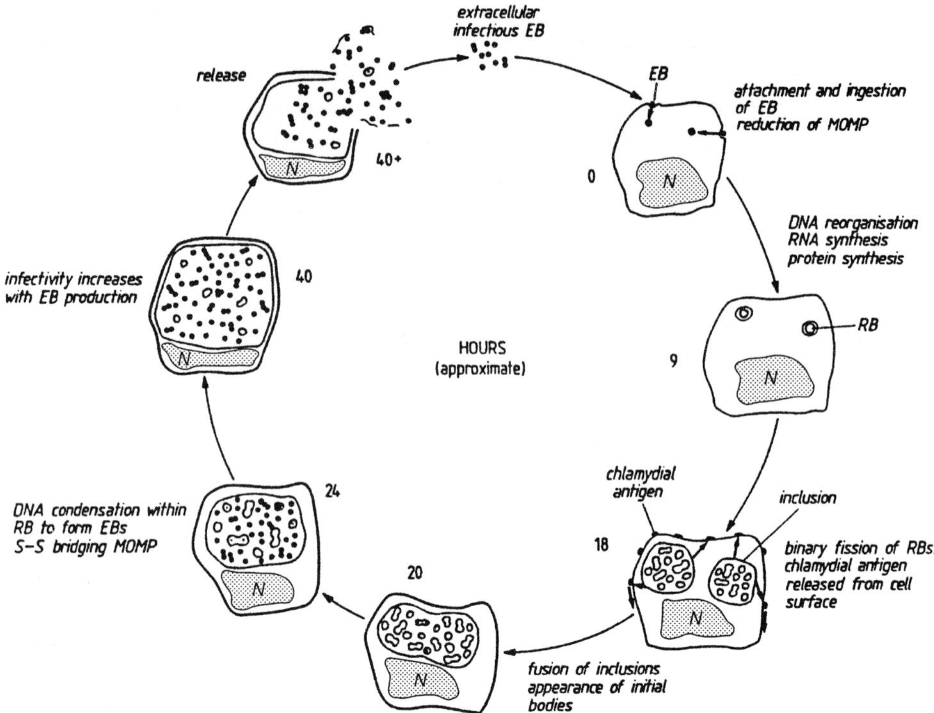

Fig. 6.1 Diagram of chlamydial development. (From Ward 1988, reproduced with permission.)

somal vesicles allows for intracellular growth and survival of the organism. The prevention of phagolysosomal fusion appears to be directed by chlamydial surface antigens and to be dependent on the presence of viable chlamydial EBs (W.L. Beatty *et al.* 1994). *In vitro*, 6–9 hours after ingestion, the EBs undergo morphological changes, increase in size, and are reorganized into the metabolically active and growing RBs. The resulting RBs multiply by binary fission within the expanding endosome, this becomes visible as a microcolony and is referred to as the stainable and recognizable chlamydial inclusion. Approximately 20–30 hours after infection of the host cell, the RBs begin again to reorganize, condensing to form infectious EBs. The reproductive cycle is complete when the chlamydiae are released by host-cell lysis or exocytosis, allowing the EBs to initiate new infectious cycles. The length of the complete developmental cycle, as studied in cell-culture models, is 48–72 hours and varies as a function of the infecting strain, host cell, and environmental conditions.

Altered and persistent chlamydial development are also observed *in vivo* and *in vitro* (W. L. Beatty *et al.* 1994). A variety of alterations in growth conditions, including the presence of antibiotics, host-elaborated factors, and deviations in the levels of essential nutrients such as host amino acids and nucleotides, can induce altered chlamydial development. These conditions generally delay RB maturation, inhibit differentiation to infectious EBs, and are associated with gross morphological alterations of RBs—typified by markedly enlarged, atypical chlamydial forms. Ultimately, the altered intracellular chlamydial development may lead to persistent infections; in the absence of overt chlamydial growth altered *Chlamydia* spp. exist in a viable but culture-negative state distinct from their typical intracellular morphological forms. The term 'inapparent' has also been used in defining the state of the chlamydial organism, connating clinical disease in the absence of a readily recognizable aetiological agent (Rahman *et al.* 1992*b*). The concept of persistent chlamydial infections has long been recognized as a major factor in the pathogenesis of chlamydial disease (Byrne 1988; Kuo 1988), but only recently has there been an attempt to define the pathobiology as well as metabolic and immunological conditions necessary to induce persistence in cell-culture models (W. L. Beatty *et al.* 1994; Nettelnbreker *et al.* 1994). Finally, the recently proposed term 'slow bacterial infection' may also be appropriate to describe the relationship between the survival and persistence of chlamydiae and the immune reactions in arthritis and other systemic chlamydial disease (M. Hammer and Zeidler 1994; Rook and Stanford 1992).

Pathology and immunopathology

Despite the prominence of synovitis in CIA, surprisingly few histological, ultrastructural, and immunohistochemical studies of the synovium have been undertaken. Early studies of Reiter's syndrome describe the synovitis, but infections causing these cases were not established. Early reports (Weinberger *et al.* 1962; Kulka 1962) described a strikingly superficial inflammatory arthritis in early Reiter's syndrome. Infiltration by polymorphonuclear granulocytes (PMN) seemed to be greater than was usual in RA, and this provided a clue to those investigators who followed to consider infection. Erythrocyte extravasation, oedema, necrosis, and vascular congestion were all noted.

Recent studies have also found a proliferation of lining cells, dramatic vascular congestion, and prominent infiltration by PMN among and below synovial lining cells (Fig. 6.2) as features of Reiter's syndrome of recent onset (Schumacher *et al.* 1988). More chronic synovitis in Reiter's syndrome can be indistinguishable from RA (Nanagara *et al.* 1995; Norton *et al.* 1966; Rahman *et al.* 1992*b*). Occasional specimens have shown haematoxyphilic cytoplasmic inclusions suggestive of those of chlamydia, but these have not been confirmed by direct immunofluorescence antibody assays (DFA) or other techniques. Note that these descriptions do not specifically identify CIA, but define a broad group that certainly includes some CIA.

Immunohistochemical studies on Reiter's synovium are few and more than 15 years old (Baldassare *et al.* 1981; Brandt *et al.* 1968). These groups reported immunoglobulins and complement intracellularly and in the interstitium during both acute and chronic synovitis. No recent studies have been performed to characterize cell subsets, adhesion molecules, and other features now amenable to study. Electron microscopic findings in early Reiter's syndrome have been described by several groups (Logroscino 1981; Nanagara *et al.* 1995; Norton *et al.* 1966; Schumacher *et al.* 1988). Dramatic vascular occlusions with platelets and fibrin (Fig. 6.3) as well as electron-dense deposits in vessel walls can be seen. These interesting vascular changes have received little attention because of the potentially more important identification of chlamydia-like bodies. Norton *et al.* (1966) described these in large synovial mononuclear cells. Schumacher *et al.* (1988) and Nanagara *et al.* (1995) noted them primarily in perivascular cells (Fig. 6.4). Confirmation by immunoperoxidase staining is essential to be certain of the organisms, and this was achieved by Nanagara *et al.* These studies also noted unidentified small, possibly viral particles (Schumacher *et al.* 1988). The question of added effects from the interaction between viruses and the chlamydia raised in 1988 is still

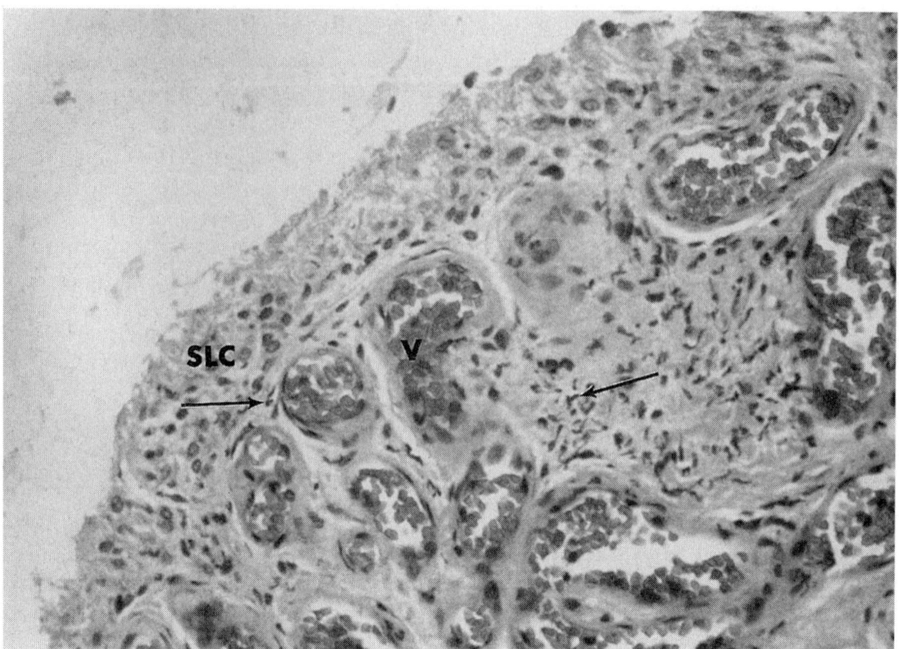

Fig. 6.2 Reiter's syndrome. Synovitis of < 4 weeks' duration. SLC, proliferated synovial lining cells; V, congested vessels; arrows, perivascular PMNs. (Haematoxylin and eosin < 300)

germaine, but aside from the case of patients with HIV and Reiter's syndrome there are no suggestions of specific viruses in 'reactive' CIA.

In more chronic Reiter's syndrome electron microscopy (EM) has shown persistent fibrin in perivascular areas. There are intracellular structures consistent with reticulate bodies, usually in small numbers in vacuoles of apparent macrophages and fibroblasts (Nanagara *et al.* 1995). Many are atypical and pleomorphic. Elementary bodies were also identified in all six patients in this study. Most EBs were extracellular and among fibrin-like material, although some were also identified in macrophages, fibroblasts, and occasionally in vacuoles of vascular endothelial cells. Immunogold staining for chlamydial LPS, MOMP, and elementary-body antigens was positive in these chronic cases (Nanagara *et al.* 1995). All signals were weaker than in positive controls produced by infecting HeLa cells with chlamydial elementary bodies *in vitro*. This can be postulated to be due to synovial generation of TH1 cytokines, such as interferon-gamma (IFN-γ) which has been shown to be one factor that is able to inhibit the metabolic activity of chlamydia (Beatty *et al.* 1993).

Still limited studies using reverse transcriptase PCR in the synovium of early arthritis confirm the prominent presence of IFN-γ (Kotake *et al.* 1995; 1997) and in this aspect support the findings of Simon *et al.* (1993). Inhibition of metabolic activity could contribute to difficulties in culturing the organism, to its protection from eradication, and to its persistence as an 'inapparent infection'.

Chlamydia trachomatis seems more easily demonstrated in synovial tissue than in synovial fluid (SF) both by PCR (Branigan *et al.* 1995) and by EM with immuno EM (IEM) (Nanagara *et al.* 1995). In the IEM study, LPS was occasionally demonstrated in SF macrophages without any identifiable elementary bodies or reticulate bodies.

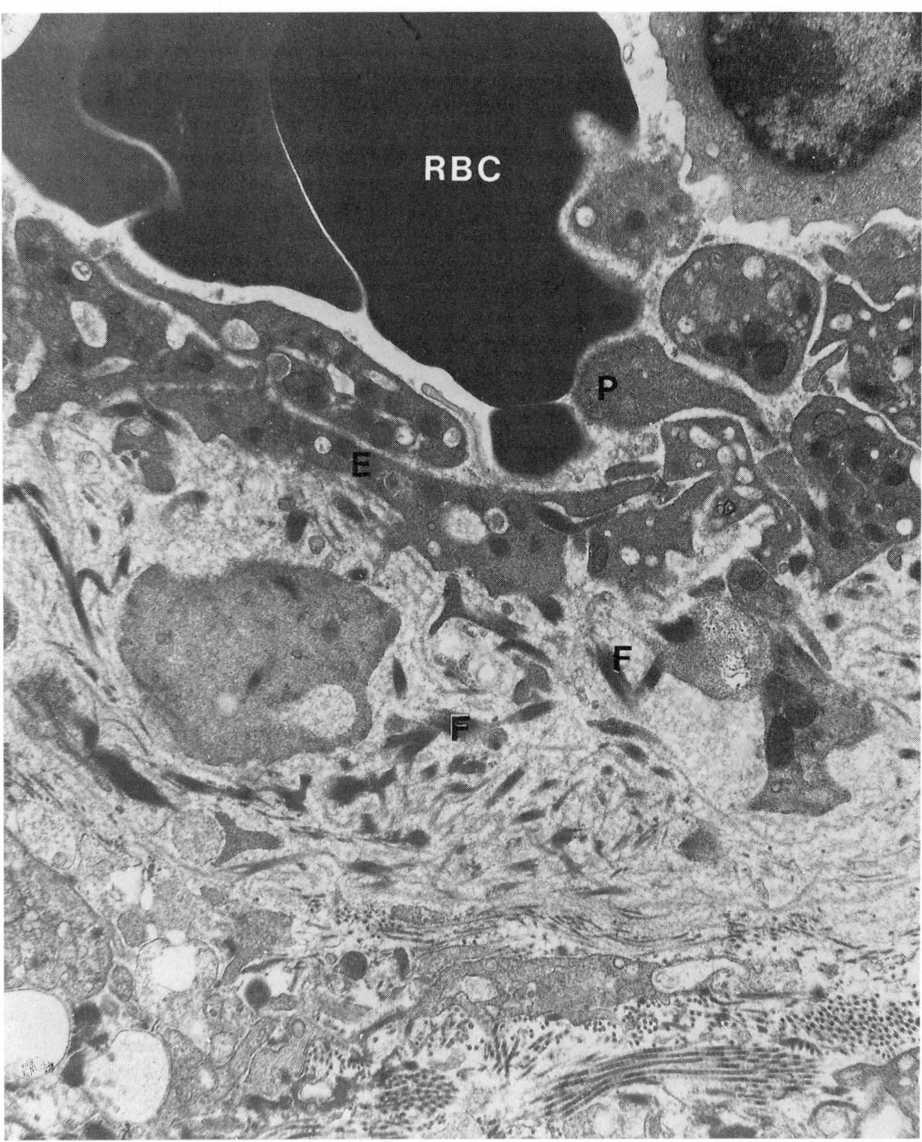

Fig. 6.3 Synovial vessel in Reiter's syndrome of < 4 weeks' duration. RBC, erythrocyte in lumen of venule; P, platelet; F, fibrin in vessel wall; E, (vascular) endothelium. (Electron micrograph < 11 700).

In-situ hybridization has now also been used to confirm a predominantly intracellular location of *Chlamydia trachomatis* 16S RNA in synovium. Interestingly, most hybridization is in the deeper synovium, not the lining cells (Beutler *et al.* 1994, 1995). These studies have not yet identified the precise cells containing the chlamydia or detailed the surrounding response, but the location in deep cells may explain why chlamydia are less readily demonstrated in SF. Exactly how chlamydia and other organisms arrive at joints remains to be addressed by further study (Schumacher 1995).

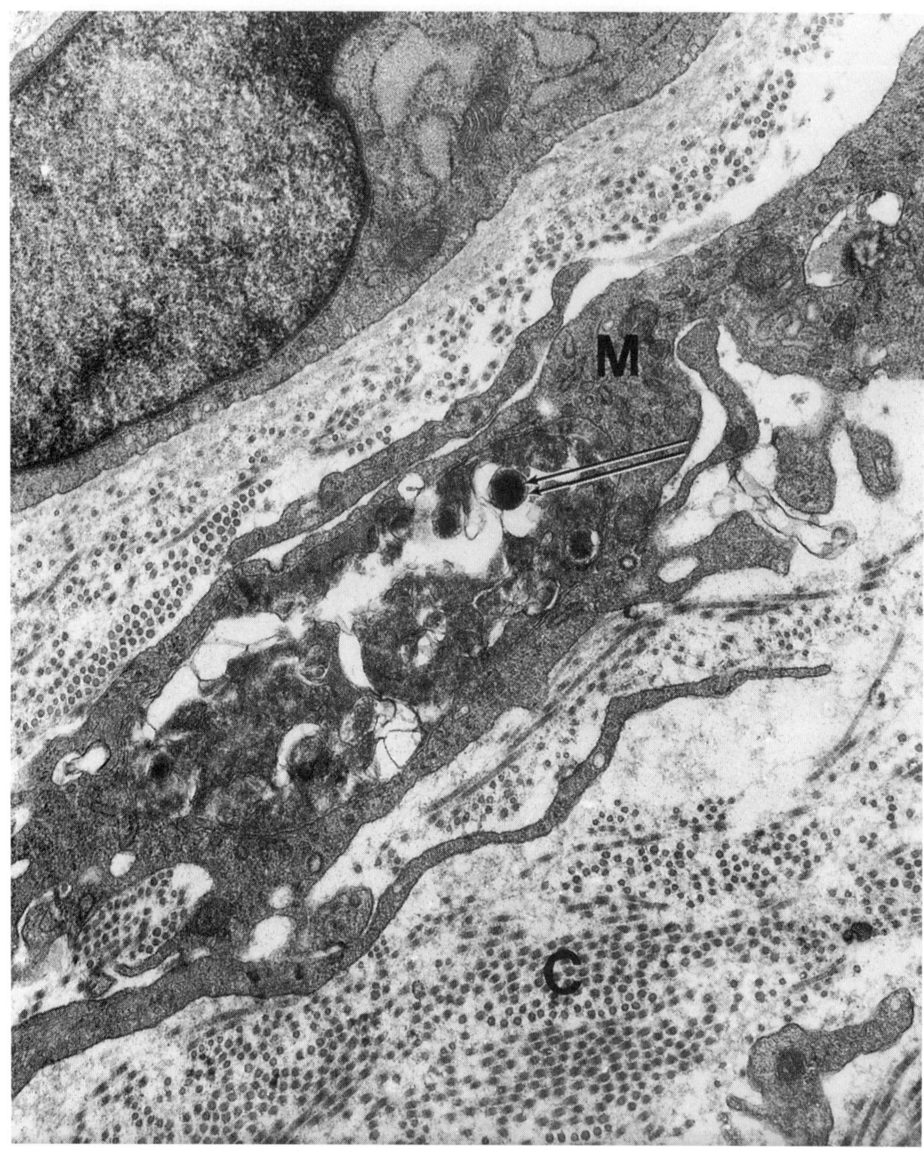

Fig. 6.4 Patient with chronic Reiter's syndrome. Presumed mass chlamydia in various stages (arrow) in vacuole of perivascular macrophage (M). C, collagen. (Electron micrograph < 19 500)

Extra-articular chlamydial lesions beyond the genitourinary tract have received extremely little histopathological study. The entheses and sacroiliac joints would seem especially important places to look for the presence of chlamydia and to examine the nature of the cellular reaction. To date, the sacroiliac joints, entheses, and skin lesions have not been examined in proven chlamydial-associated arthritis. One study of a group of incompletely classified spondylarthropathy patients who underwent sacroiliac biopsies (Braun *et al.* 1995*b*) and PCR was reported to show no evidence of chlamydia or several other organisms.

Detection of chlamydia in the conjunctiva has been discussed in a Russian report (Tarasova and Grigor'eva 1991). A vulvar rash in Reiter's syndrome showed histopathology as seen in pustular psoriasis with acanthosis, parakeratosis, and chronic inflammation (Edwards and Hansen 1992).

The keratoderma blenorrhagicum skin lesions of Reiter's syndrome have been studied histologically, but studies have not addressed whether changes are different in patients with or without chlamydia. In three patients with GU-related Reiter's syndrome but no proof of articular chlamydial involvement, biopsies showed classical keratoderma and other less typical skin lesions (Magro *et al.* 1995). Histologically, all cases showed parakeratosis, spongiform pustulation, and an absent granular layer. Capillaries and venules had perivascular and intramural mononuclear cell infiltrates mixed with neutrophils, plasma cells and rare eosinophils, with fibrin in vessel walls and leukocytoclasia leading to a histological diagnosis of leukocytoclastic vasculitis! Possibly most importantly, immunofluorescence staining with antibody against chlamydial LPS and hsp 60 was reported in vessels in two of the cases. Fibrin, IgG, IgM, and complement were found in one case. Controls were negative. No electron microscopy or other immunohistochemistry was performed. Further studies on skin and other extra-articular lesions of Reiter's syndrome would be important. The few findings noted above and the recent reports of the demonstration of *Chlamydia pneumoniae* in coronary artery lesions (Kuo *et al.* 1993) suggest that widespread dissemination is possible. In the *Chlamydia pneumoniae* study, chlamydiae were not found in normal coronary arteries. Studies are badly needed on other normal tissues to see if dissemination is always, or at least most often, associated with pathological changes, and vice-versa.

Other reports over the years suggest that *Chlamydia pneumoniae*, *C. psittaci*, and *C. trachomatis* can also cause other cardiac lesions including endocarditis and myocarditis (Odeh and Oliven 1992). *Chlamydia pneumoniae* DNA has recently been reported in the joints of patients with reactive and unclassified arthritis (Gérard *et al.* 1995*b*). This is the first direct report of identification of DNA, although the clinical association of *Chlamydia pneumoniae* with arthritis has been described as noted (see below). How much more disease is found to be associated with chlamydia may only depend on improving diagnostic techniques and interest in searching for causes in unexplained disease. *Chlamydia pneumoniae*-induced inflammation has been described in mouse lungs after experimental administration (Kimura 1994). After the initial exposure inclusion bodies, neutrophils, and macrophage infiltration were evident. After a second exposure there were few inclusions and a lymphocytic reaction.

Intravaginal administration of *C. trachomatis* in mice produced a lymphocytic infiltration of the genital mucosa (Cain and Rank 1995). The lymphocytes proliferated in response to chlamydial antigen and produced IFN-γ, but not IL-4, suggesting a TH1 local response. Chlamydia DNA has been found to persist by *in-situ* hybridization in monkey tissues with salpingitis after inoculation with the organism (Capuccio *et al.* 1994). Spread beyond the GU tract was not studied, although pelvic nodes have been found to contain chlamydia.

The triggering infection

Although a few reports have described arthritis associated with or following infections caused by *C. psittaci* (Bhopal and Thomas 1982, Lanham and Doyle 1984) and *C. trachomatis* L_1–L_3 (lymphogranuloma venereum) (see Keat *et al.* 1983), most CIA are due to infections with

Table 6.2 Sexually transmitted *C. trachomatis* diseases and sequelae

Diseases	Clinical manifestations	Sequelae
Male		
Urethritis	Dysuria, urethral discharge, and erythema	Urethral stricture
Epididymitis	Unilateral scrotal pain, swelling, tenderness	
Prostatitis	Perineal discomfort, dysuria, frequency, urethral discharge	
Proctitis	Rectal pain, bleeding and discharge, tenesmus, diarrhoea	
Female		
Urethral syndrome	Frequency, dysuria	
Cervicitis	Mucopurulent discharge, postcoital bleeding	
Endometritis/salpingitis	Pelvic/abdominal pain, abnormal uterine bleeding, fever	Infertility, ectopic pregnancy, puerperal endometritis, adhesions around the uterine appendages and liver, perihepatitis, periappendicitis
Newborn		
Conjunctivitis	Eyelid oedema, conjunctival erythema, mucopurulent discharge	
Pneumonia	Staccato pertussoid cough, tachypnoea	Asthma

C. trachomatis serotypes D to K, the most common cause worldwide of sexually transmitted chlamydial diseases. More recently, infections with *C. pneumoniae* were identified as another triggering infection for CIA; this may also be of considerable importance for rheumatology (Beaudreuil *et al.* 1995; Braun *et al.* 1994*d*; Gérard *et al.* 1995*b*; Gran *et al.* 1993; Saario and Toivanen 1993). Primary infections with *C. trachomatis* and *C. pneumoniae* cause a variety of clinical syndromes depending on the portal of entry and the patient's sex and age (see Tables 6.2 and 6.4). The main clinical aspects and risk factors are discussed in the following sections.

C. trachomatis infections

The main portal of entry for *C. trachomatis* is the urogenital tract, but the rhinopharyngeal and respiratory tract as well as conjunctivae may also be sites of primary infections in adults and newborns. Chlamydial reproduction takes place in the single-layered columnar epithelium of cervix, urethra, and paraurethral glands. Dissemination of whole bacteria from the genito-urinary tract during acute infection is well recognized. Intraluminal spread can lead to ascending infections of the upper male and female urogenital organs, and especially in females via intra-abdominal spread to cause perihepatic infection. Additionally, chlamydia can be transmitted from the genitalia to the conjunctiva by hand-to-eye contact and to the pharynx by orogenital sexual contact (Lauhio *et al.* 1991). Finally, there are good reasons to suggest that the organism can also be disseminated from the portal of entry to other tissues, including the joints, via inflammatory cells within the blood. Although the mechanisms of access to the circulation and of bacterial transport in the blood are still the subject of speculation, the *in vitro* observation of intracellular survival and persistence of chlamydia in human peripheral blood mononuclear cells and in monocytic cell lines indicates a possible pivotal role for such a dissemination within the relatively protected environment of living cells (Köhler *et al.* 1994, 1995; Manor and Sarov 1986; Schmitz *et al.* 1993).

It is important for the clinician to be aware, in detail, of the whole spectrum of triggering chlamydial infections to avoid misdiagnosis and inappropriate treatment of CIA as well as the underlying chlamydial infection. The variety of primary infections and their clinical manifestations is further complicated by the considerable frequency of asymptomatic chlamydial infections, also referred to as 'inapparent infection', 'subclinical infection', and 'latent infection'. Moreover, a recent study using PCR techniques showed a very high transmission rate with a positive test in 75% of male partners of PCR-positive women and in 58% of female partners of infected men (Viscidi *et al.* 1993).

Urogenital chlamydial infections

C. trachomatis is the most common causative agent of non-gonoccocal urethritis in males and cervicitis in females (Pearlman and McNeeley 1992; Taylor-Robinson and Thomas 1980) accounting for approximately 50–60% of cases. After an incubation period of 1–3 weeks, men develop mild dysuria and a white-to-clear urethral discharge. Sometimes, only meatal erythema may be present, and frequently physical signs are completely absent. Chlamydia urethritis is more likely to be mild or asymptomatic compared with gonococcal urethritis. Co-infection with *Neisseria gonorrheae* and *C. trachomatis* occurs in heterosexuals in up to 30% of some populations and risk groups. Approximately 80% of co-infected men develop postgonococcal urethritis if treated with penicillin or cephalosporin alone. Up to 50% of cases with postgonococcal urethritis are attributable to *C. trachomatis*. The most important complication of chlamydial urethritis is urethral stricture.

Urethral chlamydial infection in women is mostly asymptomatic, but just as in men urinary symptoms should rise suspicions. The urethral syndrome of frequency and dysuria without bacteriuria has been associated with urethral chlamydial infection in up to 60% of women examined. Haematuria and suprapubic pressure, frequently seen with bacterial cystitis, are absent.

Cervicitis is the most common genital infection caused by *C. trachomatis* in women, and 50–90% of these infections are asymptomatic. *C. trachomatis* can be recovered from the cervix in 5–35% of sexually active women, depending on the characteristics of the population. The prevalence of infection varies from 5 to 10% in sexually active college students to 35% or greater in women attending sexually transmitted disease clinics and pregnant women of lower socioeconomic status in urban centres. Risk factors for genital chlamydial infections in women are noted in Table 6.3. Approximately two-thirds of women whose partners have chlamydial urethritis will have positive cervical or urethral cultures for *C. trachomatis* (Viscidi *et al.* 1993). Mucopurulent discharge and a history of postcoital spotting may be obtained by history. On examination, ectopy, or eversion of the squamocolumnar junction is frequently observed. Oedematous, polypous swelling of the cervix with purulent mucus and

Table 6.3 Factors associated with genital chlamydial infections in women

Concomitant sexually transmitted disease
Multiple sexual partners
More than one sexual partner in preceding 6 months
Age less than 24 years
Use of non-barrier contraceptive or no contraceptive
Postcoital bleeding or clinical evidence of friable cervix
Mucopurulent cervical discharge

marked vascular injection is typical. The cervix is friable and bleeds easily with placement of the speculum or sampling of the glandular epithelium.

Other less frequent types of primary chlamydial infection are proctitis in men and bartholinitis in women. Non-LGV (lymphogranuloma venereum) serovars of *C. trachomatis* account for approximately 5% of cases of proctitis occuring more frequently in homosexual and bisexual males. These men may be asymptomatic or present with symptoms such as rectal pain, bleeding, discharge, tenesmus, or diarrhoea. On examination, the rectal mucosa is erythematous and friable.

Symptomatic and asymptomatic ascending infections of the urogenital tract are common. In men, infection ascending via the proximal urethra leads to cystitis; via the afferent prostatic ducts to prostatitis; and via the vas deferens and vasa efferentia of the epididymis to epididymitis. Epididymitis is seen mainly in promiscuous men presenting with unilateral scrotal pain, swelling, tenderness, and fever. Symptoms of acute prostatitis include perineal discomfort, dysuria, frequency, and urethral discharge.

It is mainly young women who contract ascending chlamydial infections via the uterus and Fallopian tubes causing pelvic inflammatory diseases (PID) such as endometritis and salpingitis. Symptoms of chlamydial PID are often described as atypical or mild. Endometritis is a common complication after instrumentation of the uterus and is reported to occur in up to 20% of asymptomatic woman infected with chlamydia undergoing a suction abortion. The most important risk factor associated with female Reiter's syndrome and seronegative arthritis is salpingitis. Although other microbiological agents, such as mycoplasma, ureaplasma, and gonococcus, may cause salpingitis, in one study of 73 females with reactive arthritis, evidence for *C. trachomatis* infection was found in 59% (Yli-Kerttula and Vilpulla 1988). The mean time from the first salpingitis to the onset of joint disease was one year. This long delay may explain why the diagnosis of CIA is often overlooked in females. Moreover, in individual cases, salpingitis could occur or recur even several years before or after the onset of joint disease. An additional important feature of salpingitis is the tendency to recur or run a chronic course with equivocal symptoms such as chronic abdominal pain. Altogether the careful history not only of recent gynaecological symptoms but also the diagnosis of former PID manifestations can give important indications to search for chlamydial infection.

Unfortunately, many cases of PID are asymptomatic and the first clinical manifestations are late complications. Infertility and ectopic pregnancy are the most common complications of PID, but perihepatitis, periappendicitis, puerpural endometritis, intra-abdominal adhesions, and possibly poor pregnancy outcome (preterm labour, premature rupture of membranes) have also been attributed to chlamydial infections.

In both sexes, ascending infections can cause acute or chronic cystitis. A few cases of pyelonephritis due to *C. trachomatis* has been described.

Altogether the spectrum of urogenital manifestations of *C. trachomatis* is much broader than that covered by the preliminary classification criteria for Reiter's syndrome, which only includes urethritis and cervicitis. Unfortunately, the available literature on CIA gives only limited data concerning the frequency and clinical manifestations of the triggering chlamydial infections. In one recent study urethritis was the most frequent symptom of the precipitating chlamydial infection in CIA in men with 63%, compared with 25% in women (Wollenhaupt *et al.* 1995). In women, the diagnosis of cystitis was as frequent as urethritis. From the frequency of prostatitis in men (13%) and salpingitis in women (11%), there was no apparent difference in the number of truly symptomatic infections in both sexes. But in women, in particular, the genitourinary symptoms were often subtle and only diagnosed by specific inquiry and additional urological or gynaecological examination by specialists. Silveira *et al.* (1993) assessing the prevalence of *C. trachomatis* infection in patients with spondylarthritides, obtained a history of dysuria in 31% and urethral discharge in 8% during the previous 3 months. A previous history of venereal disease was present in 25%. Nevertheless, strong future efforts and prospective studies are needed to define more precisely the frequency, the presentation, and the whole spectrum of urogenital chlamydial infections in CIA. The dissociation between the symptoms of the triggering infection and the rheumatic manifestations, best described for salpingitis (Yli-Kerttula and Vilpulla 1988) but also seen with other chlamydial urogenital manifestations (Kvien *et al.* 1994; Wollenhaupt *et al.* 1995), is a further issue to be addressed in the future. Additionally, diagnostic tools are needed to differentiate between new infection, asymptomatic chronic infection, reinfection, and activation of persistent infection as causes of the onset or relapse of CIA in individual patients.

Ocular infections

Chlamydial ocular infections can be divided into three different forms: neonatal chlamydial ophthalmia (see below), adult ophthalmia, and trachoma.

Trachoma, a chronic keratoconjunctivitis is caused by *C. trachomatis* serotypes A to C and is endemic in China, Egypt, and the Near East, but has not been described as causing CIA. In Western countries, the oculogenital strains of *C. trachomatis* belonging to the serotypes D to K have been isolated from patients with conjunctivitis. Chlamydiae can be transmitted from the genitalia to the conjunctiva by smear infection. The clinical picture shows follicular conjunctivitis and epithelial and subepithelial infiltration of the cornea with mucopurulent or serous reactions.

Upper airway and respiratory tract infections

In some patients *C. trachomatis* has been isolated from pharyngeal swabs, nasal and sinusoid discharges, and bronchoalveolar lavage. Clinical manifestations described in association were tonsillitis, sore throat, sinusitis, and atypical pneumonia.

Systemic manifestations

C. trachomatis may also cause myocarditis, endocarditis, pericarditis, and meningioencephalitis (Giordano *et al.* 1996; Hughes and Keat 1994). However, except for one case with chlamydial bacteraemia the aetiological connection was established only by the association with the clinical features of urogenital infection and a positive culture at the portal of entry. One may speculate, as with CIA, that these systemic manifestations are due to the widespread dissemination of the organism.

Neonatal infections

The organism is transmitted during delivery and the typical sites of infection are the eye and the rhinopharynx. Significant common clinical manifestations include inclusion conjunctivitis and a late-onset pneumonia occuring as late as 4 months after delivery. Although the conjunctivitis may be subclinical, symptoms usually begin within 3 to 13 days of delivery, initially are unilateral, and consist of oedema of the eyelids, conjunctival erythema, and a mucopurulent discharge. In the case of pneumonia late sequelae such as asthma cannot be excluded.

C. pneumoniae infections

C. pneumoniae is a common cause of acute respiratory tract infections. Population-prevalence antibody studies have shown that in many countries around the world at least 50% of adults have antibodies. The rate increases rapidly from 5 to 20 years of age and then increases slowly into old age. The clinical features of the human-to-human transmitted airborne infection vary from mild upper respiratory disease to primary atypical pneumonia (Table 6.4). Upper respiratory symptoms, particularly pharyngitis, often relatively severe with hoarseness and usually with fever may be seen initially without signs of pulmonary involvement. Pneumonia and bronchitis remain the most common clinical syndromes, but sinusitis and, less commonly, otitis may also accompany them or be the only manifestation (Table 6.4). The pneumonitis is commonly a single subsegmental lesion, but more extensive unilateral and even bilateral pneumonitis has been found. Rhonchi and rales are commonly heard on auscultation, even in patients with relatively mild symptoms. More recently, frequent bronchospasm and the onset of asthma has been associated with acute *C. pneumoniae* infection (Hahn *et al.* 1991). Other complications or manifestations described are myocarditis, endocarditis, and sarcoidosis (Grayston 1989; Groenhagen-Riska *et al.* 1988). Moreover, a possible aetiological role of *C. pneumoniae* in chronic obstructive pulmonary disease, coronary heart disease, and

Table 6.4 Clinical disease with *C. pneumoniae* infections in 1100 adults, diagnosed serdogically (Modified from Grayston 1992)

Disease	Symptoms	Frequency (%)
Pneumonia	Mild to severe	51
Bronchitis	Often prolonged	28
Pharyngitis	Often accompanies above	7
Sinusitis	Initial or later complication	3
Otitis	Less common	
Febrile illness	'Influenza-like'	10
Asymptomatic	Common	

Table 6.5 Evidence for arthritis triggered by *Chlamydia pneumoniae* infection

Authors	Year	Number	Infectious manifestations	Complications
Saario and Toivanen	1993	3	Pharyngitis, fever, bronchitis, pneumonia	Myocarditis, AV-conduction disturbance
Gran *et al.*	1993	1	Pharyngitis preceeding pneumonia, fever	Erythema nodosum, myocarditis
Braun *et al.*	1994	5	Pharyngitis (n = 1), bronchitis (n = 2), asymptomatic (n = 2)	
Beaudreuil *et al.*	1995	1	Asymptomatic	
Gérard *et al.*	1995*b*	5	Initial diagnosis of reactive arthritis or undiagnosed	

atherosclerosis is being increasingly discussed and investigated (Grayston 1992; Saikku *et al.* 1992; Ward 1995).

Clinical details have been described up to now in only 10 patients with CIA attributed to *C. pneumoniae* infection (Beaudreuil *et al.* 1995; Braun *et al.* 1994*d*; Gran *et al.* 1993; Saario and Toivanen 1993). Pharyngitis, bronchitis, and pneumonia are the typical clinical manifestations of the triggering infection reported, but 3 of the 10 patients were asymptomatic for preceding upper or lower respiratory infection (Table 6.5). In two cases, myocarditis and in one erythema nodosum were seen in addition to arthritis as complications of the *C. pneumoniae* infection.

The Clinical Spectrum of chlamydia-induced arthritis

CIA, like other spondylarthritides, combines four syndromes: a peripheral arthritis; enthesopathy; a pelviaxial syndrome; and extramusculoskeletal manifestations. The combination of these four varies from one patient to another, and in a given patient during the course of the disease. It is unclear which factors determine the clinical picture of CIA in an individual patient.

General clinical aspects common to CIA and other spondylarthritides are discussed elsewere in this book (see Chapter 4). We will therefore concentrate on those rather limited data described in case and cohort studies which are more specifically related to patients with CIA confirmed by microbiological diagnosis (culture, molecular biology, morphology) of chlamydial infection (Doury *et al.* 1983; Kvien *et al.* 1994; Wollenhaupt and Zeidler 1990*a*, Wollenhaupt *et al.* 1989*a*, 1995; Zeidler 1992, Zeidler and Wollenhaupt 1991). Diagnoses of CIA based on serology alone are of questionable value, as there are also high antibody titres in the normal population and in many patients with other rheumatic diseases (Erlacher *et al.* 1995). However, patients with positive urogenital smears and CIA are generally positive for chlamydial IgA-antibodies (Wollenhaupt *et al.* 1989*c*).

Only a few case reports and case series have described rheumatological features of CIA due to *C. psittaci*, *C. pneumaniae*, and *C. trachomatis* serovar lymphogranuloma venereum, and these lack description of any specific characteristics (see Braun *et al.* 1994*d*, Keat *et al.* 1983, Lanham and Doyle 1984). Most information specific for clinical manifestations is available for CIA caused by *C. trachomatis* serovar D to K infections as follows.

Presentation

While Reiter's syndrome and SARA are generally thought to occur mainly in males, CIA can affect males and females with equal frequency depending on the classification criteria, selection, and disease duration (Table 6.6). Triggering chlamydia infections in women are often asymptomatic. The urethral syndrome in females is rarely diagnosed, and other urogenital inflammatory involvement like cervicitis or salpingitis may be overlooked in the context of the rheumatic disease. In a recent cohort of CIA patients, all positive for *C. trachomatis* in urogenital smears, but 30% asymptomatic for urogenital chlamydial infection, the sex ratio was nearly equal (Wollenhaupt *et al.* 1995). Silent chlamydial infections were present in more women (11 of 18 asymptomatic patients, 61%) than men (7 of 18, 39%). In the tertiary rheumatological referral centre, more chronic cases of arthritis (mean duration 18 months, 44% with arthritis of >1 yr) were seen; but even in patients seen in an early synovitis outpatient clinic, the mean duration of arthritis was still 9 months (Wollenhaupt *et al.* 1989*a*). Other series of patients with seronegative oligoarthritis of longer duration, in which the diagnosis was made by positive urogenital culture or intra-articular chlamydial antigen, also described a considerable number of females with CIA (Taylor-Robinson *et al.* 1988; Weyand and Goronzy 1992). Altogether, females with CIA are more frequently asymptomatic in the genitourinary tract and generally present with advanced, more chronic disease. Only a thorough history or examination may evoke very mild urogenital symptoms at presentation or clinical features suggesting former chlamydial infection.

The incubation period of sexually acquired non-gonococcal urethritis is approximately 8–15 days, and the mean overall incubation period for patients with SARA was suggested to be approximately 28 days (Keat 1987). Precise data specifically for CIA are not available. Moreover, as mentioned earlier in some individuals, especially females, the interval between the infection and arthritis may be much longer in the case of asymptomatic subclinical

Table 6.6 Demographic and clinical characteristics of CIA

	Doury *et al.* 1983	**Kvien *et al.* 1994**	**Wollenhaupt *et al.* 1995**
Number of patients	86	25	60
Male/female	72/14	20/5	33/27
Mean age (years)	33	26	33
Duration of arthritis at presentation	—	2 weeks	18 months
Patients presenting with			
– first episode of arthritis (%)	—	—	53
– recurrence of arthritis (%)	—	—	3
Urogenital symptoms present	65	64	70
HLA-B27 positive (%)	62	45	57

infection, relapsing infection, and reinfection (Yli-Karttulla and Vilpulla 1988). It also appears possible that chronic persistent chlamydial genital infections may remain asymptomatic for long periods and only become complicated by CIA much later due to additional factors (for example, childbirth, gynaecological manoeuvres, reduced resistance).

Acute peripheral synovitis is usually the first rheumatic symptom, although, as in other spondylarthritides, presentation may be as painful enthesopathy, low-back pain, or other less common musculoskeletal manifestations.

Arthritis

The pattern of joint involvement in CIA resembles that of other reactive arthritides with monoarticular, asymmetrical arthritis and preferential involvement of the large joints of the lower limb (Table 6.7) (Doury *et al.* 1983; Kvien *et al.* 1994; Wollenhaupt *et al.* 1995). Approximately 10% of patients remain monoarthritic. Knee and ankle joints are most commonly affected, but any joint may be involved (Fig. 6.5). When small joints are affected, characteristically only one or two of the group are involved but a polyarthritis of the small joints has also been seen. The joint pattern is the same in patients with silent vs. symptomatic urogenital chlamydial infection (Wollenhaupt *et al.* 1995). The arthritis in the few patients with CIA caused by *C. pneumoniae* also seems to fit into this typical joint pattern of reactive arthritis and spondarthritis (Table 6.8).

Although long-standing and chronic arthritis is not rare (see below, p. 90), the persistence of synovitis leads only infrequently to articular erosions. Most patients have non-erosive joint

Table 6.7 Rheumatological manifestations of CIA

	Doury *et al.* 1983	**Kvien *et al.* 1984**	**Wollenhaupt *et al.* 1995**
Mono-/oligoarthritis (%)	76	68	68
Polyarthritis (%)	21	32	32
Enthesopathy (%)	23	4	28
Inflammatory low-back pain (%)	26	28	35
Sacroiliitis (X-ray) (%)	—	—	33
Erosive bone lesions (X-ray) (%)	—	—	7

Table 6.8 Arthritis due to *Chlamydia pneumoniae*

Authors	**Year**	**Number**	**Involved joints**	**HLA-B27 positive**
Saario and Toivanen	1993	3	Knee, ankle, finger, shoulder	1/2
Gran *et al.*	1993	1	Ankle, wrist	—
Braun *et al.*	1994	5	Knee, elbow, wrist, Achilles tendon	2/4
Beaudreuil *et al.*	1995	1	Ankle, knee	—

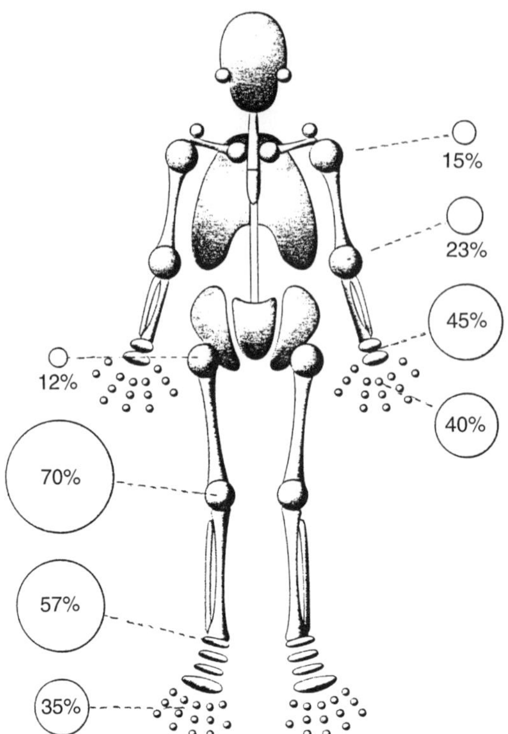

Fig. 6.5 Frequency of joint manifestation in CIA. (From Wollenhaupt *et al.* 1995, reproduced with permission.)

involvement (Table 6.7). Erosive bone lesions were observed in one CIA cohort in only four patients (12%) with oligoarthritis associated with symptomatic chlamydial infection and were seen at the metatarsophalangeal joints (three patients) and radioulnar joint (one patient) (Wollenhaupt *et al.* 1995).

Enthesopathy

Inflammatory involvement of ligaments and tendinous insertions, that is to say inflammatory enthesopathy, is reported in 4–28% of patients with CIA (Table 6.7). As in other reactive arthritides the sites of attachment of the Achilles tendon and the plantar fascia to the calcaneus are most commonly involved, but it may also occur at other sites. In one study most patients had Achilles tendinitis ($n = 9$), a few plantar fasciitis ($n = 3$), heel pain ($n = 3$), and pain at the pelvic crest ($n = 2$) (Wollenhaupt *et al.* 1995). Enthesopathy was observed in 39% of patients with silent and in 24% of the patients with overt urogenital infection, although the difference was not statistically significant. There was no difference between HLA-B27 positive and negative patients or between male and female patients.

Enthesopathic lesions can be visualized at an early stage by focal isotopic uptake on 99mTc-methylene diphosphanate scintigraphy. Complete skeletal scintiscan may lead to the identification of enthesitis not apparent or overlooked by physical examination (Lin *et al.* 1995). Advanced enthesopathies are characterized radiographically by bone erosions and new bone formation, namely large, fluffy bone spurs as is well described in Reiter's syndrome and other spondylarthritides.

Axial involvement

Inflammatory low-back pain is reported in 28–35% of patients with CIA. In two reports all patients were positive for chlamydia urogenital smears (Kvien *et al.* 1994, Wollenhaupt *et al.* 1995). In the earlier French study diagnosis was based on the direct microbiological testing in only 22% of patients' and in 77% on indirect methods (serology or synovial lymphocyte transformation test), but in 77% of cases clinical features of chlamydial urogenital infection preceded the arthritis by not more than 1 month (Doury *et al.* 1983). Radiological sacroiliitis was observed in 33% of patients (Table 6.7) (Wollenhaupt *et al.* 1995), which indicates more destructive involvement of this axial joint than of the peripheral joints. There is no difference in inflammatory low-back pain and radiological sacroiliitis in patients with silent vs. symptomatic chlamydial infection (Wollenhaupt *et al.* 1995). However HLA-B27 is significantly associated with radiographic sacroiliitis. Of 28 B27-positive patients, 15 (54%) had sacroiliitis in contrast to only 5 of 32 B27-negative patients (16%; $p < 0.0005$) (Wollenhaupt *et al.* 1995). Nevertheless, as in other reactive arthritides, development into the full picture of ankylosing spondylitis may be rare. Cases of AS with definite chlamydial aetiology have not been described. Long-term follow-up studies of CIA are hoping to answer the question of the frequency of development into AS. These seems to stand in contrast to documented cases of AS following Shigella-induced reactive arthritis (Sairanen *et al.* 1969).

Cervical spine manifestations have been reported only rarely in Reiter's syndrome, either as a presenting feature or in severe chronic cases (Halla *et al.* 1988). However, one unusual observation will serve to illustrate that cervical spine manifestations should also be included in the clinical spectrum of CIA (Zeidler and Wollenhaupt 1991). A 54-year-old woman presented with severe occipital neck pain, restricted head rotation and fever. The history was negative for urogenital infection but 2 weeks before the beginning of the disease she had a 'flu-like' illness with sore throat. The sedimentation rate (Westergren) was 106 mm/h; rheumatoid factor and HLA-B27 antigen were negative; serology for *C. trachomatis* antibodies (Ipacyme, Medac) were positive with an IgG titre of 1:256 and an IgA titre of 1:32; cervical smears were positive for chlamydia with the immunofluorescence test (Syva, Darmstadt). Bone scintigraphy showed high tracer activity in the right craniocervical region. Erosive changes were noted in the right C1–C2 lateral facet joint on plain X-ray. The diagnosis was made of a CIA with isolated acute craniocervical arthritis, and the patient was treated with diclofenac 50 mg, three times per day, physiotherapy, and a 3-month prescription of doxycycline at 200 mg per day. Over the next several months, she achieved total remission with disappearance of cervical pain, only slight residual limitation of head rotation, normal sedimentation rate, negative urogenital smears for chlamydia, and normalization of the serology with negative IgA and IgG.

Extramusculoskeletal manifestations

Features of CIA outside the musculoskeletal system can be classified into (1) local symptoms from the urogenital infection with *C. trachomatis* and (2) systemic manifestations. Such a differentiation takes into account the presence of chlamydia in a replicative, infective form of the developmental cycle in most genitourinary manifestations, with corresponding identification in some cases by routine microbiological culture methods; whereas in cases with only systemic manifestations, the isolation of chlamydia is generally impossible. Conjunctivitis may be present in both groups: in some patients with acute inflammation the organism may be grown from conjunctival scrapes, although cultures are mostly negative in chronic conjunctivitis. From a practical point of view one must further consider that ascending urogenital infections often elude microbiological diagnosis because of the impracticality of gaining material for an appropriate investigation.

Urethritis and cervicitis are reported in 57–65% of patients with CIA (Table 6.9), with features of ascending infection less frequent: salpingitis (5%), prostatitis (8%), epididymitis (3%), and pylonephritis (2%) (Amor *et al.* 1983, Doury *et al.* 1983, Kvien *et al.* 1994, Wollenhaupt *et al.* 1995). In these series, most patients had mild to moderate genitourinary symptoms and were only diagnosed by specific inquiry and additional urological or gynaecological examination. In addition to actual manifestations of urogenital chlamydial infection present at the clinical visit, approximately 50% of patients with silent and asymptomatic urogenital chlamydial infection reported earlier genitourinary disease (Wollenhaupt *et al.* 1995). In this series, all patients were in complete clinical remission from genital disease for more than 3 months before their arthritis developed. This further underlines the dissociation between clinical symptomatology of the urogenital chlamydial infection and the presence of long-standing or recurrent asymptomatic, culture-positive infection at the entry site. An additional important clinical aspect is the high degree of sexual promiscuity and high proportion of new sexual partners described in one study of patients with spondylarthropathies and positive *C. trachomatis* culture (Silveira *et al.* 1993).

Ocular involvement, usually in the form of bilateral conjunctivitis, is a further common accompanying feature reported in approximately one-third of patients with CIA, but in one study the frequency was 73%. Although conjunctivitis is an essential constituent of the classical triad of Reiter's syndrome, the complete syndrome may only be present in at most

Table 6.9 Extra-articular manifestations in CIA

	Doury *et al.* 1983	**Amor *et al.* 1983**	**Kvien *et al.* 1994**	**Wollenhaupt *et al.* 1995**
Urethritis/cervicitis (%)	63	65	64 (Urethritis/cervicitis to Pyelonephritis combined)	57
Salpingitis	—	—		5
Prostatitis	—	—		8
Epididymitis	—	—		3
Pyelonephritis	—	—		2
Uveitis	12	5	28 (Uveitis and Conjunctivitis combined)	13
Conjunctivitis	73	21		30
Keratitis	—	2	—	—
Balanitis	19	24	—	6
Stomatitis	7	11	24 (Stomatitis and Skin abnormalities combined)	—
Skin abnormalities	—	—		10
Diarrhoea	39	39	8	0

10–20% of patients with CIA (Zeidler 1992, Zeidler and Wollenhaupt 1991). Acute anterior uveitis (AAU) is reported in 5–13% of patients. AAU usually presents with more severe symptoms, whereas conjunctivitis often may be asymptomatic with such mild symptoms that patients rarely consciously link them with the arthritis and the musculoskeletal symptoms.

Skin and mucous membrane involvement, in the form of circinate balanitis, keratoderma blenorrhagicum, or gingivostomatitis, is a familiar phenomenon in patients with Reiter's syndrome. Balanitis has also been encounted in CIA in 6–24% of cases, while stomatitis and skin abnormalities were observed in 7–20%. Most interestingly, gastrointestinal symptoms and diarrhoea were reported in 39% of the patients in two older series, but in only 0–8% in the two more recent studies (Table 6.9).

From the observations that *C. trachomatis* may cause myocarditis, endocarditis, hepatitis, meningoencephalitis, perihepatitis, and periappendicitis, there is a suggestion that these systemic manifestations may also accompany or follow CIA. Most recently, the case of a 38-year-old woman was reported, who developed continued fever and pericarditis caused by *C. trachomatis* infection while under treatment with oral corticosteroids for classic sicca syndrome (Giordano *et al.* 1996). Repeated blood cultures revealed a *C. trachomatis* bacteraemia, and ocular as well as vaginal swabs were also positive for *C. trachomatis.* A 2-months oxytetracycline treatment induced complete remission of pericarditis and the eradication of chlamydia. Future studies and observations are awaited to show the role of such clinical features in *C. trachomatis*-induced CIA.

In two patients with CIA due to *C. pneumoniae* infection, myocarditis was diagnosed in association with the acute course of the arthritis (Gran *et al.* 1993; Saario and Toivanen 1993). In one of these patients, chest radiograph and echocardiography revealed cardiac dilatation. A cardiac systolic mumur was heard in the other patient, and sick sinus node syndrome with severe bradycardia and later atrioventricular block was found. Chest radiographs revealed cardiac failure and echocardiogram showed mitral regurgitation and prolapse of mitral valve leaflets with some pericardial effusion.

Course and prognosis

Less information is available on the course of CIA, compared with the faster evolving pathological, diagnostic, and clinical characterization of this rheumatological condition. Only limited data are available from the short-term follow-up (2–3 years) of patients with CIA defined by laboratory diagnosis of the triggering chlamydial infection; as yet no long term studies have been performed. The picture of the natural history and prognosis must therefore be drawn from the literature reviewing the course of patients with postvenereal Reiter's syndrome not proven to be chlamydia associated.

In two very important studies, Csonka specifically addressed the question of the risk of a recurrence in relation to urethral infections occurring during the period following the initial attack of postvenereal Reiter's syndrome (Csonka 1958, 1960). From 185 consecutive patients attending a venereal disease clinic, the vast majority of the 80 patients observed for less than 1 year had a single attack, whereas 97 of 105 patients followed for more than one year experienced multiple episodes of the disease (Csonka 1958). These findings emphasize the need for a long observation period.

Some 30 patients could be followed for 10 years or more. Although this group was not representative of the whole series and certainly contained the more seriously and chronically involved cases, the analysis demonstrated several interesting features. Recurrence of urethritis did not inevitably lead to further arthritic attacks. There was no obvious reason why some episodes of urethritis in the same patients were followed by arthritis and others were not. Later attacks of arthritis were not always preceded by urethral infection, unlike the first attacks in this group. In a data analysis of 144 patients followed for more than 2 years, no urethral infections were found in 42% of the recurrent attacks (Csonka 1960). The author suggested that a high proportion of recurrences without preceding urethritis are relapses rather than new attacks because they occurred during periods of sexual abstinence. On the other hand, some of the episodes were apparently provoked by sexual intercourse. The intervals between the episodes were extremely variable, ranging from 3 months to 18 years.

The experience from patients with CIA diagnosed in an university out-patient, early synovitis clinic and followed for a mean of 30 months indicates that a remitting or chronic form of arthritis or spondylarthritis develops in a considerable proportion of individuals (Wollenhaupt *et al.* 1989*b*, 1990). More than half of the patients showed a chronic disease with arthritis (55%), enthesopathy (41%), and inflammatory axial symptoms (28%), and only 45% were in remission. Extra-articular manifestations were seldom seen: only one patient had urethritis and two patients had conjunctivitis. In contrast, Glennas *et al.* (1994), in a 2-year follow-up of patients with CIA of very short duration (median 2 weeks) at entry, described a somewhat more favourable outcome. As many as 40% of the patients still had arthritis after 1 year in contrast to the general view that most reactive arthritis is in remission after 6–9 months' disease duration, but after 2 years all patients were free of clinical signs of arthritis in peripheral joints. No flares of arthritis following recovery were observed and the mean time to resolution of arthritis was 24 weeks (range 12 to 52). A much earlier diagnosis, and consequently early treatment, including oral tetracyclines in nearly all patients, may be one explanation for the more favourable outcome. It should further be noted that although at the final follow-up visit none of the patients had arthritis, 25% still complained of joint pain and 10% reported back pain, whereas about 5% reported enthesopathies. Finally, it has recently been reported that some patients classified as having rheumatoid arthritis may in fact have CIA (Pando *et al.* 1995). This suggests a poorer prognosis and underestimation of the chronicity of this rheumatological condition.

Diagnosis and differential use of laboratory tests

One of the problems with accepting a role for disseminated chlamydia causing arthritis and for evaluating different series of patients is the wide variety of diagnostic tests in use (Genc and Mardh 1991).

Antibodies to *Chlamydia trachomatis* were used as supportive evidence of diagnosis in some early studies, but these antibodies, especially the IgG antibodies, are present in many people as a result of past infection and do not correlate with disease. In one recent study of patients with undifferentiated oligoarthritis, in only half of chlamydia IgG-antibody titre-positive patients could a chlamydia infection be confirmed by urogenital swab culture (Erlacher *et al.* 1995). Moreover, epidemiological studies have revealed a prevalence of a positive antibody test in approximately 5% of the normal population (Schachter 1978).

Therefore, the determination of specific isotypes of anti-chlamydia antibodies of the IgM and especially IgA class were suggested to yield further diagnostic information in patients with suspected CIA (Wollenhaupt *et al.* 1989*c*). The short duration of the IgM antibody response should indicate a recent or current chlamydial infection. The detection of IgA antibodies indicates a persistent agent since their half life is only 5–6 days in normal subjects. Recently, evidence was found for the intra-articular production of IgA anti-chlamydia antibodies (Bas *et al.* 1996*b*). Nevertheless, the sensitivity and positive predictive value of these specific isotypes in the rheumatology clinic is rather low (Bas *et al.* 1996*a*, Sieper *et al.* 1992*a*). Using single isotypes (IgG, IgM, IgA) only very high antibody titres indicate a diagnosis of CIA. With two different isotypes and their combination, the best sensitivity (63%) was obtained for IgM and/or IgA, with a specificity of 81% (Bas *et al.* 1996*a*). The negative predictive value was 84%; therefore the absence of IgM and/or IgA could be helpful in eliminating suspicion, but is not sufficient since there would be 19% false-positives and 33% false-negatives. Also, as noted below, chlamydia can clearly be found in synovium in a number of patients who are negative serologically.

Direct immunofluorescent (DIF) antibody studies were used by several investigators (Ishikawa *et al.* 1986; Keat *et al.* 1987) to attempt to demonstrate chlamydial antigens in synovium or SF. Both found evidence for chlamydia. The latter group found chlamydia in 5 out of 8 sexually acquired reactive arthritis patients, but this technique is not being widely used on synovium. DIF or culture has not been found to be as sensitive as PCR or nucleic acid hybridization in GU specimens (Oh *et al.* 1996; Wong *et al.* 1988), and presumably is not as sensitive in the joint.

Identification of chlamydial elementary and reticulate bodies by electron microscopy, with confirmation by immunohistochemistry, stimulated some of the renewed interest in the role of direct invasion of chlamydia into the joint (Schumacher *et al.* 1986, 1988), but this is a time-consuming, expensive, and unwieldy tool for most laboratories. False-positive results have not been reported, but the sensitivity of this technique is not known. Sampling can be a problem with EM as only very small areas of tissue are examined.

Hybridization was able to identify the 16S rRNA of *Chlamydia trachomatis* in RNA extracted from synovial fluid (Hammer *et al.* 1992) or synovium (Rahman *et al.* 1992*a*). This was positive in 6 out of 8 patients studied by Rahman *et al.* with Reiter's syndrome who had been negative by urethral and synovial cultures; only 1 of the 4 tested had serum antibodies to chlamydia. Interestingly, in this study chlamydial RNA was also found in patients with an acute septic monoarthritis picture, hypogammaglobulinaemia, and undiagnosed synovitis. Hammer *et al.* (1992) found chlamydial rRNA in 1 of 11 patients diagnosed clinically and serologically as CIA, in 3 patients with undifferentiated arthritis, and in the synovium of 1 patient with CIA. Clearly, testing for chlamydia not only identifies patients with classic Reiter's syndrome, spondylarthropathy, or reactive arthritis, but suggests that chlamydia may also be involved in other clinical situations. In-situ hybridization using the same probes (Beutler *et al.* 1994) can confirm the precise localization in the tissue, and seems very convincing. Recent reverse transcriptase PCR studies which have identified primary transcripts of the 16S rRNA may be most convincing, since these primary transcripts persist only seconds after cell death (Hudson *et al.* 1995), and their detection strongly supports the presence of viable organisms.

By far the most common diagnostic testing is performed by PCR targeting a variety of chlamydial genes. After a few initial reported failures, possibly because of the use of only synovial fluid or the use of primers for antigens which may be less common, most groups now seem to be successful in finding PCR evidence of chlamydia in high percentages of joints with post-GU infection 'reactive' arthritis or undiagnosed arthritis suspected to be related to chlamydia (Bas *et al.* 1995; Branigan *et al.* 1995; Li *et al.* 1996; Taylor-Robinson *et al.* 1992).

In our opinion the diagnosis of CIA can be most definitively established by the various techniques for identifying chlamydia in the lesion of interest, most often the synovium. Direct visualization by EM or *in-situ* hybridization adds important confirmation.

Cultures of joint material for chlamydia have occasionally been successful in the past (Dunlop *et al.* 1968; Engleman *et al.* 1969; Schachter *et al.* 1966), and work should continue on improving culture techniques. Schachter *et al.* (1966) isolated chlamydia from the synovium or SF, or both, in 5 out of 8 RS patients, whereas the results from all of the 15 non-RS control patients were negative. Engleman *et al.* (1969) reported culturing chlamydia from the SF and/or synovium of 6 out of 34 RS patients. Dunlop *et al.* (1968) reported isolating chlamydia from four of the eight RS patients they studied; in three cases, it was from SF and in one case from synovium; however, they advised that the possibility of laboratory contamination should be considered in interpreting these results. On the other hand, a later study (Gordon *et al.* 1973) failed to isolate chlamydia from the SF of 12 patients and 6 synovial biopsy samples. Although Keat *et al.* (1987) showed chlamydial particles in the joints of ReA patients, they failed to culture chlamydia from those joints. Importantly, the development of better techniques to culture chlamydia, namely the tissue-culture system, has not yielded any recent success in isolating chlamydia from joints.

Successful chlamydial culture primarily reflects one phenotypic characteristic of the organism: the presence of titreable levels of infective, viable elementary bodies in any given clinical sample. A negative culture cannot exclude the possibility of some form of latent organism or inactivation of the organism by cytokines or antichlamydial antibodies usually present in the inflammatory SF and tissue. The striking inconsistency in results for the many isolation attempts may well reflect as yet incompletely understood biological peculiarities of the chlamydia life cycle. For example, it is quite possible that under certain conditions, such as can prevail in joints, chlamydia enter a phase of their life cycle during which extremely low levels of the infectious extracellular elementary body form are produced. Screening clinical samples containing such organisms would thus give a false-negative culture result.

As pioneered by Ford, use of synovial lymphocytes to demonstrate preferential transformation to chlamydial antigens can be a powerful but indirect method to support the presence of chlamydia in joints (Ford and Schulzer 1994). Many such studies were performed using crude antigens. Gaston *et al.* (1996) have now used two specific antigens, the 57 kDa heat-shock protein and a 18 kDa histone-like peptide. Evaluation of the cellular immune response to chlamydia may be helpful in understanding disease mechanisms as well as providing clues to diagnosis. Clearly, it is no longer acceptable to simply classify arthritis as 'venerally associated reactive'; several groups have found similar arthritis due to *Ureaplasma urealyticum* (Li *et al.* 1996), and there may possibly be other GU causes.

More studies have been done comparing different techniques for the identification of chlamydia in the GU tract and in the conjunctivae in trachoma. Cultures as currently performed may be inadequate. A significant proportion of men treated for non-gonococcal urethritis, a majority of which is caused by chlamydia, go on to develop persistent or recurrent symptoms of urethritis. Although these patients are culture-negative for all known pathogens, about 50% of them become asymptomatic after an empirical 3-week course of antibiotics effective against chlamydia (Wong *et al.* 1988).

Chlamydial infection in the genitourinary tract has been shown to persist for at least 15 months in women who showed no signs or symptoms of genital disease (McCormack *et al.* 1979). In this study, women who were culture-negative but antichlamydial antibody positive at initial screening, were as likely to be culture-positive at follow-up as women who were culture-positive from the start. Although the possibility of reinfection could not be excluded, the investigators raised the issue of whether subclinical (that is to say inapparent or possibly latent) chlamydial infections in women may account, in part, for the relatively lower numbers of women diagnosed with RS since they lack one of the important diagnostic features of RS.

Although reinfection is widely accepted as the cause of recurrence for trachoma, reactivation of latent/inapparent infection as a possible factor cannot be ruled out. Work in a monkey model of trachoma suggests that chlamydial RNA is present in the conjunctivae of experimentally infected animals long after both culture and DFA screening tests are negative (Hudson *et al.* 1990). Recurrent conjunctivitis occurred in three German patients who had persistent chlamydial DNA after therapy (Haller *et al.* 1991).

Standard non-culture laboratory screening methods to detect chlamydia are not always particularly sensitive (Schachter *et al.* 1988), and essentially all such methods are also based on either phenotypic characteristics of the organism or host-response characteristics. Since the monoclonal antibodies used in DFA, for example, are targeted to the chlamydial, major outer-membrane protein, results of chlamydial screening by way of DFA would be profoundly affected by any differential or aberrant antigen production as a function of the chlamydial life cycle.

PCR on urine for *Chlamydia trachomatis* identified three times as many cases as did cultures in an urban, adolescent female clinic (Oh *et al.* 1996). A ligase chain reaction on urine for chlamydial DNA was nearly as sensitive as cultures in another study. A DFA identifying chlamydial elementary bodies in cervical smears requires experience in distinguishing chlamydia from artefacts and gives results similar to an enzyme immunoassay. DFA is time-consuming and not generally available. The rapid enzyme immunoassay is commercially available and can be run in 1 hour in the laboratory, but it may be only about 50% sensitive when used in an asymptomatic population with a 6.6% infection rate (Genc and Mardh 1991, Hoak *et al.* 1994).

Therapy

The widely quoted study of Lauhio *et al.* (1991) has encouraged many clinicians to propose, or try, aggressive antibiotic therapy in chlamydia-associated 'reactive' arthritis, Reiter's syndrome, or unclassified arthritis. Lauhio *et al.* compared lymocycline, a long-acting tetracycline, comma for 3 months with placebo in reactive arthritis patients in a double-blind prospective study. Benefit in the form of a modest, but significant, decrease in duration of symptoms was noted in those patients thought to have chlamydia-associated disease, but not in those with other suspected triggers. Neither this study, nor most others, checked for the eradication of organisms. One recent report describes quinolones as effective treatment in 5 patients with monoarthritis or dactylitis occurring 2–4 weeks after acute genitourinary inflammation (Palazzi *et al.* 1997). Triggering organisms were not identified.

Previously, most of the attempts to treat suspected CIA with empirical antibiotics failed to show any benefit. Popert *et al.* (1964), in a controlled study, treated patients with Reiter's syndrome with oxytetracycline at a dose of 2 g per day for only 5 days and failed to see significant improvement of the patients. However, this fell short of the recommended regimen of between 7 and 14 days for even uncomplicated chlamydial urethritis. Another study (Williams *et al.* 1989) using long-term treatment with doxycycline, also failed to demonstrate any beneficial effects. The subjects of this study, however, were Navajo Native Americans, who usually develop Reiter's syndrome in association with shigella infection rather than chlamydia or other venereal infection. This might explain why the Williams *et al.* (1989) study produced negative results. Bardin *et al.* (1990) suggested that prolonged treatment of urethritis with tetracycline or erythromycin significantly reduced the frequency of post-venereal and recurrent episodes of arthritic exacerbation in RS patients. It would be important to know if the eradication of organisms was directly related to the prevention of arthritis. As early as 1984 Martin *et al.* showed that the *in-vitro* chlamydia-specific lymphocytic response of Reiter's patients is decreased after antibiotic treatment and they recommended effective antibiotic therapy to all patients with clinical syndromes associated with *C. trachomatis* as well as treatment of their sexual partners.

New regimens of antibiotic treatment for CIA may well have to be developed. Some physicians are using chronic antibiotic therapy for various types of apparent reactive arthritis, but there is little supporting evidence for this approach (Toivanen *et al.* 1993). Even if this is effective, the mechanisms of action could be other than antimicrobial. Different forms of tetracycline or other antibiotics may have variable effects on patients with different sets of clinical features. The dosage and duration of optimal therapy need to be evaluated before any consensus on optimal therapy can be advised. There is an important need for continued systematic and well-controlled studies and collaboration wherever sufficient numbers of patients and facilities are available. If an important role for chlamydia in arthritis and a variety of other diseases continues to be demonstrated, vaccination may ultimately be useful (Schachter 1985).

A number of patients in the growing series in Philadelphia and the National Institutes of Health have been shown to have evidence of persistent *Chlamydia trachomatis* in their synovium by PCR for 16S rRNA and MOMP, in-situ hybridization for 16S rRNA, EM, and immunoEM despite fairly aggressive antibiotic treatment, although none of these were in formal protocols (Beutler *et al.* 1997). Organisms persisted after 1 month of doxycycline and 3 months of ciprofloxacin treatment (Nanagara *et al.* 1995). A formal study of azithromycin therapy with pre-and posttreatment synovial biopsies is planned. Nevertheless, these initial observations raise concern that the organism may be difficult to eradicate from joints.

Therapy of genital infections has been recently studied in several comparison studies. Azithromycin, which can be given as a single dose for uncomplicated GU infection, was deemed to give better cure rates than the standard 7-day course of doxycycline, in part, because of compliance problems with the doxycycline (Genc and Mard 1996; Magid *et al.* 1996). Culture-proven *C. trachomatis* cervical infections responded clinically in 100% of patients to 100 mg doxycycline, twice a day, and in 93% to 300 mg ofloxacin per day (Hooten *et al.* 1992).

Criteria for cure vary from symptomatic cure to conversion to DFA-negative status. More sensitive techniques, such as hybridization for 16S rRNA suggest that some DFA-negative patients and animals still harbour chlamydia (Hudson *et al.* 1990; Rahman *et al.* 1992*a*).

Results of antibiotic therapy almost certainly are influenced by host features and the properties of different strains of organisms. As yet, we know of no studies examining the effects of human HLA or other genes on response. In mice, there are chlamydia resistant and susceptible strains, with one key difference appearing to be that the C56BL/6 resistant mice mount a better early production of TNF-alpha that may help control infection (Darville *et al.* 1996). Some unusual manipulations may need to be considered. Might combinations of antibiotics and immunosuppresives be effective? Could corticosteroids or methotrexate allow organisms to resume growth and be more susceptible to antibiotics? Might some sort of stimulation of macrophage function help to rid the host of the chlamydia? Interestingly, in adjuvant arthritis in the rat elimination of macrophages by clodronate-containing liposomes ameliorated the arthritis (Kinne *et al.* 1995). Studies examining not just symptoms and signs but the state of the organism in the joint and elsewhere will be of interest.

Since *C. trachomatis* has also been identified in synovium in a number of patients with RA (Pando *et al.* 1995; Branigan *et al.* 1996) as well as isolated cases of sarcoidosis, Henoch–Schonlein purpura and psoriatic arthritis, as well as in unclassified arthritis, the question must be raised whether antibiotics might merit a trial in such patients. Minocycline has recently been reported to show some benefit in RA (Alarcon 1995; Kloppenburg *et al.* 1994), but whether this is due to antimicrobial effects or other actions such as inhibition of matrix proteases is not yet known.

In addition to the PCR and molecular hybridization evidence for chlamydia in joints of patients with classical RA, there is supportive evidence that synovial fluid lymphocytes from some patients with RA respond primarily to chlamydial antigens (Ford and Schulzer 1994; Ford *et al.* 1985). Once the role for chlamydia in these cases is determined, we may need to broaden our concepts of 'CIA'.

A variety of other treatments have been successful in groups of patients with Reiter's syndrome. Although in these series there has been no definitive identification of chlamydia as the triggering or persisting factor, one must suspect that some are chlamydia related.

Sulphasalazine has been reported to be effective in Reiter's syndrome (reactive arthritis) in a large Department of Veterans Affairs study in the USA (Clegg *et al.* 1996), in studies of reactive arthritis (Peliskova *et al.* 1991), and in a series of spondarthropathies that included Reiter's cases (Dougados *et al.* 1995*a*) and in four cases of Reiter's syndrome associated with HIV infection (Disla *et al.* 1994). In the latter study CD4 lymphocyte counts rose after sulphasalazine without any specific antiretroviral therapy. Mesalamine was effective in a patient with Reiter's syndrome where distal ileum inflammatory disease was present (Thomson *et al.* 1994*b*). Detailed studies of intestinal lesions and the nature of triggering organisms are still needed in therapeutic trials.

Methotrexate (Lally and Ho 1985) and azathioprine (Calin 1986) have been used with success in severe Reiter's syndrome, but in no cases was the relationship to chlamydia evaluated carefully. If the immune response rather than the presence of live organisms is the cause of disease, drugs such as those used for rheumatoid arthritis may be appropriate.

Gold was given in one study, with improvement in laboratory parameters in 172 men with Reiter's syndrome (Kovalev 1991). Relapses were reported in only 8.3%. Non-steroidal anti-inflammatory drugs (NSAIDs) and intra-articular steroids often seem to be beneficial in Reiter's cases in general, but these have not been studied in patients with proven chlamydia. In chlamydial salpingitis the addition of an NSAID had no apparent benefit (Landers *et al.*

1993). Etretinate has been reported to be effective for the arthritis of Reiter's syndrome associated with HIV (Louthrenoo 1993; Williams and DuVivier 1991).

Therapy of extra-articular lesions in chlamydia-associated arthritis or Reiter's syndrome usually receives little comment. Uveitis is generally treated with mydriatics and local or systemic steroids (De Ancos *et al.* 1994) or with cyclosporin. We could find no descriptions of antibiotic therapy in patients with uveitis, although it is obviously used with at least a temporary effect in trachoma.

The successful treatment of *C. pneumoniae* respiratory tract symptoms has been reported with erythromycin, clarithromycin, doxycycline, and azithromycin (Della Santa *et al.* 1994; Hahn 1995). Whether such treatments completely eradicate chlamydia is not known. There have been no organized trials of the treatment of arthritis or other systemic complications of *C. pneumoniae* disease.

7 Psoriatic arthritis and spondylitis: a clinical approach

L. R. Espinoza and M. L. Cuéllar

Definition and historical background

Psoriatic arthritis (PsA) can be defined as a chronic inflammatory disorder affecting the musculoskeletal system in psoriatic patients. This definition encompasses a broad spectrum of clinical articular manifestations, including monoarthritis, distal interphalangeal inflammatory joint involvement, asymmetric and symmetric polyarthritis, and axial or spondylitic involvement (Espinoza *et al.* 1992*a*).

The association of psoriasis with arthritis was first described by the French physician Baron Jean Luis Alibert (1818), although the term 'psoriasis arthritique' was introduced by another French physician, Pierre Bazin (1860). Bourdillon (1888) extensively described it in 34 patients in his doctoral thesis. Nevertheless, its existence as a unique disorder distinct from rheumatoid arthritis remained controversial until 1964, when psoriatic arthritis was classified separately from rheumatoid arthritis by the American College of Rheumatology, formerly the American Rheumatism Association (ARA) (Blumberg *et al.* 1964).

Several important contributions, including the seminal work of Wright (1956, 1959) and Wright and Moll (1976*b*), and the later recognition of the association of certain HLA antigens, particularly HLA-B27, with arthritis and spondylitis, lend support to the concept of psoriatic arthritis as a distinct entity belonging to a larger group—the so-called seronegative spondyloarthropathies (Brewerton *et al.* 1974).

Epidemiology

Several population studies suggest that the prevalence of psoriasis in the general population is approximately 1–2% in North American and Northern European whites (Baker 1966; Ingram 1964). The existence of geographical and racial differences has been clearly shown, however, with a much lower prevalence in certain ethnic groups, including African and African-Americans, Latin American Indians, and Orientals (Convit 1962; Kenney 1971; Yui Yip 1984). The prevalence of psoriasis is similar in both men and women, although women develop psoriasis earlier than males, especially when there is a positive family history (Holgate 1975).

The incidence of various forms of inflammatory articular involvement in psoriatic patients is approximately 5–7%, but has been reported to be as low as 0.2% and as high as 40% (Espinoza 1985; Little *et al.* 1975; Reed and Becker 1960). Several factors, including patient selection, duration and extent of skin disease and severity, account for this wide variability. A recent study in 205 unselected Italian psoriatic patients showed a frequency of arthritis of 36% (Salvarani *et al.* 1995). The prevalence of PsA in the general population is estimated to be 0.1%, or

10–20 times lower than that of rheumatoid arthritis, and it is equally distributed between males and females (Wright and Moll 1976*b*). However, the National Arthritis Data Workgroup suggested a good estimate for the prevalence of psoriatic arthritis in the USA to be 0.67%, a prevalence close to the 1% prevalence of rheumatoid arthritis (Lawrence *et al.* 1989).

Psoriatic arthritis can also occur in children, but its frequency is much lower than in adults. This estimate is confounded by the fact that arthritis in children often precedes the onset of psoriatic skin involvement by several years. The prevalence of PsA in children has been estimated at 10–15 cases per 100 000 population, approximately 20% of the prevalence of juvenile rheumatoid arthritis (Cassidy and Petty 1990). In a study from Italy, 5 patients with PsA were found in juvenile 425 psoriatic patients, for a prevalence of 1% (Biondi *et al.* 1994). All five patients had a family history of psoriasis and onset of skin disease between the ages of 10 and 20 years. Arthritis preceded psoriasis in two cases, and the interval between the onset of cutaneous and articular involvement was ≤8 years.

Pathogenesis

The interplay of multiple factors including genetic, immunological, and environmental, most likely lead to the full development and clinical expression of this disorder (Cuéllar and Espinoza 1995). The genetics of both psoriasis and PsA are complex, but the polygenic, multifactorial characteristics of inheritance are well established with variable penetrance, familial occurrence, and age of onset. Moreover, exacerbation by a variety of environmental factors are well recognized, including infection with beta-haemolytic streptococci and human immunodeficiency virus (Cuéllar *et al.* 1994; Espinoza *et al.* 1978, 1988, 1994*a,b,c*; Gerber *et al.* 1982; Gladman *et al.* 1986, 1992; Gladman and Espinoza 1992; Veale *et al.* 1995).

A high concordance among monozygotic twins, familial aggregation, and high prevalence of certain HLA antigens, provide a strong support for a role of genetic factors. Several HLA antigens, both class I and II, have been shown to be associated with PsA. These include HLA-B13, B16 and its splits B38 and B39, as well as B17, B7, B27 Cw6, DR4, and DR7 (Espinoza *et al.* 1978; Gerber *et al.* 1982; Gladman *et al.* 1986). In addition, it is possible that genetic factors outside the HLA system play a role, as has been recently demonstrated for psoriasis. Studies in two large kindreds, in which members were affected with psoriasis in several generations, found an association with a gene localized in the distal end of human Chromosome 17q (Tomfohrde *et al.* 1994). The latter finding may explain the complexity of the inheritance pattern seen in this disorder and demonstrates that, in some families, psoriasis susceptibility is the result of variation at a single major genetic locus other than the HLA locus.

Evidence accumulated also provides support for the participation of immunological factors, both humoral and cellular, in the pathogenesis of PsA. The presence of circulating immune complexes, particularly of the IgA isotype, depressed lymphocyte response to specific and non-specific antigens, predominance of activated CD4+ memory T cells in the synovial membrane, and the more recent findings of increased expression of the platelet-derived growth factor (PDGF)-β receptor in the psoriatic fibroblast and the upregulation of certain pro-inflammatory cytokines, especially IL-6, support the concept that immunological factors play a role in the pathogenesis of PsA (Espinoza *et al.* 1994*a,b*).

Environmental factors, particularly streptococcal and HIV infections, may trigger and/or exacerbate psoriasis and PsA (Espinoza *et al.* 1988). Other retroviral agents may also play a role. Trauma and stress have also been suggested to be potential triggering agents (Scarpa *et al.* 1992*b*).

Clinical manifestations

Most patients have an insidious onset of this disease, although the onset may be acute in approximately one-third of patients. Constitutional complaints such as fever, weight loss, and/or malaise, are uncommon. The age of onset peaks around 40 years, and, in contrast to rheumatoid arthritis, there is a male: female ratio of approximately 1:1. In approximately 60–75% of patients with PsA, joint involvement occurs years after the onset of skin involvement. In approximately 10–15%, both skin and joint involvement appear simultaneously, and in the remaining 10–15%, arthritis appears prior to the onset of skin involvement. In juvenile PsA, articular involvement may precede the onset of cutaneous involvement by several years—up to 20 in approximately 50% of cases.

Classification

The lack of a uniform, validated criteria for the classification of PsA has hampered progress in its investigation (Gladman 1995). Several attempts have been made in the past to classify patients with PsA into different clinical subsets (Tables 7.1 and 7.2) (Moll and Wright 1973; Vasey and Espinoza 1984). The subgroups shown in Table 7.2 have had the widest recognition and acceptance, although some problems limit their utility and a modified version has recently been introduced (Table 7.3) (Helliwell *et al.* 1991*a*). In this new version, patients with PsA may have all three skeletal manifestations, although they may occur separately. This is an improved version, but some authors have found the utility of this classification scheme poor compared with the original criteria of Moll and Wright (1973).

Table 7.1 Classification criteria for psoriatic arthritis[a]

1. **Mandatory**: Psoriatic skin or nail involvement
2. One other feature from the following:
   (a) Pain and soft-tissue swelling of distal interphalangeal joints for more than 4 weeks
   (b) Pain and soft-tissue swelling of peripheral joints in an asymmetric pattern for more than 4 weeks
   (c) Symmetrical peripheral arthritis for more than 4 weeks in the absence of rheumatoid factor or subcutaneous nodules
   (d) Peripheral radiological features: 'pencil in cup' deformity, erosion of terminal phalanges, 'fluffy' periostitis, and bony ankylosis
   (e) Spinal pain and stiffness with restriction of motion for more than 4 weeks
   (f) Spinal radiological features; grade 2 bilateral sacroiliitis, or grade 3 or 4 unilateral sacroiliitis

[a] Reproduced from Vasey and Espinoza (1984)

Table 7.2 Clinical subgroups of psoriatic arthritis[a]

1. Predominant distal interphalangeal joint involvement
2. Arthritis mutilans
3. Symmetrical polyarthritis indistinguishable from rheumatoid arthritis but with negative serology
4. Asymmetrical oligoarthritis or the involvement of a single joint
5. Ankylosing spondylitis as predominant feature

[a] Reproduced from Moll and Wright (1973)

Table 7.3 Classification of psoriatic arthritis[a]

1. Peripheral arthritis resembling rheumatoid arthritis but commonly involving the distal interphalangeal joints. Other characteristic findings include dactylitis, unilateral limb oedema, enthesopathy, and arthritis mutilans
2. Sacroiliitis and spondylitis may be asymmetrical and the spondylitic features include chunky syndesmophytes and paravertebral ossification
3. Extra-articular osseous manifestations include the SAPHO (synovitis, acne, pustulosis, hyperostosis, and osteomyelitis) syndrome

[a] Reproduced from Helliwell *et al.* (1991*a*)

Table 7.4 'Vancouver' criteria for the classification of juvenile psoriatic arthritis[a]

Definite juvenile PsA	
Arthritis beginning before 16 years of age	Joint swelling, or at least two of the following: limited range of motion of the joint(s), pain on movement of joint, or joint margin tenderness, persisting for at least 6 weeks
and **either**:	
Typical psoriasis	Unmistakable psoriatic rash observed by the physician or diagnosed as such by a dermatologist; rash not necessarily coincident with arthritis
or:	
At least three or four minor criteria, as follows:	
Dactylitis	Diffuse digit swelling, extending beyond the margin of the joint capsule
Nail pitting	More than 2 pits on the fingernails at any examination
Psoriasis-like rash	Historical or examination features of a psoriatic rash, but evidence inconclusive.
Family history of psoriasis	Diagnosis of psoriasis in a first- or second-degree relative
Probable juvenile PsA	
Arthritis beginning before 16 years of age	As defined above
and	
Any two of the minor criteria described above	As defined above

[a] Reproduced from Southwood *et al.* (1989)

In the past several years, other groups have also introduced criteria for the classification of spondyloarthropathies, with the main goal of discriminating patients with spondyloarthropathy from those without (Amor *et al.* 1990; Dougados *et al.* 1991*a*). Juvenile PsA is classified separately from adult disease (Table 7.4) (Southwood *et al.* 1989). As with the adult criteria, there is a need for prospective, multicentre studies to validate these criteria.

Articular manifestations

In over half of patients with PsA, arthritis is polyarticular, either symmetrical or asymmetrical (Figs 7.1(a), (b). Differential diagnosis with rheumatoid arthritis rarely presents a problem, and several clinical aspects are useful for distinguishing between these two entities (Table 7.5). Our experience in this respect agrees with that reported by others (Gladman *et al.* 1987; Roberts *et al.* 1976; Scarpa *et al.* 1984).

Gladman *et al.* (1987) analysed 220 patients with PsA at their first visit to a PsA clinic, and found that the majority of the patients presented with polyarthritis, which was asymmetrical in half the cases. Scarpa *et al.* (1984) also found that the majority of their patients with PsA presented with polyarthritis. Asymmetrical oligoarticular involvement is the second most common form of PsA, seen in approximately 30–40% of patients.

There is disagreement in the literature about the frequency of oligoarthritis in PsA (Kammer *et al.* 1979; Torre Alonso *et al.* 1991; Veale *et al.* 1994). A number of authors have reported this form as the most common type of arthritis seen in PsA. Kammer *et al.* (1979) found that over half of their patients (54%) with PsA presented with asymmetrical oligoarthritis. Similarly, Torre Alonso *et al.* (1991) found that the majority of their 180 patients

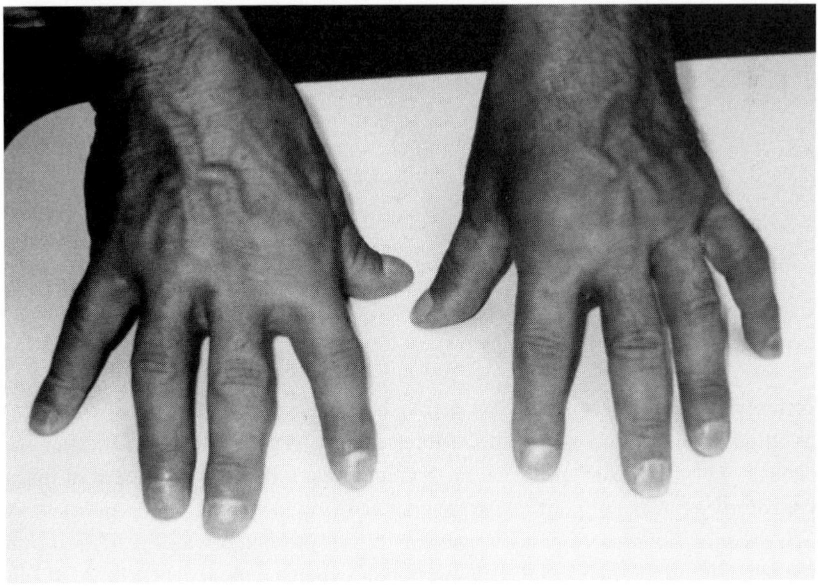

(a)

Fig. 7.1a Psoriatic arthritis involving metacarpophalangeal and proximal interphalangeal joints in a symmetrical fashion.

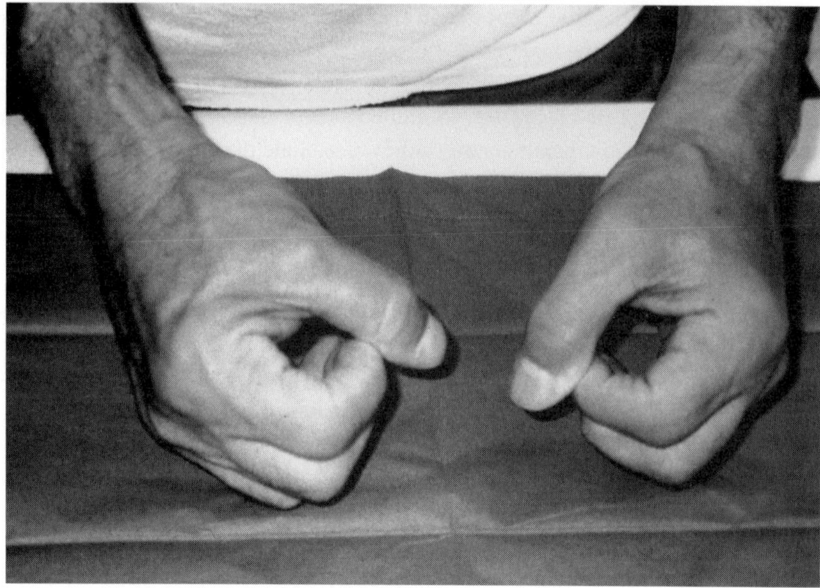

(b)

Fig. 7.1b Hands of the same patient with psoriatic arthritis as in Fig. 7.1*a*, showing marked inability to make a fist due to symmetrical polyarthritis (patient is a surgeon).

Table 7.5 Psoriatic arthritis vs rheumatoid arthritis: differential diagnosis

Feature	Psoriatic arthritis	Rheumatoid arthritis
Sex distribution	Male = female	Female > male
Rheumatoid factor	Unusual; low titre	Usual; 80%
Skin involvement	Characteristic	Rare
Nail involvement	Common: > 60%	Rare
Subcutaneous nodules	Rare < 1%	Common: 40–50%
Joint pattern	Asymmetrical	Symmetrical
DIP[a] involvement	Common > 50%	Uncommon < 5%
Back involvement	Common	Unusual

[a] DIP, distal interphalangeal.

prospectively followed over an 8-year period had oligoarthritis, followed in order of frequency by polyarthritis and spondylitis. More recently, Veale *et al.* (1994), after analysing their patients with PsA, concluded that an asymmetrical oligoarthritis pattern of disease was the most common pattern of joint involvement, occurring in 43% of PsA patients. A symmetrical polyarthritis was present in 33%, and this subset presented with the highest number of erosions and deformities, and a higher proportion of patients with grade III/IV ACR functional disability. In our experience, a significant proportion of these patients with oligoarthritis eventually evolve into a polyarticular form, usually asymmetrical. This has previously been reported by Gladman (1994) and Jones *et al.* (1994).

The so-called typical PsA form of distal interphalangeal (DIP) arthritis rarely presents alone or in isolation (1–2% in our experience), but is commonly seen in combination with either polyarthritis or oligoarthritis in 40–50% of cases overall. Torre Alonso *et al.* (1991) found no patients with isolated DIP involvement. In contrast, Veale *et al.* (1994) reported predominant DIP involvement in 16% of their patients with PsA, and 46% in combination with other patterns. They suggested that DIP joint disease may represent recent or early PsA.

Axial or spondylitic involvement is the third major subset of PsA and occurs in approximately one-third of patients. This subset is seldom the dominant pattern of joint involvement in PsA patients and, when present, its severity is typically milder than that seen in ankylosing spondylitis (AS). Gladman *et al.* (1993) found a higher frequency of inflammatory neck and back pain and stiffness, limitation of back movement, grade 4 sacroiliitis, and syndesmophytes in patients with idiopathic AS, whereas peripheral arthritis was more common and more severe in PsA. A lower frequency of HLA-B17, and a higher frequency of HLA-B27 and Cw2, was found in AS, compared with PsA. A higher incidence of symptomatic cervical spondylitis (45%) was found by Jenkinson *et al.* (1994*a*). They only found radiological evidence of cervical spondylitis in 36% of their patients. In general, symptoms tend to be more severe in males than in female patients with PsA (Gladman *et al.* 1993), and the prevalence of HLA-B27 is higher in this subset as compared to the other forms of PsA (Table 7.6). More unusual subsets, including arthritis mutilans, SAPHO, and Charcot-like arthropathy, occur in less than 2–3% of patients with PsA.

In general, children may exhibit inflammatory articular involvement similar to that seen in the adult form of PsA. Southwood *et al.* (1989) have described two distinct groups of juvenile PsA: earlier onset in young girls, and a later onset in adolescence in boys. Tenosynovitis of the tendon sheaths of digits or toes is highly characteristic as an initial presentation, and early diagnosis is important because progression to an asymmetrical destructive polyarthritis is not unusual.

Extra-articular manifestations

Skin

Cutaneous involvement is characterized by the presence of well-delineated erythematous papules and plaques covered with layers of flaking, or adhering, thick silvery-white or grey scales, preferentially localized along extensor surfaces. There are multiple forms of psoriasis, and any of them can be associated with PsA. By far the most common form associated with PsA is psoriasis vulgaris, which accounts for over 90% of PsA patients. Guttate psoriasis is more commonly seen in children, consisting of multiple erythematous papules which develop in a 'droplike' generalized distribution, and tends to occur following a streptococcal pharyngitis.

The morphology of the skin lesions is modified by their location. For example, lesions in flexures do not exhibit the thick silverywhite or grey appearance that is seen at less occluded sites. Lesions on the palms and soles are much more hyperkeratotic and thickened (Fig. 7.2).

Table 7.6 Characteristics of axial involvement in spondyloarthropathies

	Axial/ sacroiliac involvement (%)	M/F ratio	HLA-B27 (%)	Vertebral squaring	Syndesmophytes (type)	Apophyseal joint involvement	Thoracolumbar mobility
Ankylosing spondylitis	100	⩾ 2.4:1	85–90	Usual	Marginal, symmetrical, bilateral, orderly spread	Common	Limitation
Enteropathic arthritis	10	3:1	33–75	Usual	Similar to AS	Similar to AS	—
Psoriatic arthritis	40–50	3:1	40–50[a]	Occasional	Marginal and non-marginal, asymmetrical, Uni/or bilateral, no orderly spread	Occasional	Less limitation
Reiter's syndrome	2–20	50:1[b]	60–75	Occasional	Similar to PsA	Similar to PsA	—

AS, ankylosing spondylitis; IBDS, spondylitis of inflammatory bowel disease; RS, Reiter's syndrome; PsA, psoriatic arthritis. [a] When spondylitis is present. [b] Postvenereal RS.

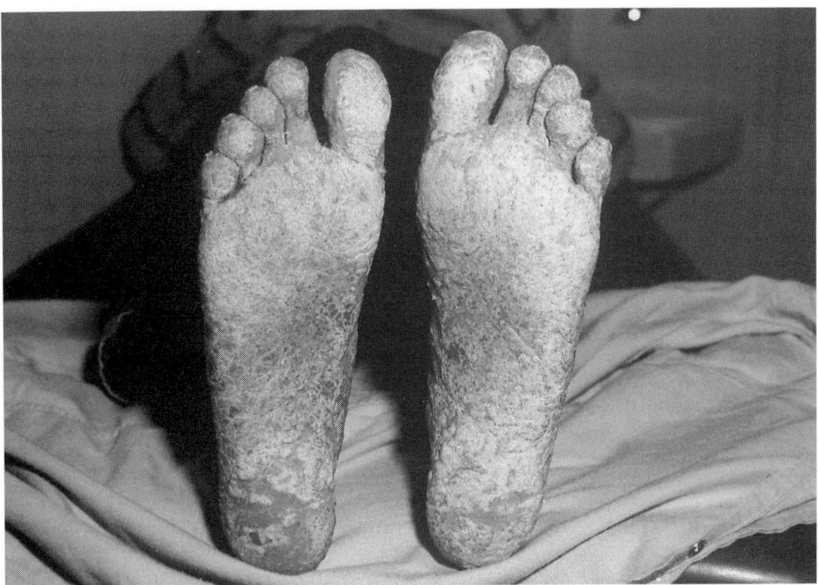

Fig. 7.2 Extensive lesions of keratoderma blenorrhagica on the soles of a patient with psoriatic arthritis.

Often, individual lesions may be non-scaly, although it is possible to induce scaling by gently scratching the plaque with a fingernail. In addition, a characteristic finding, the so-called Auspitz sign, can be induced by gentle scraping (pinpoint bleeding from the dilated and proliferating blood vessels in the papillary dermis, where there is little protection by the overlying atrophic epidermis).

Other forms of cutaneous involvement, such as pustular and erythroderma forms, may all be seen in association with PsA. In general, there is some degree of association between the severity of skin involvement and joint disease. However, the exact relationship between the extent of cutaneous involvement and the severity of joint disease remains to be established.

Nails

Nail involvement is commonly seen in psoriasis, particularly in those patients with joint involvement, and this may be a better predictor of arthritic involvement than the severity of skin disease. Nail lesions were the only clinical manifestation that identified patients with psoriasis destined to develop arthritis (Gladman *et al.* 1986).

Involvement of the nail matrix produces the characteristic pitting of the nail, while nailbed involvement induces separation of the nail from the underlying nailbed (onycholysis) or subungual hyperkeratosis (Fig. 7.3). The latter can be easily confused with fungal disease, which may need to be excluded.

None of the nail lesions are unique to psoriasis, and may be present in other chronic dermatitides and normal individuals. However, the combination of pitting and onycholysis or the presence of more than 20 pits is highly suggestive of psoriasis.

Jones *et al.* (1994) found nail involvement in 67% of PsA patients and that it was more common in DIP involvement (27% of total) and significantly associated with adjacent DIP

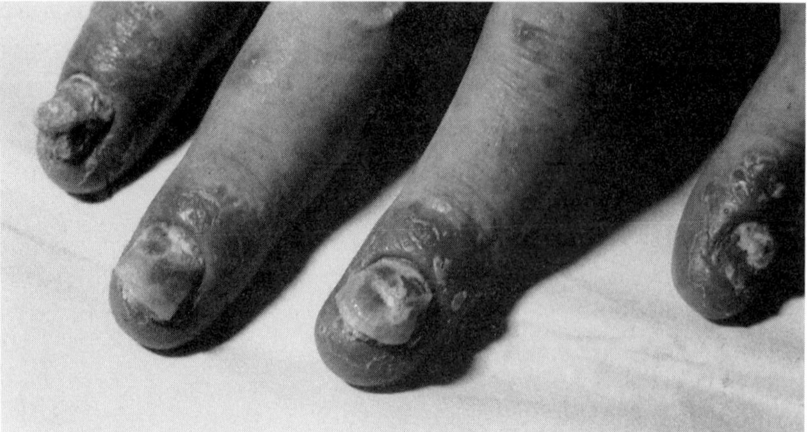

Fig. 7.3 Extensive subungual hyperkeratosis in a patient with asymmetrical oligoarthritis.

joint disease. Skin and nail disease severity, however, did not correlate with joint severity, joint activity, or functional status, or differ between subgroups, and it was concluded that the mode of onset does not predict outcome in the majority of patients. Lavaroni *et al.* (1994) reported nail changes in 86.5% of patients with PsA, with subungual keratosis being the most common toenail alteration, while the most frequent fingernail change was pitting.

Enthesopathies

Inflammatory changes at the tendon–bone junction (enthesis) is a characteristic finding in the spondyloarthropathies, including PsA. It may be the presenting manifestation in some patients, and its exact prevalence in PsA is not well defined.

Ocular involvement

Psoriasis and its related arthritis are systemic disorders, and involvement of any organ system may occur. The ocular involvement seen in psoriatic arthritis resembles that of the other seronegative spondyloarthropathies, and includes primarily anterior uveitis. This occurred in 7% of patients with psoriatic arthritis and in 4% of patients with uncomplicated psoriasis (Gladman *et al.* 1986). Conjunctivitis, episcleritis, and keratoconjunctivitis are not common among these patients. Cabral *et al.* (1994) found the risk of developing uveitis 5 years after the onset of juvenile PsA small, and although ocular complications were relatively frequent—33%, among patients with uveitis, normal vision was maintained or correctable in over half of the patients.

Other extra-articular manifestations

Cardiopulmonary involvement, including subclinical pulmonary alveolitis, aortic regurgitation, and mitral valve prolapse, has been described in PsA (Scherak *et al.* 1993).

An increased prevalence (11%) of renal involvement including haematuria, proteinuria, or cylindruria, has been described in PsA (Omdal and Husby 1987). The development of myopathy (Thomson *et al.* 1990), leukocytoclastic vasculitis (Barlon and Schulz 1991), and Sjögren's syndrome in PsA have been well documented, as has amyloidosis. Bianchi *et al.* (1993) have reported the presence of significant thyroid gland involvement such as enlargement, antimicrosomal antibodies, and increased T4 levels in patients with active PsA.

Of great interest and intriguing significance is the association of gut involvement with spondyloarthropathies including PsA. Schatteman *et al.* (1995) performed ileocolonoscopy in 64 PsA patients. Inflammatory lesions were found in 10 of the 64 patients (16%), in 3 of the 15 (20%) with oligoarthritis, and 7 of the 23 (30%) with spondyloarthritic involvement. In contrast, none of the 26 patients exhibiting polyarthritis had the lesions. In this group of patients, HLA-B27 and Bw62 were significantly more prevalent in patients with gut inflammation, 60 and 50% respectively. The prevalence of gut inflammation in psoriatic spondylitis is significantly lower than in non-psoriatic spondyloarthropathies. These findings thus apparently suggest that the skin and the gut may be independent portals of entry for causative antigens in the SpA.

Gouty arthritis may occur in 5–7% of PsA patients. The extraordinary association of HIV infection with psoriasis and PsA is well established. Both psoriasis and PsA may occur *de novo* or be exacerbated by the presence of underlying HIV infection (Espinoza *et al.* 1988). A wide spectrum of psoriatic lesions including vulgaris, guttate, pustular, and exfoliative erythrodermic forms of skin involvement, may be seen in HIV infection. Both skin and joint involvement may be widespread and extremely severe, despite aggressive therapy.

Laboratory findings

There is no single laboratory abnormality specific for psoriasis and/or psoriatic arthritis, nor laboratory marker that could predict the development of PsA in patients with psoriasis.

In general, the erythrocyte sedimentation rate may be an indicator of disease activity, but it is only elevated in half of the patients. It may reflect, however, the degree of skin inflammation. C-reactive protein correlates well with radiographic joint destruction and overall disease severity, but not with the type of joint involvement (Helliwell *et al.* 1991*b*). Low titre rheumatoid factor may be seen in 10–15% of patients. Antinuclear antibodies may be seen in approximately 10% of patients, and the appearance of DNA antibodies following phototherapy has also been described. Mild normochromic, normocytic anaemia may be seen in patients with progressive polyarticular disease. Elevated levels of serum immunoglobulins, particularly IgA, may be seen, as well as circulating immune complexes. Hyperuricaemia may be increased in 10–15% of patients and reflects overall increased skin activity. Analysis of synovial fluid reveals inflammatory changes with an increase in the number of leuckocytes, predominantly polymorphonuclear cells. Elevated levels of haemolytic complement in synovial fluid may be found. Azzini *et al.* (1995) have described a significant increase in C16:0 total saturated fatty acids, a lower level of serum selenium, an increased level of plasma copper, and a significant decrease in C18:2, C20:4, and omega-6 polyunsaturated fatty acids. Borg *et al.* (1994) found increased IgA antibodies to cytokeratins in patients with psoriasis and PsA, but not in the sera from patients with ankylosing spondylitis or Reiter's syndrome, or in controls.

Radiographic findings

Radiological manifestations may be seen in up to two-thirds of patients with PsA, and can be seen in the synovial and cartilaginous joints, and in tendon and ligament attachments to bone in the appendicular and axial skeleton. In general, the frequency of joint involvement in PsA depends on what techniques are used for their study. More sensitive techniques such as sonography, scintigraphy, computed tomography (CT), and magnetic resonance imaging (MRI) yield a higher incidence of joint involvement than conventional radiography (Azouz and Duffy 1995; Bissoli and Sansone 1994; Jevtic *et al.* 1995; Rubatelli *et al.* 1994). However, the plain radiograph remains the primary and most important modality for assessing these disorders.

In peripheral joints as seen in rheumatoid arthritis, plain radiographs of the hands and feet yield the most characteristic findings. Soft-tissue swelling is perhaps the most common radiological finding in these areas. A sausage-like swelling of the entire digit may also be seen. A propensity for less pronounced osteopenia, especially in the hands, compared with RA, is also a characteristic feature. Other findings include periarticular erosions (Fig. 7.4), joint-space narrowing or widening, periostitis, and bony proliferation. In contrast to RA, however, PsA patients may exhibit a more aggressive radiological course, including the presence of acro-osteolysis (pencil-in-cup deformity), subluxation and dislocation, or bony fusion. In the spine, the most common site of involvement is the sacroiliac joints, followed by the cervical spine. The thoracolumbar spine is involved much less commonly. Radiological findings at these levels are somewhat similar to those seen in AS, but with less severity. Sacroiliac joint involvement is usually bilateral, but unilateral or markedly asymmetric involvement is more often seen than in AS, and fusion is unusual. Osteitis and squaring of the vertebral bodies are not as common as in AS. Syndesmophyte formation appears in the thoracolumbar spine, tends to be paramarginal,

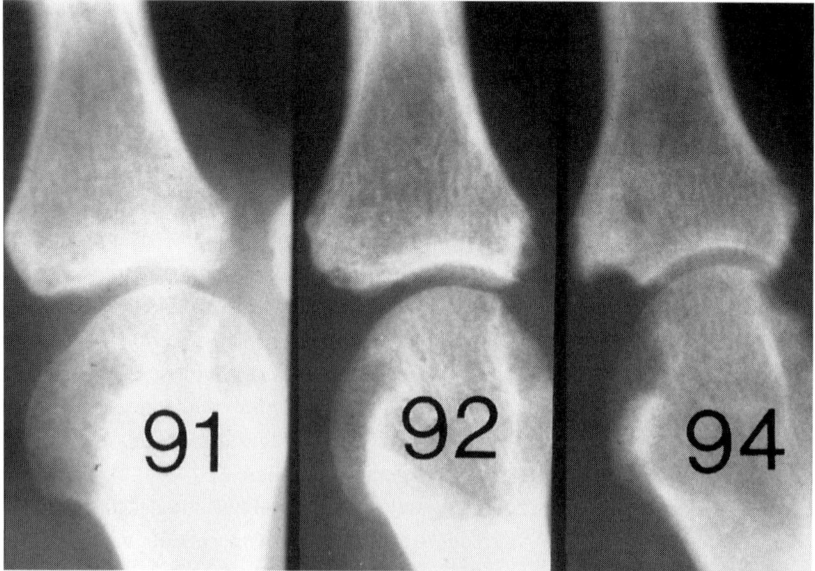

Fig. 7.4 Progression of articular erosion in a patient with symmetrical psoriatic polyarthritis.

bulky, and asymmetrical, and may appear in the absence of sacroiliac joint disease. Erosion of the odontoid process leading to atlantoaxial instability and subluxation may also occur, as in RA, but is unusual in patients with psoriatic arthritis.

The temporomandibular, manubriosternal, and sternoclavicular joints are relatively commonly involved in PsA. Subchondral erosions similar to those seen in RA are found in these joints (Scutellari *et al.* 1993).

Natural course and prognosis

During the past several years it has become well established that PsA is not as benign as was once thought. It is increasingly recognized that a sizeable proportion of patients present a clinical course characterized by severe disease activity and deforming, destructive arthropathy (Gladman 1994; Gladman *et al.* 1990*b*). In view of our existing knowledge, PsA should be considered as a clinical spectrum, at one end of which patients may present with enthesitis, nail and cutaneous involvement, and monoarthritis, with oligoarthritis taking up a middle position, and at the other end either asymmetrical or symmetrical polyarthritis. Axial or spondylitic involvement may be seen at any stage, as well as other extra-articular manifestations. The most severe forms of joint involvement, including arthritis mutilans, are seen at the end of the spectrum that includes the polyarticular form. The transformation of the monoarthritis into asymmetrical oligoarthritis or polyarthritis is well recognized (Jones *et al.* 1994; Sesztak *et al.* 1995). Gladman (1994) has recently reviewed her experience with 415 PsA patients followed at the University of Toronto Psoriatic Arthritis Clinic. The average length of follow-up was 5.25 years (ranging from a single visit to a follow-up of 18.5 years). In all, 96 patients were followed for 1 year or less, 139 for 1–5 years, 116 for 6–10 years, and 64 for more than 10 years. Over the course of follow-up, 35 patients died from causes unrelated to PsA. Furthermore, over the same period, the majority of the patients (62%) continued to demonstrate polyarthritis, with or without back involvement, while 21% demonstrated oligoarthritis and 10% distal involvement. Only 4% of patients had an isolated spondylitis. As previously reported, the number of patients with deformities and radiologically evident damage increased over time, as did the average number of deformities or radiologically damaged joints per patient. The majority of her patients (50–71%) had no deformities at presentation, however 58% of those followed for more than 10 years demonstrated more than five deformities at their last clinic visit. Of interest, seven patients went into complete remission of joint disease during this period of follow-up.

In the past few years, several risk factors for disease progression and poor prognosis in PsA have been identified. Gladman *et al.* (1995) found that a high number of effusions and past medications predict damage progression, whereas a low sedimentation rate correlates with lack of progression; they concluded that evidence of significant inflammation at the first visit predicts the progression of joint damage in the future. Further univariate analysis of data from the same group revealed that HLA antigens B27, B39, and DQw3 were associated with disease progression, whereas HLA-DR7 was protective. Similarly, multivariate analysis identified the HLA antigens B27, when DR7 was present, and DQw3, when DR7 was absent, as predicting disease progression across all transitions, whereas HLA-B39 was associated with progression in the early stages of disease (Gladman and Farewell 1995). An association between high IgA levels and disease severity has also been described (Piazzini *et al.* 1995).

Pregnancy does not have an adverse effect on the course of PsA. Østensen (1992) reported that the symptoms of patients with PsA improved or even remitted in 80% of pregnancies, whereas 80% of AS patients had unaltered or aggravated disease symptoms. Fetal outcome was not adversely affected by PsA. In addition, delivery was uncomplicated in PsA, but a postpartum flare during the first 3 months after delivery occurred in 70% of mothers with PsA.

More recently, the health status of patients with PsA has been assessed with the aid of psychosocial scales such as the Health Assessment Questionnaire (HAQ) and the Arthritis Impact Measurement Scale (AIMS) (Husted *et al.* 1995). Further work is needed to fully ascertain their impact in PsA.

Patients with psoriatic erythroderma, generalized pustular psoriasis, and psoriatic polyarthritis, have a worse prognosis, and may die from complications directly related to the disease, including metabolic disorders, amyloidosis, cardiovascular failure, cachexia, or complications of specific immunosuppressive treatment (Husted *et al.* 1995; Roth *et al.* 1991).

Therapeutic management

Most PsA patients respond well to most NSAIDs, although salicylates seem to be less effective than in RA. The response in those with polyarthritis and/or spondylitic involvement leaves a lot to be desired (Bulbul *et al.* 1995; Cuellar *et al.* 1994*a*). In the latter groups, it appears that phenylbutazone and/or oxyphenbutazone are effective, as in ankylosing spondylitis. NSAIDs should be used at full dosage for a minimum of 4 weeks to fully evaluate their efficacy. At times, it may be necessary to try more than one NSAID before switching to another class of agents.

The use of combination and/or more aggressive therapy at earlier stages of PsA is gaining wider acceptance, as in RA (Amor *et al.* 1995*a*; Gubner *et al.* 1951). Accumulated evidence, demonstrating the progression of disease and/or the development of deformities and disability in over half of PsA patients after several years of follow-up, provides support for a more aggressive therapeutic approach during the early stages of the disease. The prompt institution of an adequate therapy programme should result in better protection from musculoskeletal complications that lead to functional disability, although data from controlled trials demonstrating efficacy are largely lacking for most of the common treatments.

Several second-line or disease-modifying drugs have been used in the treatment of PsA including methotrexate, gold compounds, antimalarials, sulphasalazine, azathioprine, penicillamine, and cyclosporin A (Black *et al.* 1964; Dorwat *et al.* 1978; Dougados *et al.* 1995*a*; Farr *et al.* 1990; Gladman *et al.* 1992; Levy *et al.* 1972; Marks 1988; O'Brien *et al.* 1962; Palit *et al.* 1990; Price and Gibson 1986; Seideman 1990; Steinson *et al.* 1990; Wagner *et al.* 1993). Other less frequently used compounds include retinoids, vitamin D_3 derivatives, somatostatin, PUVA (psoralen plus ultraviolet A), bromocriptine, anti-CD4 monoclonal antibodies, and 2-chlorodeoxyadenosine (Cuéllar *et al.* 1994*a*; Eibschutz *et al.* 1995; Huckins *et al.* 1990; Klinkhoff *et al.* 1989; Pearlman *et al.* 1979; Sayrat 1992).

Methotrexate is the second line agent of choice used in our population of PsA (Espinoza *et al.* 1992*b*). Our own experience and that of others point to its efficacy (Gutierrez-Ureña and Espinoza 1995). especially when given early, although radiological improvement has not been demonstrated (Abu-Shakra *et al.* 1995). The starting dose is somewhat higher than that for patients with RA, averaging about 11.5 mg per week for most patients (range 5 to

30 mg per week). PsA patients tolerate methotrexate relatively well and in only a few will treatment need to be discontinued. Careful patient selection, and more importantly perhaps, a close monitoring of concomitant medication, particularly NSAIDs, diuretics, and anti-hypertensive agents, and of liver and renal function, are mandatory. Liver biopsy is not required before therapy, and should be reserved for patients with persistent liver–function test abnormalities. The most frequent side-effects are gastrointestinal, including stomatitis, nausea, and abdominal pain. The addition of folic acid, 1 mg once or twice daily, decreases and ameliorates the side-effects without altering efficacy. The use of mouth washes containing allopurinol may prevent the appearance of oral ulcerations. Liver–function test abnormalities occur in approximately 25% during the first 3–4 months of therapy, but subsequently subside. Significant liver damage, including cirrhosis, is rare, but may occur. Bone marrow aplasia resulting in pancytopenia and death is a concern (Gutierrez-Ureña *et al.* 1996).

Sulphasalazine is a promising therapeutic agent for both psoriasis and PsA, and has been shown to be effective in two large controlled trials (Dougados *et al.* 1995; Clegg *et al.* 1996). The recommended dose is 2–3 g per day. GI intolerance is a limiting factor (Dougados *et al.* 1995; Gupta *et al.* 1995; Seideman 1990), although its use in combination with methotrexate deserves further study. The effect of sulphasalazine on the radiographic progression of psoriatic asthritis has not been examined.

Cyclosporin A is extremely efficacious for the treatment of both psoriasis and PsA. Improvement is seen within a few weeks after initiation of therapy. Discontinuation of therapy is usually followed by exacerbation of both skin and joint involvement in a matter of weeks. Limiting factors regarding its widespread use are the high incidence of side-effects—liver, renal, and lymphoproliferative disorders—and cost. It has been suggested as the ideal agent to be used in combination with methotrexate (Marks 1988; Steinson *et al.* 1990; Wagner *et al.* 1993).

Corticosteroids should be used only in special circumstances such as severe exacerbation of cutaneous and/or joint involvement. A psoriatic rash often flares up when corticosteroids are reducted and/or discontinued; an erythrodermic rash is a secondary effect of withdrawal. Topical steroids are effective in controlling skin involvement, and intra-articular use in selected joints can be of great benefit.

Surgical procedures and rehabilitative management of the psoriatic arthritis patient are similar to those performed in patients with rheumatoid arthritis and ankylosing spondylitis (Hakkinen *et al.* 1994; Hicken *et al.* 1994; Linschoten and Krachkow 1993), although results tend to be less gratifying than in these disorders.

8 Spondyloarthropathies in children and adolescents

Alan M. Rosenberg and Ross E. Petty

With the emergence of rheumatology as an established paediatric subspecialty, it has become increasingly apparent that a wide spectrum of rheumatic diseases afflict children more frequently than had been appreciated previously. The spondyloarthropathies, once believed to occur almost exclusively in adults, are now recognized as frequently having their onsets during childhood and adolescence. In this chapter the clinical characteristics of childhood spondyloarthropathies are discussed and advances in diagnosis and management are considered.

Overview of childhood spondyloarthropathies

The concept of childhood spondyloarthropathies is adopted from that of Wright and Moll, based initially on the presence of chronic arthritis and the absence of rheumatoid factor (Wright and Moll 1976*a*). As it has evolved, the term seronegative spondyloarthropathy is now used to designate those arthropathies in which, in addition to seronegativity and chronic appendicular joint arthritis, there is a tendency towards axial arthritis, enthesitis, and an association with the histocompatibility antigen HLA-B27. The discrete clinical entities comprising the spondyloarthropathy class of childhood rheumatic disease include juvenile ankylosing spondylitis, certain subsets of arthritis that exist in association with psoriasis or inflammatory bowel disease, and most postinfectious reactive arthritides. In addition, there are those children whose evolving disease suggests a spondyloarthropathy, but in whom a specific diagnosis cannot be made because the early clinical manifestations are insufficiently differentiated. The disorders comprising the spondyloarthropathy class of childhood rheumatic disease are more similar than their apparently disparate clinical features might initially suggest. Most of the childhood spondyloarthropathies are typified by onset in later childhood, oligoarthritis predominantly of large joints of the lower limbs in an asymmetrical pattern, axial and sacroiliac arthropathy, enthesitis, male predominance, acute iritis, family histories of similar disorders, associations with HLA-B27, and seronegativity for both antinuclear antibodies and rheumatoid factors (Fig. 8.1).

The presenting manifestations in children with spondyloarthropathies do not always satisfy adult diagnostic criteria. Consequently, these children might remain undiagnosed or have their complaints ascribed to other causes. When used to identify children with a spondyloarthropathy, currently available adult criteria, such as the criteria of Amor (Amor *et al.* 1991) and of the European Spondyloarthropathy Study Group (Dougados *et al.* 1991*a*), provide comparable diagnostic sensitivities (74 and 79% respectively) and specificities (98 and 92%) (Prieur *et al.* 1990). These criteria, however, do not differentiate among the spondyloarthropathies.

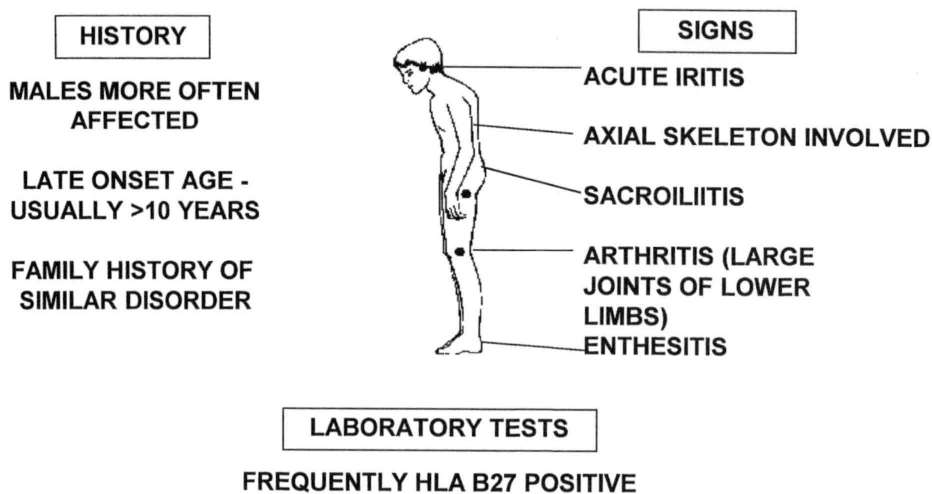

Fig. 8.1 The characteristics of spondyloarthropathies in children and adolescents.

Criteria proposed recently for identifying specific forms of spondyloarthropathies in children require validation before they can be confidently employed (Fink 1995; Hochberg 1995; Prieur *et al.* 1993).

Studies of paediatric rheumatology clinic populations in the United States and Canada have provided a clearer indication of the prevalence of spondyloarthropathies relative to other childhood arthropathies. Of a total of more than 16 000 paediatric patients in two independent disease registries, 41% had a rheumatic disease and of these, 30% (12% of the total) were diagnosed as having a spondyloarthropathy. In comparison, 38% were diagnosed as having one of three juvenile rheumatoid arthritis subtypes (as defined by American College of Rheumatology criteria (Brewer *et al.* 1977). Thus, as reflected by these clinic populations, the spondyloarthropathies are among the most common arthritides of childhood.

A syndrome of seronegative, enthesopathy, and arthropathy: SEA syndrome (undifferentiated spondyloarthropathy)

The early recognition and differentiation of childhood spondyloarthropathies from other chronic arthritides of childhood is difficult. SEA syndrome, which accounts for up to 20% of the paediatric rheumatology clinic population, defines a group of children who are distinguishable from children with other arthritides and whose disease usually evolves into a pattern characteristic of one of the spondyloarthropathies (Cabral *et al.* 1992; Rosenberg and Petty 1982). Affected children are seronegative for antinuclear antibodies and rheumatoid factors, and have enthesitis and arthralgia or arthritis. Most (more than 70%) have the HLA-B27 antigen.

Enthesitis is a prominent feature of childhood spondyloarthropathies and is a key feature of the SEA syndrome. It is not specific, however, and occasionally occurs in children with juvenile rheumatoid arthritis and even systemic lupus erythematosus, and the signs of the osteochondroses of Osgood–Schlatter, Sindig–Larsen, and Sever can mimic those of enthesitis.

Follow-up of children with SEA syndrome indicates that most represent patients who have the earliest manifestations of an evolving spondyloarthropathy, usually anklyosing spondylitis (Cabral *et al.* 1992). Evolution into a discrete spondyloarthropathy is more likely in the presence of HLA-B27, a family history of a spondyloarthropathy, arthritis (rather than arthralgia) at onset, and an older onset age (more than 5 years). Different eventual outcomes of children with SEA syndrome are evident when different populations are evaluated. Ethnicity, geography, or environment could account for the poorer eventual outcome in Mexican children with SEA syndrome, most of whom (92%) developed progressive ankylosing spondylitis within 5 years of onset (Burgos-Vargas and Clark 1989; Burgos-Vargas *et al.* 1997).

A set of criteria for identifying atypical spondyloarthropathy in children has been proposed by Hussein and colleagues (Hussein *et al.* 1989). Major criteria include:

(1) family history of spondyloarthropathy or oligoarthritis;

(2) enthesopathy;

(3) digital joint arthritis;

(4) sacroiliitis;

(5) presence of HLA-B27; and

(6) recurrent arthritis or arthralgia.

Minor criteria included:

(1) onset after the age of 10 years;

(2) male gender;

(3) involvement of lower extremities only;

(4) acute iritis or conjunctivitis;

(5) hip arthritis, and

(6) an antecedent history of enteritis.

When these criteria were evaluated in a group of 26 children, 96% were correctly classified as having atypical spondyloarthropathy, with a sensitivity of 85% and a specificity of 100%. The diagnostic accuracy was comparable when either four of six major criteria or three major and three minor criteria were present.

Juvenile ankylosing spondylitis

Juvenile ankylosing spondylitis is the prototypical childhood spondyloarthropathy. Ironically, it is seldom that children and adolescents, at onset, unambiguously satisfy adult diagnostic criteria for the disease. For several reasons, neither the Rome (Kellgren *et al.* 1963) nor the New York (Bennett and Burch 1968*b*) criteria, used for diagnosing adult ankylosing spondylitis, is appropriate for use in children and adolescents: axial skeletal involvement appears relatively later in the course of the disease in children, well-established normal values for axial spine flexion and chest expansion that correlate with age, gender, and height are unavailable, and sacroiliac imaging studies cannot reliably distinguish changes due to inflammation from those of a normally developing joint. In most children, the diagnosis is provisionally suspected but cannot be established until the disease eventually evolves into a more characteristic pattern. For the purposes of this discussion, juvenile ankylosing spondylitis refers to an onset before the age of 17 years as defined by the New York criteria (Bennett and Burch 1968*b*). In the absence of validated criteria, age at onset is the sole criterion that distinguishes juvenile ankylosing spondylitis from the adult disease. As early juvenile ankylosing spondylitis may be difficult to differentiate from other forms of chronic juvenile arthritis (particularly oligo-articular onset subtypes), many of these children may be imprecisely classified as having pauciarticular juvenile chronic (EULAR 1977) or pauciarticular juvenile rheumatoid (Brewer *et al.* 1977) arthritis. It should be pointed out, however, that prepubertal children have been observed with unequivocal AS that ostensibly meets adult criteria (Burgos-Vargas *et al.* 1996).

Epidemiologic and demographic characteristics of juvenile ankylosing spondylitis

Based on the prevalences of ankylosing spondylitis in populations of various racial origins and the percentage of adults who had a childhood onset of their disease, it has been estimated that the prevalence of ankylosing spondylitis in Caucasian children is 12–33 per 100 000 (Burgos-Vargas and Petty 1992). Other racial groups, in particular North American aboriginals, have higher prevalences of HLA-B27 and correspondingly higher estimated prevalences of ankylosing spondylitis, ranging from 13–69 per 100 000 (Boyer *et al.* 1988; Burgos-Vargas and Petty 1992; Gofton *et al.* 1975; Oen *et al.* 1986; Rosenberg *et al.* 1982).

By one estimate, ankylosing spondylitis may occur in as many as 0.4–1.8% of the adult Caucasian population (Gran and Husby 1993). In retrospective analyses of adult ankylosing spondylitis patients, as many as 20% of Caucasians (Bennett and Burch 1968*b*; Riley *et al.* 1971) and 50% of Mexican mestizos (Burgos-Vargas *et al.* 1989; Jiménez-Baldaros *et al.* 1989) had their disease onset during childhood. Even if 10% of adults are conservatively estimated to have had the onset of ankylosing spondylitis during childhood, the extrapolated prevalence in children is as high as 40–150 per 100 000.

Juvenile ankylosing spondylitis is recognized in males predominantly. Male-to-female ratios of 5:1 to 9:1 have been documented, but it is possible that the observed male predominance is not a true reflection of the occurrence of the disease in females. That there is no gender disparity with respect to the HLA-B27 antigen and that radiographic evidence of sacroiliitis may be as common in B27-positive women as men (Calin and Fries 1975*a*), suggest that although clinical expression of the disease is more apparent in males than in females, the actual prevalence may not differ appreciably.

Characteristically, juvenile ankylosing spondylitis begins in later childhood or during adolescence, and in this regard it is distinctly different from the young peak age at onset of pauciarticular juvenile chronic arthritis.

Genetic factors

The frequent occurrence of ankylosing spondylitis or another spondyloarthropathy in family members suggests a genetic basis for the disease. The striking association between the HLA antigen B27 and ankylosing spondylitis and other spondyloarthropathies is as well established in children as it is in adults. Of the recognized HLA-B27 subtypes (B*2701 to B*2712), five (HLA- B*2701, B*2702, B*2704, B*2705, B*2707) have known associations with spondyloarthropathies (Khan 1995). Specific subtypes are known to predominate in certain ethnic populations, but none is known to be especially associated with childhood-onset ankylosing spondylitis. However, in one study a class II HLA molecule, DR8, has been linked with juvenile onset ankylosing spondylitis (Ploski *et al.* 1994). It was detected in 39% of patients with onset of ankylosing spondylitis prior to age 16 years and in only 20% of those with an adult onset. A higher frequency of the LMP allele 2h was also observed in those with juvenile onset (Ploski *et al.* 1994). Further studies are required to confirm these findings.

Clinical manifestations

The prototypical child with ankylosing spondylitis is male, over the age of 10 years at onset, and frequently with a family history of spondyloarthropathy. Appendicular joint involvement is characteristically oligoarticular, predominantly affecting large joints of the lower extremities, although any joint, including the temporomandibular joint, can be affected. Isolated hip-joint arthritis is not an uncommon presenting feature of juvenile ankylosing spondylitis, whereas it is distinctly uncommon in other forms of chronic childhood arthritis. Arthritis affecting the intertarsal or the metatarsophalangeal joints is also typical of juvenile ankylosing spondylitis but uncommon in other chronic childhood arthritides. Characteristically, lumbosacral and sacroiliac joint involvement occurs late in the course of the illness in children, but careful examination may reveal early signs, including axial skeleton tenderness, limitations of spine movement, and flattening of the flexed lumbosacral spine. Ankylosing spondylitis is an unlikely diagnosis if arthritis predominantly affects the upper extremities or small joints. Of the upper limb joints, the shoulder is the most commonly affected. Enthesitis, although not diagnostic, is highly characteristic of juvenile ankylosing spondylitis. Affected entheses are usually those around the foot, ankle, and knee; occasionally entheses of the pelvis and upper extremities are symptomatic (Figs. 8.2 A,B,C).

Children with ankylosing spondylitis seldom present with axial skeleton symptoms or signs, a notable distinction from adults. Fewer than 25% of children have axial pain, stiffness, or restricted motion, or symptoms and signs of sacroiliitis. Children with ankylosing spondylitis seldom have measurable restriction of chest expansion, and sternoclavicular, costosternal, and manubrialsternal joints are uncommonly involved (Burgos-Vargas *et al.* 1993).

Extra-articular manifestations include acute, recurrent, symptomatic iritis (in contrast to the chronic asymptomatic uveitis typical of pauciarticular juvenile arthritis) in approximately 15–20% of children (Ansell 1980; Häfner 1987). Aortic valve insufficiency, a feature in approximately 5% of adults with long-standing disease, is rare in children, possibly reflecting the shorter disease duration (Kean *et al.* 1980; Reid *et al.* 1979). Amyloidosis occurs in less than 5% of children with the disease in the United Kingdom, and even less frequently in North America. The association of spondyloarthropathies with both overt and subclinical inflammatory bowel disease is well known in adults, and subclinical bowel inflammation may also commonly exist in children with ankylosing spondylitis, an observation that might prove important in understanding the pathogenesis of the disease (Mielants *et al.* 1993*c*).

Diagnosis

The patient's history and findings on physical examination are cornerstones of the diagnosis of juvenile ankylosing spondylitis. Laboratory and radiographic studies may also provide useful information. Laboratory evaluation of the child with ankylosing spondylitis reveals

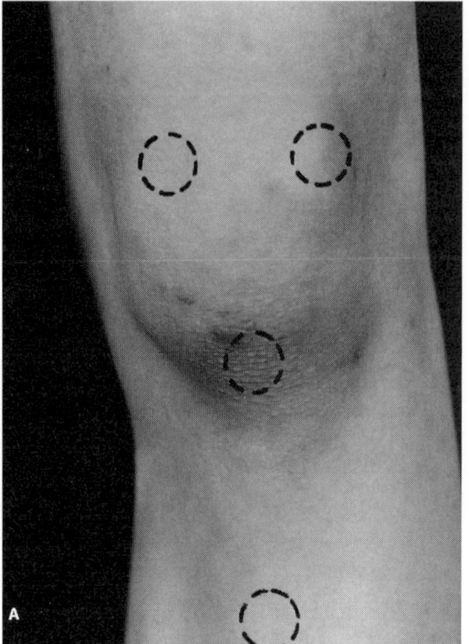

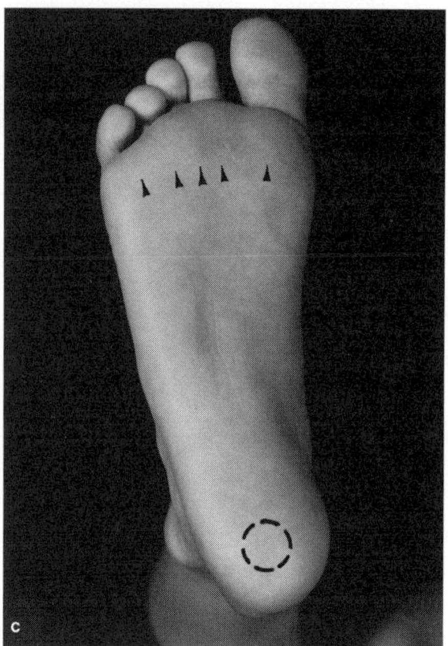

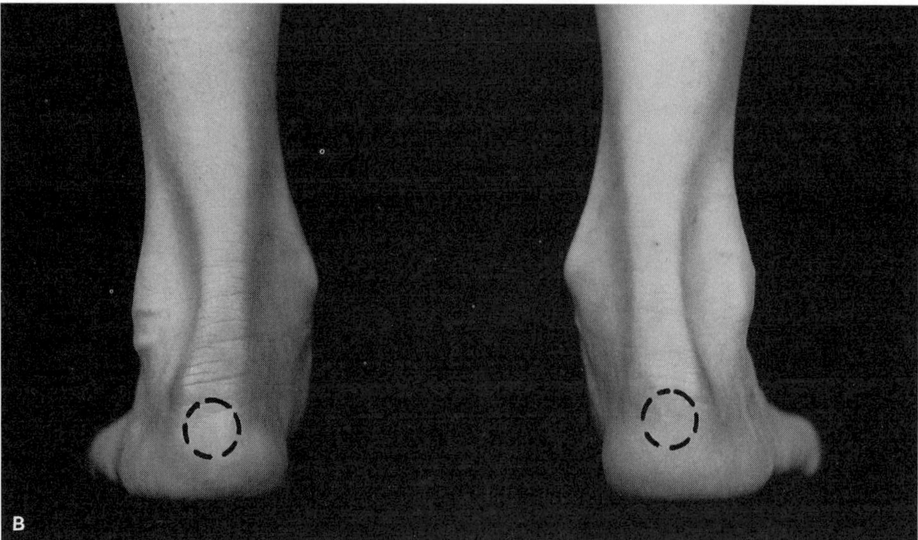

Fig. 8.2 Typical enthesopathic sites involved in spondyloarthropathies in children and adolescents. (A) Insertions of the quadriceps onto the superior margin of the patella, at the origin of the infrapatellar ligament on the patella and at the insertion of the infrapatellar ligament onto the tibial tuberosity. (B) At the insertion of the Achilles' tendon onto the calcanei. (C) At the insertions of the plantar fascia onto the calcaneous and onto each of the metatarsal heads.

mild to moderate abnormalities of the inflammatory indices, including elevations of white blood cell and platelet counts and the erythrocyte sedimentation rate. Normocytic, normochromic or hypochromic anaemia and mild hypoalbuminaemia can occur. Tests for antinuclear antibodies and rheumatoid factor are negative. HLA-B27 is demonstrable in more than 90% of children with ankylosing spondylitis, but it should not be regarded as a diagnostic test: it is not abnormal, merely characteristic.

Radiographic changes, which constitute important diagnostic markers of ankylosing spondylitis in adults, develop later in the course of a child's disease and, therefore are seldom useful in diagnosing early juvenile ankylosing spondylitis. Radiographic characteristics of arthritis in the appendicular joints do not differ predictably from those of other chronic arthritides, although erosions are less likely, and ankylosis, particularly of the intertarsal joints, is more frequent (Burgos-Vargas *et al.* 1989). Enthesitis may be associated with radiographic findings including erosions, hyperostosis, calcification, or accelerated growth of the affected site (Figs 8.3 and 8.4). Radiographic evidence of lumbosacral spine disease is unusual in childhood spondylitis but loss of the normal lumbar lordosis can be seen. Occasionally, there is evidence of osteitis of the anterior corners of the vertebral bodies resulting in reactive

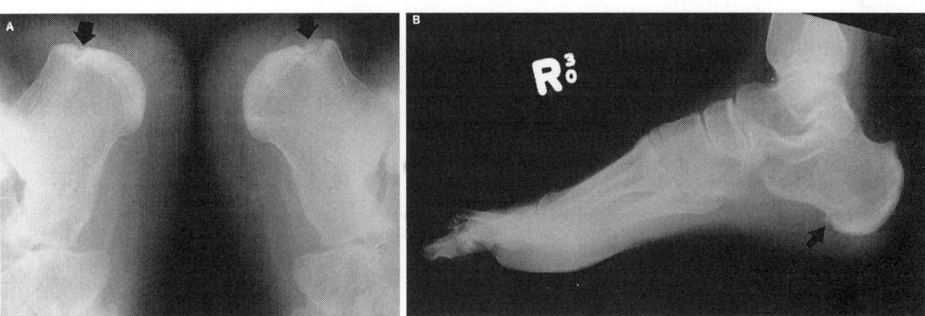

Fig. 8.3 Radiographs demonstrating erosive (A) and hyperostotic changes (B) at enthesopathic sites on the calcanei.

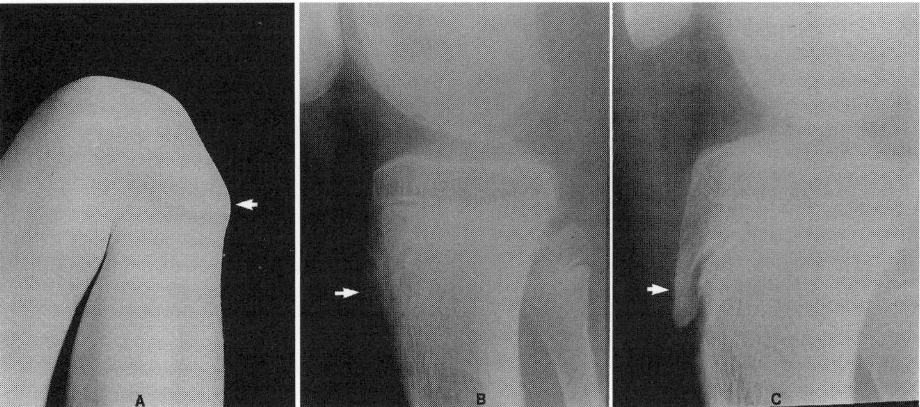

Fig. 8.4 Bony overgrowth (A) and premature fusion of the epiphysis (B) of the tibial tuberosity in an adolescent with unilateral enthesitis at this site. The uninvolved, normal side is shown for comparison (C).

sclerosis ('shining corners'), but progression to syndesmophyte formation is rare during childhood or adolescence. Radiological evaluation of sacroiliac joints is notoriously difficult in the immature skeleton, and radionuclide scans are difficult to interpret until fusion of the sacroiliac joint has occurred. Computed tomography of sacroiliac joints, although not generally required or recommended in the investigation of children, can demonstrate erosions which tend to predominant on the iliac side of the joint and are usually accompanied by sclerosis of the adjacent bone. Later, changes occur on both sides of the joint, and, ultimately, fusion of the sacroiliac joints can occur, although rarely in the child or adolescent.

Management of juvenile ankylosing spondylitis

The optimal management strategy for the child or adolescent with ankylosing spondylitis is one in which pharmacotherapy is incorporated into a multidisciplinary, comprehensive treatment plan (Fig. 8.5). Compliance with pharmacological and physical and occupational therapy is optimized if both patient and family are educated about the disease and its implications, and if psychological and social factors are recognized and dealt with. Attention to vocational aspirations is especially important for the adolescent patient.

Physical therapy is focused on maintaining or regaining joint range of motion and minimizing pain and disability. Particular attention should be paid to posture, chest expansion, and motion of the spine. Occupational therapy assessments are important to attend to the ever-changing needs of the growing and developing child in the home, school, and recreational settings. Splinting, to minimize joint contractures or provide symptomatic relief by temporarily immobilizing the painful joint, is occasionally indicated. Custom-moulded orthoses can help alleviate tenderness associated with enthesitis of the foot.

There are no validated protocols for managing juvenile ankylosing spondylitis, but guidelines can be proposed (Fig. 8.6). Initial pharmacological therapy consists of non-steroidal anti-inflammatory drugs (NSAIDs). There is no convincing evidence that one NSAID is superior to any other for treating children with ankylosing spondylitis. Tolmetin sodium (15–30 mg kg^{-1} day^{-1}) and naproxen (10–15 mg kg^{-1} day^{-1}) have been satisfactorily evaluated in the paediatric population and, therefore, are the NSAIDs of choice. Indomethacin (1–2 mg kg^{-1} day^{-1}) is often effective for older children and adolescents, but its gastrointestinal toxicity, in particular, may limit its use.

Failure of NSAIDs to control inflammation should prompt the institution of glucocortocoids or other second-line drugs such as sulphasalazine. Intra-articular triamcinolone hexacetonide (1–2 mg kg^{-1} $joint^{-1}$) is effective when control of a small number of joints is required, and can be considered as initial therapy especially when only one or two joints are affected. More widespread disease occasionally requires the use of oral glucocortocoids (prednisone or prednisolone 0.5–1 mg kg^{-1} day^{-1}), on an interim basis only, until long-acting agents such as sulphasalazine take effect. Sulphasalazine (50 mg kg^{-1} day^{-1} to maximum of 2.5 g day^{-1}) is a useful second-line agent in the management of juvenile ankylosing spondylitis (Suschke 1992). Methotrexate (10 mg/m^2 per week) can be considered in resistant disease (Creemers *et al.* 1995). None of the therapeutic options used for the management of juvenile ankylosing spondylitis is curative; at best they control inflammation, minimize disability, and help to promote normal growth and development.

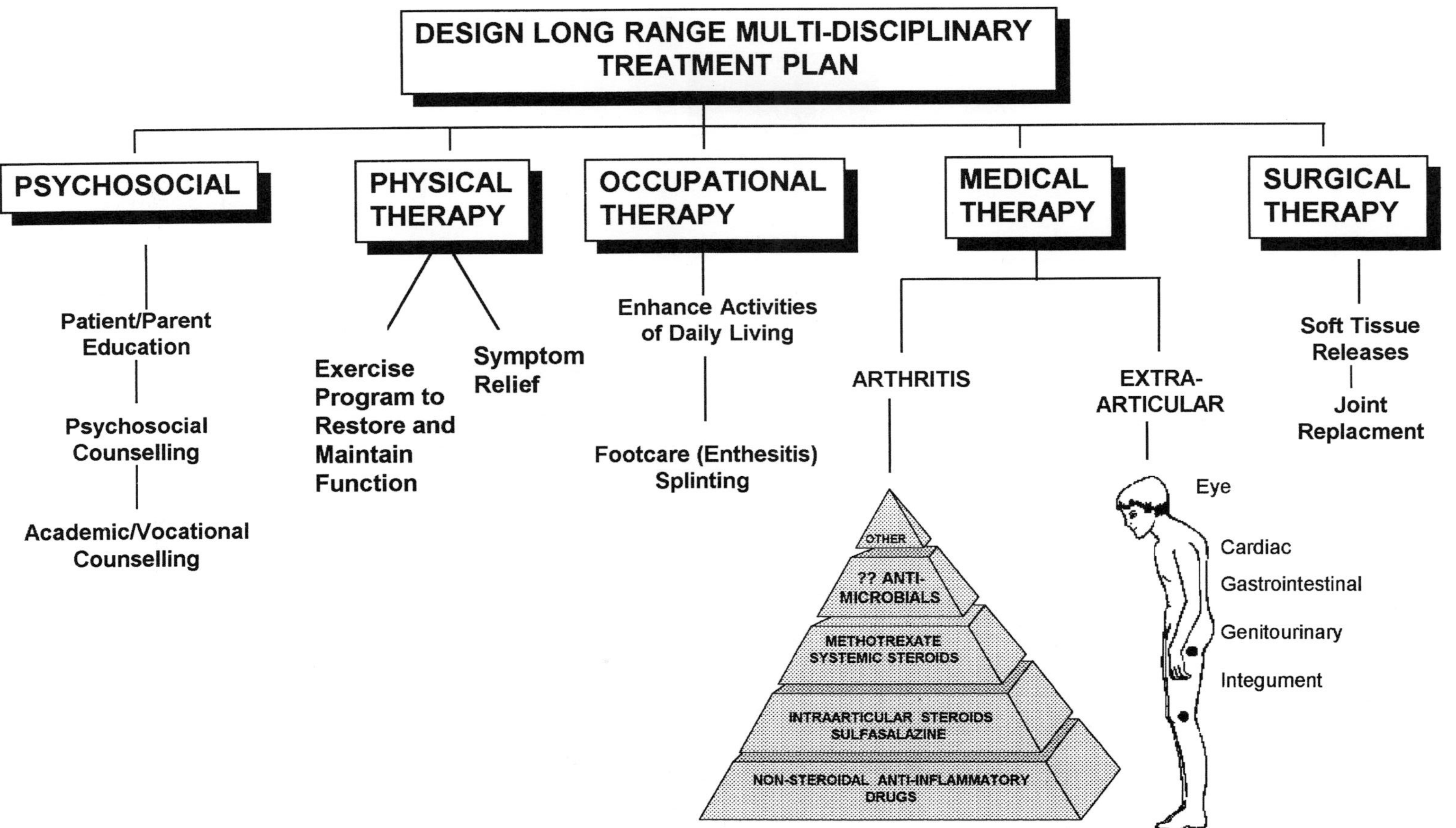

Fig. 8.5 The multi-faceted, multi-disciplinary approach to managing the spondyloarthropathies in children and adolescents.

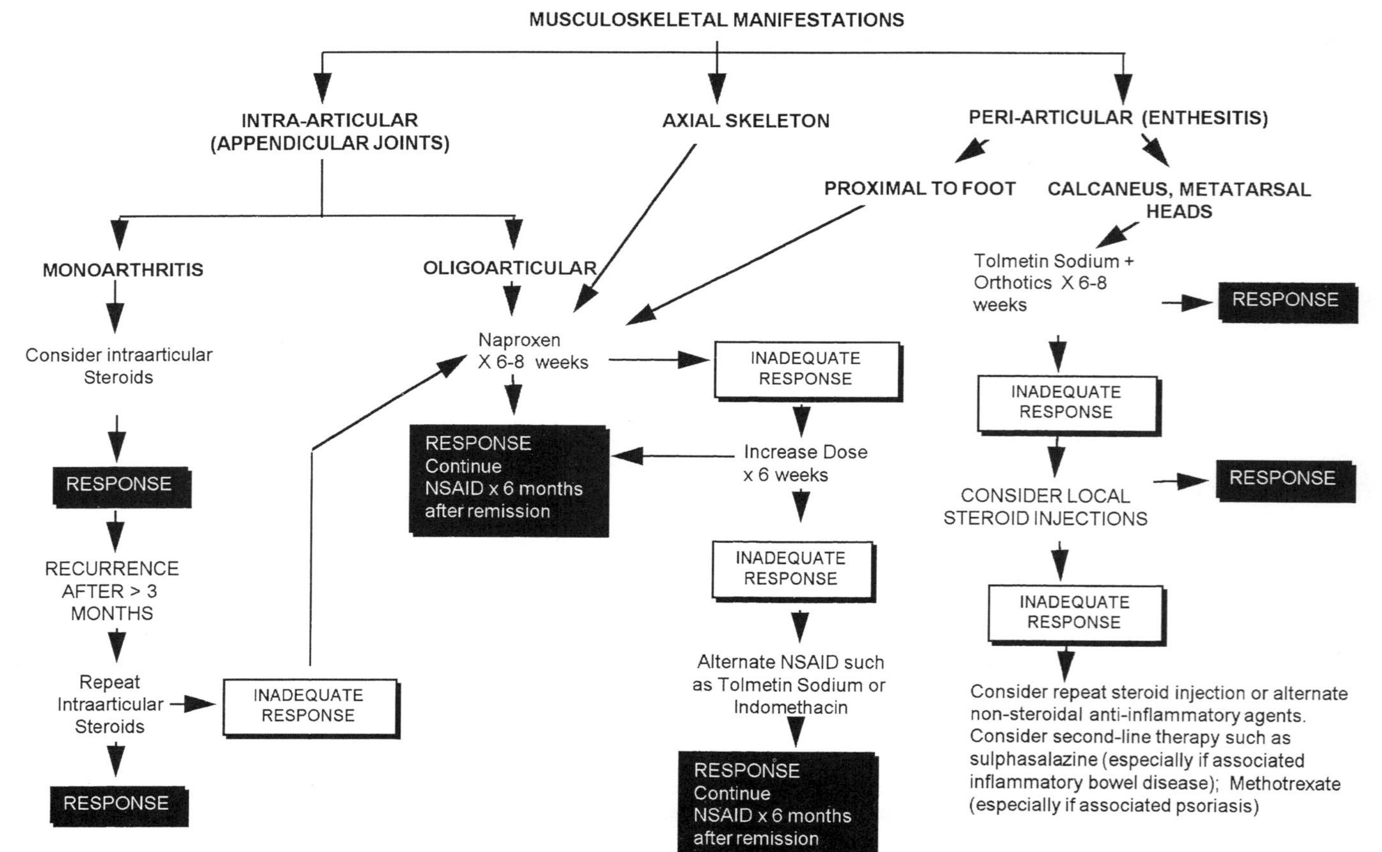

Fig. 8.6 Pharmacotherapeutic approach to management of spondyloarthropathies in children and adolescents.

Course and prognosis

The course of juvenile ankylosing spondylitis is prolonged, often chronic. Frequently, it is characterized by a stuttering onset with symptomatic periods followed by intervals during which there is no clinical or laboratory evidence of inflammation, and during which drug therapy may not be required. Usually, however, the disease eventually becomes more continuously active, requiring longterm anti-inflammatory therapy.

Long-term outcome studies of juvenile ankylosing spondylitis are limited. In a retrospective survey of 22 adults with onset of ankylosing spondylitis before the age of 16 years and who were followed for a mean of 13 years, 20 had low-back pain and morning stiffness and 7 had unremitting disease; one of these patients required total knee-joint replacement, and 95% still required anti-inflammatory drugs (Marks *et al.* 1982). At follow-up, 73% were either at school or employed. In a group of 24 patients with juvenile ankylosing spondylitis followed for 15 years, none had retained normal function, 50% were in Steinbrocker functional class II and the other 50% were in functional classes III or IV (Garcia-Morteo *et al.* 1983). A high frequency of hip-joint replacement among these patients was noted. In general, early axial spine involvement and hip disease may be important indicators of a poor prognosis.

Reactive arthritis

The term reactive arthritis refers to the development of arthritis following infection in the gastrointestinal, genitourinary, or upper respiratory tracts.

Infectious agents such as salmonella, shigella, yersinia and chlamydia typically are associated with reactive spondyloarthritides. While generally thought to be reactive, the discovery of intra-articular organisms and particles of organisms suggests that, in some instances of reactive arthritis, a putative inciting microorganism can be found in the affected joint (Arnett 1993). Why these 'arthritogenic' bacteria produce a spondyloarthropathy-like disease, whereas other bacteria produce a different type of arthropathy (such as acute rheumatic fever secondary to streptococcal infection) is unclear, but might reflect the characteristics of the organism itself, the host's immunogenetic predisposition, or other host factors. Although acute rheumatic fever and post-streptococcal arthritis are classic examples of reactive arthritis, they are not associated with spondyloarthritis, and will not be further considered.

Arthritis, including spondyloarthritis, has been described in children and adolescents following gastrointestinal infection with *Yersinia enterocolitica, Salmonella* species, *Shigella flexneri*, and *Campylobacter* species. Reactive arthritis following genitourinary tract infection with *Chlamydia trachomatis* or *Mycoplasma tiny* has also been described in children. In contrast to adults, in whom genitourinary tract infection is the most common preceding site of infection, children with reactive arthritis usually have an antecedent gastrointestinal infection.

Reiter's syndrome is a characteristic reactive arthritis syndrome that comprises a tetrad of arthritis, conjunctivitis, urethritis, and mucocutaneous lesions (keratoderma blenorrhagicum, circinate balanitis, and oral mucous membrane ulcers) (Reiter 1916). Reiter's syndrome is uncommonly reported in the paediatric age group (Rosenberg and Petty 1979). The condition, however, can be overlooked unless specific findings such as balanitis, urethritis, and keratoderma blenorrhagicum are searched for, and the asynchronous development of the components of the syndrome considered.

Most children with reactive arthritis do not have inflammation of the joints of the axial skeleton, and in reported cases, fewer than 50% have HLA-B27. It is possible that, as is the case with arthritis of inflammatory bowel disease, reactive arthritis should be thought of as two syndromes: one a peripheral polyarthritis occurring principally in children who lack HLA-B27; and an axial arthropathy, like ankylosing spondylitis, in children who are HLA-B27 positive. Further data are required to substantiate or refute this possibility.

Yersinia enterocolitica (serotypes 3 or 9) has been reported to be the aetiological organism in one-third of children with reactive arthritis (Taccetti *et al.* 1994). The gastrointestinal manifestations are often mild and characterized by gastroenteritis in young children, but may simulate appendicitis or an acute abdomen in the older child. After an interval of 1–2 weeks, monoarthritis or asymmetrical oligoarthritis or polyarthritis develops, predominantly in the large joints of the lower extremities. Signs of lumbosacral spine and sacroiliac joint involvement are present in approximately 25% of affected patients. Associated features can include fever, rash, acute iritis, erythema nodosum, and myocarditis. Laboratory examinations reveal abnormalities in indices of inflammation and the presence of HLA-B27 in approximately 50% of the affected patients.

The diagnosis of yersinia-related reactive arthritis is based on the clinical presentation and the presence of high or increasing titres of IgM antibodies to the organism. Stool cultures are almost always negative at the time arthritis begins.

Treatment is usually limited to the use of NSAIDs; antibiotic therapy is not indicated. The arthritis is usually self-limiting, lasting an average of 6 months, but occasionally lasting as long as 2–3 years.

Reactive arthritis following infection with *Salmonella typhimurium* or *S. enteriditis* is less frequent than that following Yersinia. The gastrointestinal symptoms may be mild. Lower extremity oligoarthritis, sometimes associated with fever, occurring 1–2 weeks later is typical. In contrast to Yersinia, stool cultures for salmonella are usually positive and serum antibodies to the organism can be detected in 50% of the affected patients. Treatment of the joint disease is not required if the arthritis is mild and of brief duration. NSAIDs are indicated for more protracted arthritis.

Brief (24–72 hours) but intense abdominal pain, watery or mucoid diarrhoea, and high fever characterize the initial manifestations of *Shigella flexneri* gastroenteritis. Oligoarthritis of the large joints of the lower extremity can follow in 1–3 weeks. Circulating antibodies to *Shigella flexneri* serotype 2 or 2a are present, but the stool culture is often negative when arthritis is first manifested. NSAID therapy, while not always required, can be used to treat protracted arthritis. The prognosis for complete disease remission is excellent.

Arthritis associated with inflammatory bowel disease

Arthropathy is the most common non-intestinal manifestation of chronic inflammatory bowel disease, present in 20% of children (Cassidy and Petty 1995; Passo *et al.* 1986). Peripheral arthritis occurs in 10–20% of children with ulcerative colitis, and in 10–15% of those with regional enteritis (Lindsley and Schaller 1974). Axial skeletal inflammation resembling ankylosing spondylitis is less common, comprising approximately 25% of all children with both inflammatory bowel disease and associated arthritis. Secondary hypertrophic osteoarthropathy is a rare cause of musculoskeletal manifestations associated with childhood inflammatory bowel disease (Ansell 1992).

Oligoarthritis, or limited polyarthritis, characteristically affects large joints of the lower extremities. It may be abrupt in onset and intermittent in course, reflecting, in general, the degree of activity of the gut disease. Arthritis may be the first indication of underlying bowel inflammation and, together with marked elevations of the erythrocyte sedimentation rate, anaemia, hypoalbuminaemia, weight loss, fever, and occasionally erythema nodosum or pyoderma gangrenosum, should suggest the diagnosis of inflammatory bowel disease, even in the absence of abdominal symptoms or signs.

Sacroiliac joint and axial skeleton inflammation, sometimes with peripheral enthesitis, can occur in children with inflammatory bowel disease who have HLA-B27. It is usually more subtle than the peripheral arthritis, but occasionally causes severe pain and limitation of motion. The axial arthritis appears to be associated with gut inflammation, but does not reflect its activity, and may progress even with optimal control of enteric inflammation.

Management of peripheral arthritis is usually contingent upon adequate control of gut inflammation, and responds to the short-term use of NSAIDs or low-dose oral prednisone. Sulphasalazine is effective in controlling both the gastrointestinal and joint inflammation, and is particularly indicated in those children with sacroiliac and lumbosacral spine disease. Physical therapy is indicated for the management of the spondylitic component of the disease.

Juvenile psoriatic arthritis

Traditionally, psoriatic arthritis is classified as a spondyloarthropathy. In children, however, this categorization is not always appropriate. Although some children with psoriasis have features typical of a spondyloarthropathy (including older onset age, male gender, axial skeleton involvement, and an association with HLA-B27), most are young females with oligoarthritis who may have antinuclear antibodies and chronic asymptomatic uveitis (Roberton *et al.* 1996). In children, therefore, psoriatic arthritis represents a clinically heterogeneous class of chronic arthropathy. Furthermore, some children undoubtedly have arthritis and psoriasis coexisting coincidentally.

Diagnostic criteria for juvenile psoriatic arthritis have been proposed (Southwood *et al.* 1989) (Table 8.1). Using these and similar criteria the prevalence of psoriatic arthritis in children has been estimated at 10–15 per 100 000 (Cassidy and Petty 1995).

The cause and pathogenesis of psoriasis and of psoriatic arthritis are unknown. Anecdotal reports have suggested an antecedent infection with varicella or streptococcus as possible inciting factors (Shore and Ansell 1982; Vasey *et al.* 1982). A familial aggregation of psoriasis indicates a genetic predisposition to developing the disease (Gladman *et al.* 1986).

Joint manifestations of juvenile psoriatic arthropathy are characterized by a predilection for large and small joints in an asymmetrical distribution (Roberton *et al.* 1996) (Fig. 8.7). Tenosynovitis of flexor tendon sheaths of the digits, when associated with intra-articular inflammation, results in characteristic dactylitis. Sacroiliac and lumbar spine joints are the least likely to be affected.

Nail pitting, dactylitis, and a family history of psoriasis are features that help to identify those children with, or destined to develop, definite psoriatic arthritis. Uveitis in children with psoriatic arthritis is similar to, but often more severe, than the chronic asymptomatic anterior uveitis associated with pauciarticular juvenile rheumatoid arthritis (Cabral *et al.* 1994). Although there may be an association between the severity of arthritis and the severity of psoriasis, no synchrony between the activity of skin and joint disease is usually evident.

Table 8.1 Vancouver criteria for the diagnosis of juvenile psoriatic arthritis[a]

Definite juvenile psoriatic arthritis
Arthritis[b] with typical psoriatic rash
or
Arthritis with three of the four following minor criteria:
Dactylitis
Nail pitting[c] or onycholysis
Psoriasis-like rash
Family history (first- or second-degree relatives) of psoriasis
Probably juvenile psoriatic arthritis
Arthritis with two of the four minor criteria listed

[a] These clinical criteria need not be present simultaneously.

[b] Arthritis defined as joint swelling or at least two of the following: limited range of motion of the joint(s), pain on movement, or tenderness persisting for at least 6 weeks.

[c] Defined as ≥ two pits on the fingernails at any examination.

Laboratory indices of inflammation may be normal or elevated. Antinuclear antibodies are present in 50% of children, but rheumatoid factor is absent. Radiographic studies, when abnormal, may show a characteristic predilection to distal interphalangeal joint involvement and periostitis.

The initial management of psoriatic arthritis is generally the same as the management of other spondyloarthopathies (Fig. 8.6). The efficacy of methotrexate in the management of both psoriasis and arthritis supports the use of this agent in the treatment of psoriatic arthritis. No controlled studies, however, have been performed to confirm the usefulness of methotrexate as a second-line agent in the management of juvenile psoriatic arthritis.

Active joint disease often requires continuing anti-inflammatory therapy, but the functional outcome is usually favourable; 70% of children with psoriatic arthritis retain normal, or only mildly limited, function (Roberton *et al.* 1996). Of the two-thirds of children who have a polyarticular onset or course, the prognosis is less satisfactory (Roberton *et al.* 1996).

Future directions

Further refinement and validation of criteria for identifying spondyloarthropathies in children are required. Such criteria will permit an earlier diagnosis and a more precise classification of the childhood spondyloarthritides and will aid in achieving a better understanding of clinical courses, responses to therapy, and outcomes. Consensus amongst paediatric rheumatologists worldwide with respect to diagnostic criteria will facilitate the international collaboration required for comprehensive epidemiological, demographic, microbiological, and immunogenetic studies. It is especially important that undifferentiated forms of spondyloarthropathies in children are more discretely characterized. Guidelines to distinguish between certain clinical subsets within the same disease category (for example, psoriatic arthropathy and arthropathies associated with inflammatory bowel diseases) are necessary.

A clearer and more complete understanding of the aetiopathogeneses of childhood spondyloarthropathies will be achieved if clinical, immunogenetic, microbiological, and

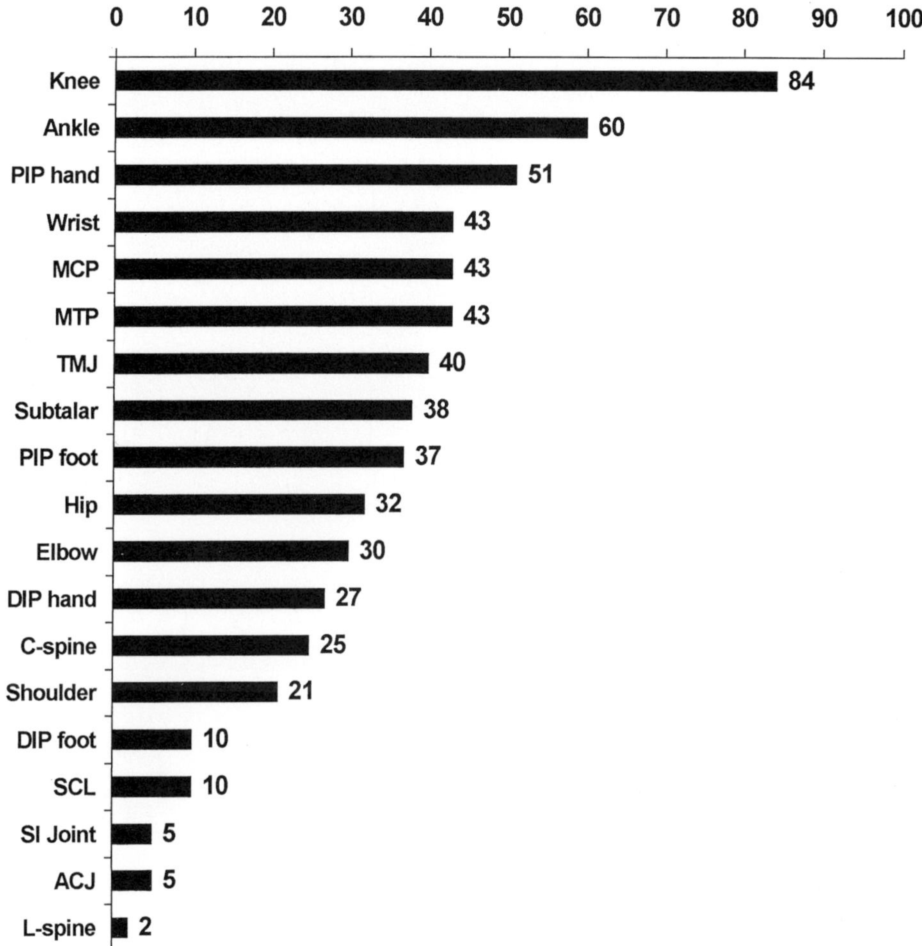

Fig. 8.7 The frequencies of specific joint involvement in juvenile psoriatic arthritis. PIP = proximal interphalangeal; MCP = metacarpalphalangeal; MTP = metatarsalphalangeal; TMJ = temporomandibular joint; DIP = distal interphalangeal; C-spine = cervical spine; SCL = sternoclavicular; SI = sacroiliac; ACJ = acromioclavicular joint; L-spine = lumbar spine

epidemiological factors are comprehensively evaluated by multidisciplinary collaborators. Especially important is the need to explore the conjoint roles of infection and major histocompatibility antigen repertoires in the pathogenesis of spondyloarthropathies.

Effectively predicting and evaluating the long-term outcomes of childhood onset spondyloarthropathies will require prospective studies conducted collaboratively by paediatric and adult rheumatologists.

9 The bowel and spondylarthritis: a clinical approach

H. Mielants and E. M. Veys

The close relationship between the bowel and the locomotor system (peripheral joints, enthesis, sacroiliac joints, and axial skeleton) is suggested by many clinical observations and several experimental animal models. Gastrointestinal abnormalities can be present in several rheumatological diseases. Among the inflammatory connective tissue diseases, these are largely restricted to scleroderma. In most other rheumatic diseases (for example, rheumatoid arthritis, polyarteritis nodosa, systemic lupus erythematosus, Henoch–Schönlein purpura) the intestinal manifestations are either restricted to a systemic arteritis involving intestinal blood vessels or related to drug toxicity.

A strong relationship between bowel inflammation and involvement of the locomotor system is most evident in the idiopathic inflammatory bowel diseases (IBD)—Crohn's disease (CD) and ulcerative colitis (UC). Recently, however, bowel inflammation has been demostrated in most of the other diseases considered as spondylarthropathies (SpA): ankylosing spondylitis (AS), urogenital and intestinal reactive arthritis (ReA), undifferentiated spondylarthropathies (undiff SpA), and some forms of psoriatic arthritis (PsA), juvenile chronic arthritis (JCA), and acute anterior uveitis (AAU) (Fig. 9.1).

Three other diseases, not belonging to the concept of SpA, are particularly attractive human models of the relationship between the altered bowel and rheumatic disease: Whipple's disease, coeliac disease, and intestinal bypass disease. The pathogenetic mechanism of these diseases is rather well defined, and eradication of the causative agent or correction of the altered bowel physiology is followed by amelioration or remittance of the arthritis. These will be considered briefly at the end of this chapter.

Bowel involvement in the spondylarthropathies

Inflammatory bowel disease (IBD)

Bargen (1929) recognized that arthritis was a complication of ulcerative colitis. Previously, the relationship between the gut and arthritis had been postulated by Smith (1922) who performed segmental bowel surgery to treat patients with rheumatoid arthritis. Hench (1935) described a peripheral arthritis in patients with IBD, and observed the tendency of the arthritis to flare with exacerbation of the colitis and to subside with remission of the gut symptoms. The introduction of the concept of spondylarthropathies by Wright and Moll (1976*a*) revealed that IBD might belong to this construct. The pauciarticular asymmetrical joint involvement in IBD, the occurrence of sacroiliitis and spondylitis, the presence of peripheral enthesitis, and the absence of rheumatoid factor and subcutaneous nodules are all characteristics of the SpA (Wright 1978*a*).

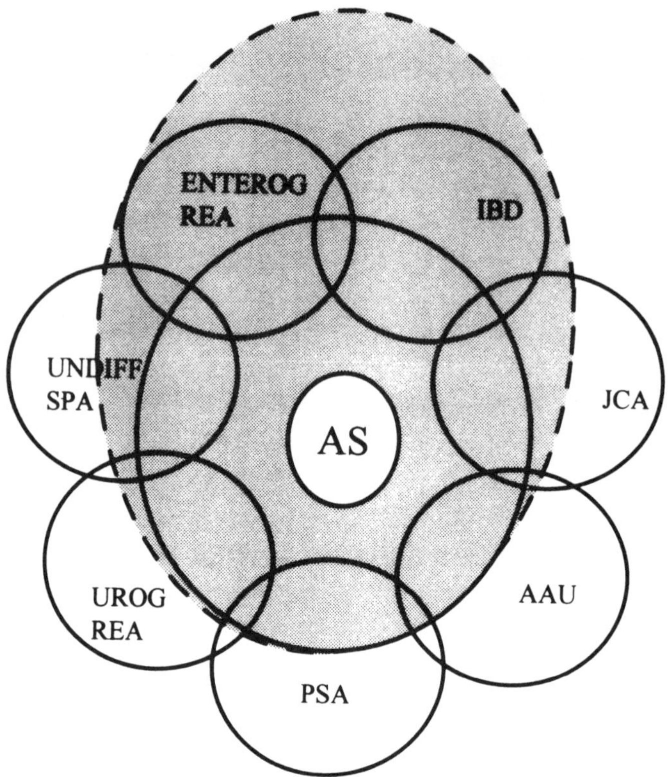

Fig. 9.1 Schematic representation of the prevalence of histological gut inflammation in the different diseases belonging to the spondylarthropathy concept (AS, ankylosing spondylitis; IBD, inflammatory bowel disease; JCA, juvenile chronic arthritis; AAU, acute anterior uveitis; PsA, psoriatic arthritis; Urogen. ReA, urogenital reactive arthritis; Undiff. SpA, undifferentiated spondylarthropathy; Enterog. ReA, enterogenic reactive arthritis).

Crohn's disease and ulcerative colitis are grouped together since they have comparable rheumatological and other associated features, and also because they show familial co-incidence, although the immunopathogenic mechanisms of the two seem to differ.

Epidemiology

The prevalence of UC ranges between 50 and 100/100 000 in the general population and seems to be higher in Caucasians. The prevalence of CD has increased during the last few decades to about 75/100 000 in the general population. A recent epidemiological study during a screening programme for colorectal cancer on an asymptomatic population suggested that the true prevalence of these diseases can be underestimated by ~ 30%. Indeed, 8 out of 481 individuals with a previously undiagnosed IBD were identified (Mayberry *et al.* 1989), confirming the existence of patients with subclinical IBD.

Intestinal symptoms

Crohn's disease is characterized by the classic triad of abdominal pain, weight loss, and diarrhoea. Disease onset may be insidious and disease progression may be subclinical. Abdominal

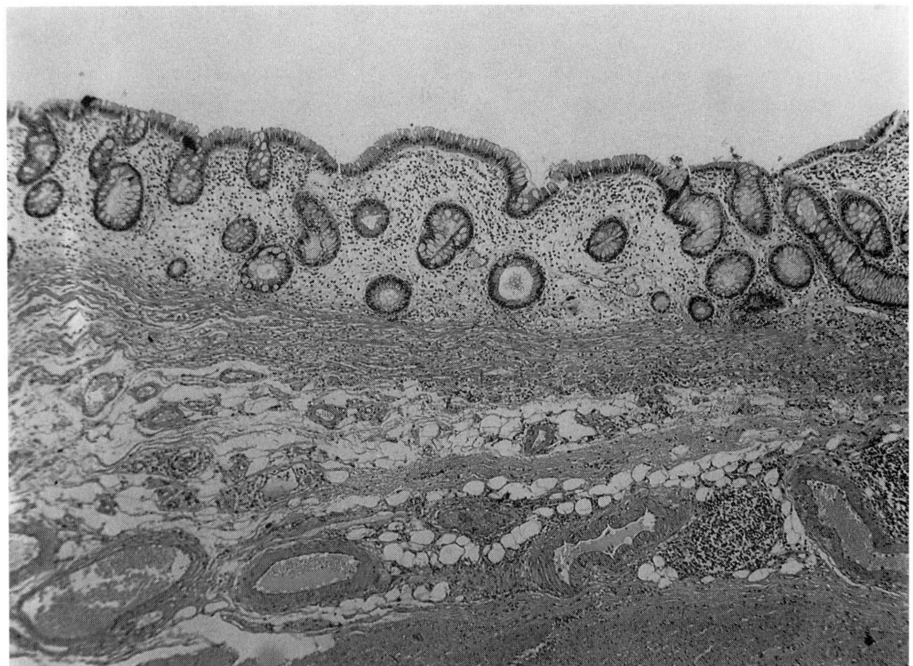

Fig. 9.2 Ulcerative colitis: chronic ulcerative colitis in a quiescent phase: the colonic mucosa is atrophic, crypts are irregular and distorted. The muscularis mucosa is widened (haematoxylin and eosin, × 64).

pain is frequent but is generally not severe. Weight loss in the range of 10–20% of bodyweight is common during disease exacerbation. Low-grade fever is common. At a later stage, fistulae and abscesses may appear. In UC, diarrhoea and intestinal blood loss are the most common abdominal manifestations. Diarrhoea is almost always present, while fever and weight loss are less common.

In UC gut lesions are confined to the colonic mucosa, which is diffusely and continuously involved, and include superficial ulcerations, oedema, friability, and microabscesses (Fig. 9.2). In CD, the lesions may occur along the entire gastrointestinal tract, although the terminal ileum and colon are predominantly involved. The distribution of the lesions is patchy, that is to say normal mucosa alternates with ulcerative lesions. These lesions are frequently transmural and granulomatous (Fig. 9.3). Aphthoid ulceration, pseudopyloric metaplasia, and sarcoid-like granulomas are virtually pathognomonic findings. The distinction between UC and CD when involvement is confined to the colon can be difficult, since the histological appearance in both may be comparable.

Peripheral arthritis

Peripheral arthritis, which occurs in 10–25% of the patients, with a higher prevalence in CD (Gravallese and Kantrowitz 1988), is the most common extraintestinal manifestation of IBD. Sex distribution is equal. Peak age at onset is between 25 and 44 years. The arthritis is pauciarticular, asymmetrical, involving large and small joints predominantly of the lower limbs. The arthritis is frequently transient and migratory. Symptoms persist for less than 4 weeks in 50% of the

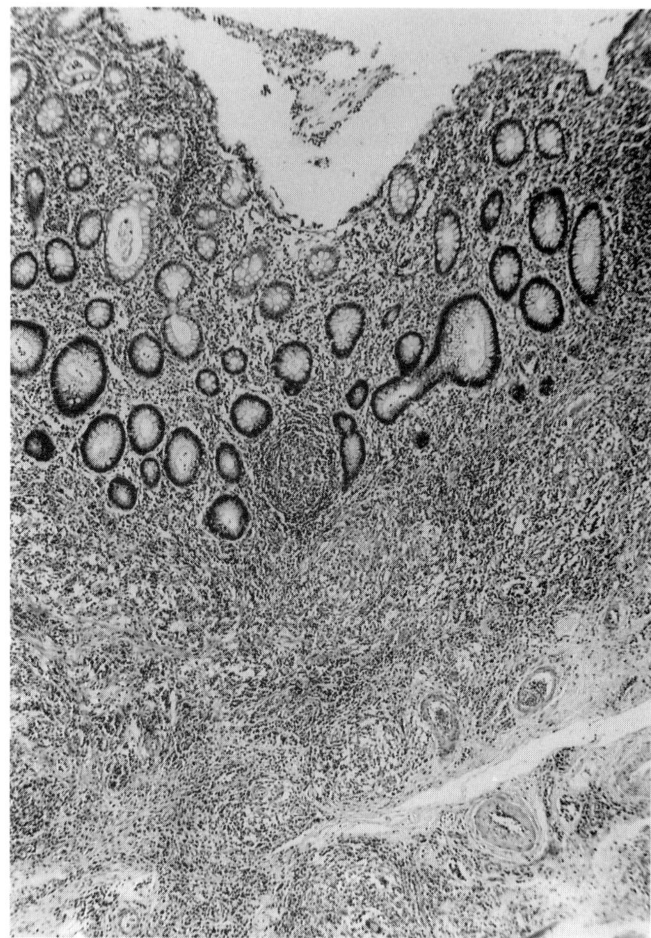

Fig. 9.3 Crohn's disease: bowel wall is thickened by fibrosis and a granulomatous inflammatory infiltrate is present (haematoxylin and eosin × 64).

patients, 5–8 weeks in 30%, 8–26 weeks in 10%, and it may become chronic in 10% of the patients (Mc Ewen *et al.* 1962). Recurrences, however, are common. Sausage fingers and toes (dactylitis) may occur.

Synovial fluid analysis is consistent with an inflammatory arthritis, with leucocyte counts ranging from 1500 to 50 000/ml, predominantly neutrophils. Synovial histology reveals only nonspecific inflammation (Bywaters and Ansell 1958; Soren 1966), although granulomatous synovitis (Hermans *et al.* 1984) has been described.

Enthesopathies, especially of the Achilles tendon and the insertion of the plantar fascia, may occur. Clubbing and rarely periostitis may occur in some cases.

Radiographs of the peripheral joints only rarely show erosions. Erosive lesions, mainly of the metacarpophalangeal and metatarsophalangeal joints, have been described (Tomlingson and Jayson 1991), differing from the arthritis seen in rheumatoid arthritis only by their pauciarticular and asymmetrical distribution (Genth *et al.* 1978) (Fig. 9.4). In some cases, reactive

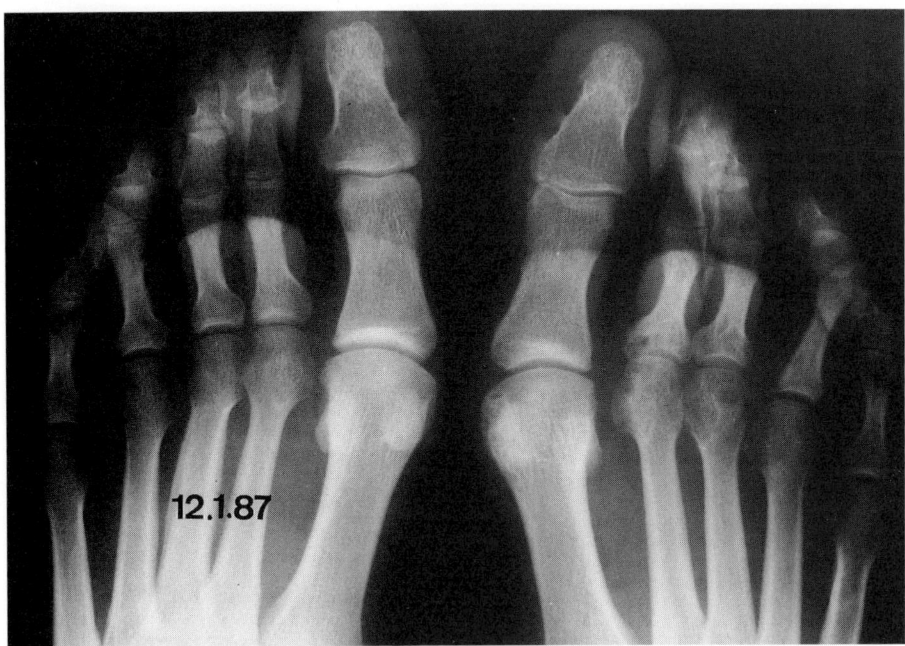

Fig. 9.4 Erosive joint lesions at the metatarsophalangeal joints (MTP II, III, and V, right side) in inflammatory bowel disease: lesions resemble the erosions found in rheumatoid arthritis, but differ in their asymmetrical distribution.

bone formation is seen in involved joints as a sign of repair, suggesting that local inflammatory episodes are repetitive but of relatively short duration (figs. 9.5(a),(b)).

In juvenile-onset CD, atypical forms of arthropathy, with symmetrical finger and gut involvement, including bouttonière deformity, MCP-, MTP-, and sacroiliac joint erosions, have been described (Norton *et al.* 1993). Erosive and destructive lesions of the hip have also been reported (Mielants *et al.* 1990*a*).

Relationship between peripheral arthritis and gut manifestations (Table 9.1)

In most cases the intestinal manifestations antedate or coincide with the joint manifestations. Nevertheless, articular symptoms may precede the intestinal symptoms by years (Haslock 1973; Scarpa *et al.* 1992*a*).

In a recent prospective study on the evolution of patients with spondylarthropathy who did not meet the classification criteria for AS, 4 out of 71 patients (5%) not presenting any clinical or histological manifestations specific for IBD at first examination developed this disease 2–9 years later (Mielants *et al.* 1995*a*). These four all subsequently developed AS; they had all shown nonspecific inflammatory gut lesions on ileocolonoscopy at the first examination (Mielants *et al.* 1995*b*). These findings clearly indicate that SpA patients can have a form of subclinical IBD in which joint and tendon inflammation is the only clinical manifestations (Mielants and Veys 1990).

Although unproven, the site and the extent of gut involvement in IBD may be important in the potential for developing rheumatological manifestations, since arthritis has been reported to be more common in patients with extensive UC than in those with the disease limited to the left colon or the rectum (Wright and Watkinson 1959). Moreover, peripheral arthritis occurs

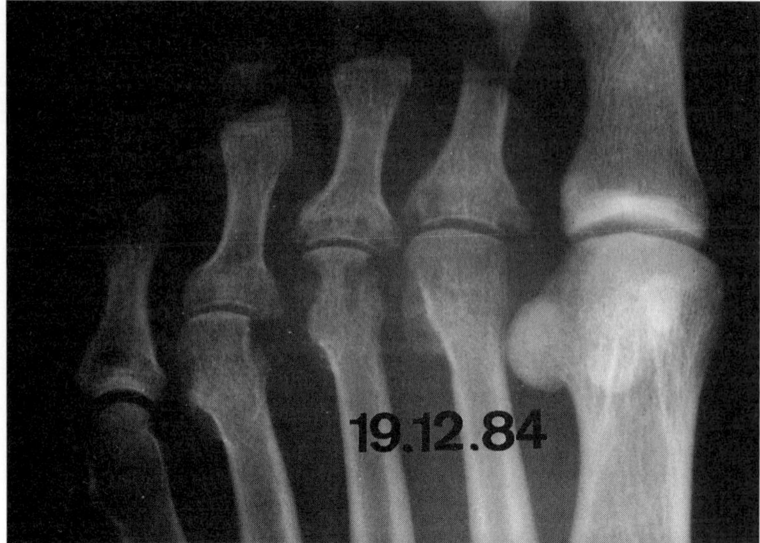

(a)

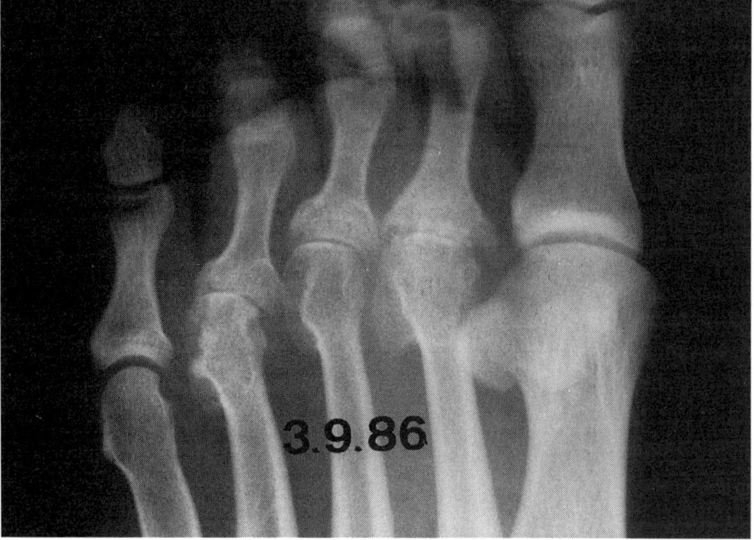

(b)

Fig. 9.5 Erosive joint lesions in spondyloarthropathies. (a) Erosive lesions (MTP II, III, IV) (19/12/84); (b) bone apposition as consequence of repair caused by remission of joint inflammation (3/9/86).

more often in CD patients with colonic localization than in those with lesions confined to the small bowel (Farmer *et al.* 1975; Greenstein *et al.* 1976), although ileal involvement alone can be associated with joint disease. However, Scarpa *et al.* (1990) reported a reverse relationship between the number of joints affected and the extent of intestinal inflammation.

The activity of the arthritis frequently runs parallel to the activity and the extent of the colonic involvement (Greenstein *et al.* 1976; Moll 1985; Selby *et al.* 1979). However, in one

Table 9.1 Extraintestinal manifestations of IBD: relation to activity of intestinal inflammation

Activity related
Peripheral arthritis
Enthesitis
Erythema nodosum
Aphthous oral ulcerations
Finger clubbing
Anaemia
Activity possibly related
Acute anterior uveitis (AAU)
Amyloidosis
Activity unrelated
Sacroiliitis
Spondylitis
Pyoderma gangrenosum
Psoriasis
Primary sclerosing cholangitis
Nephrolithiasis

study, in 55% of cases, arthritis in children with CD occurred when the bowel disease was symptomatic (Passo *et al.* 1986). Moreover, exacerbations of bowel disease in patients who previously had arthritis were unaccompanied by joint complaints. Moreover, features reflecting activity or severity of the bowel disease were more common in patients with arthritis than in those without.

In UC, there is a more distinct temporal relationship between attacks of arthritis and flares of bowel disease. Surgical removal of the diseased part of the colon, or total proctocolectomy, usually induces remission of the peripheral arthritis (Wright and Watkinson 1965*a*). Restorative proctocolectomy, with the construction of an ileal reservoir and ileal–anal anastomosis, is now widely accepted as a definitive surgical procedure in ulcerative colitis (Williams 1989). A number of papers have described the development of an acute symmetrical peripheral arthritis in patients with UC who underwent this type of surgery and who previously had never show joint symptoms (Axon *et al.* 1993; Lohmuller *et al.* 1990). This form of arthritis seems to be more related to the arthritis commonly associated with bowel bypass than to the arthritis connected with UC, and bacterial overgrowth with dissemination of high molecular weight immune complexes containing bacterial products as in bypass arthritis (Wands *et al.* 1976) could be the pathogenetic event in this situation. In CD, colonic involvement increases the susceptibility to peripheral arthritis, but surgical removal has little effect on the joint disease (Isdale and Wright 1989). By performing repetitive ileocolonoscopies in adults with SpA, a close relationship was found between gut inflammation and locomotor manifestations; in patients with resolved peripheral joint disease, gut lesions had disappeared. In those with persisting joint inflammation, gut inflammation mostly persisted; 20% of these patients developed IBD (Mielants *et al.* 1995*c*). Moreover, clinical remission of the joint inflammation together with an improvement in gut histology was induced by treatment with sulphasalazine (Mielants *et al.* 1996; Simenon *et al.* 1990).

Finally, arthritis seems related to other extraintestinal manifestations of IBD, since uveitis and erythema nodosum tend to cluster in those patients with bowel disease and active arthritis (Mayer and Janowitz 1983).

Axial involvement (sacroiliitis and spondylitis)

There is no difference between the axial involvement in UC and in CD. The true prevalence of sacroiliitis is difficult to estimate since the onset is frequently insidious. Depending on the imaging technique used, prevalence rises from 11% by X-ray (Haslock 1973) to 30% by computed axial tomography (Scott *et al.* 1990). Sacroiliitis has been reported in first-and second-degree relatives at a frequency of 8.3% (Haslock 1973) and 1.9% (Weiner *et al.* 1991). The prevalence rate for spondylitis has been estimated at 7–12% (Schorr-Lesnick and Brandt 1988), although the real prevalence may be higher. Recently, ankylosing spondylitis and unclassifiable spondylarthritis were found in 43% of the patients with ulcerative colitis (Scarpa *et al.* 1992*a*). Axial disease in IBD is 30 times more common than in the general population and 36 times more common in the relatives of IBD patients than in control families (Levine 1994). In review studies of AS, clinical proven IBD was present in 4% (Kennedy *et al.* 1993*b*) and 6% (Edmunds *et al.* 1991*a*) of the patients. Although it is generally accepted that men are more likely to develop AS than women, in these studies the sex ratio was 1:1. Moreover, women with associated IBD and AS were shown to have the youngest age of onset of AS of all groups, especially when the disease ran in the family, and to have the worst prognosis. In general, the disease was more severe in patients with associated IBD and AS than in those with uncomplicated AS, as defined by the intake of non-steroidal anti-inflammatory drugs and the decrease of spinal mobility.

The clinical picture is indistinguishable from uncomplicated AS. The patient complains of inflammatory low-back pain, thoracic or cervical pain, alternate buttock pain, or chest pain. Limitation in motion in the lumbar or cervical region and reduced chest expansion are characteristic clinical signs. As in uncomplicated AS, the limitation of cervical spine mobility is a hallmark of progression of the disease to generalized ankylosis.

Radiologically, the axial involvement of IBD is almost indistinguishable from that of uncomplicated AS, although the frequency of asymmetrical sacroiliitis seems to be higher.

Relationship between axial involvement and gut manifestations

The onset of axial involvement is independent of the bowel disease and frequently precedes it (Gravallese and Kantrowitz 1988), sometimes by as much as 20 years (Wright and Watkinson 1959). In a prospective study on the clinical evolution of spondylarthropathies, 4 out of 52 (7.7%) AS patients in whom IBD was excluded at first examination developed IBD 2–9 years later (Mielants *et al.* 1995*a*). However, all showed nonspecific gut inflammation at first ileocolonoscopy (Mielants *et al.* 1995*b*). The course of the axial involvement is usually independent of the course of intestinal disease. Nevertheless, as noted previously, four of 71 SpA patients not fulfilling the criteria for AS, and in whom IBD was excluded at first examination, developed both IBD and AS 2–9 years later (Mielants *et al.* 1995*a*). Bowel surgery has not been shown to alter the course of sacroiliitis or spondylitis. Consequently, it has been suggested that the peripheral arthritides and enthesitides are manifestations of IBD, whereas the spondylitis is an associated disease (Schorr-Lesnick and Brandt 1988).

IBD and arthritis in children

Arthritis occurs in children with IBD (Lindsley and Schaller 1974), with an estimated frequency of 12% (Passo *et al.* 1986). The arthritis is typically pauciarticular involving mostly the large joints. It is mostly benign and occurs in attacks; evolution to chronicity is rare. The arthritis frequently coincides with, or follows, intestinal disease onset, but sometimes can precede it. The attacks often coincide with flares of bowel disease, but the duration and severity of bowel disease are no worse in patients with arthritis than in those without (Passo *et al.* 1986). Sacroiliitis and spondylitis can occur in a few cases.

Other extraintestinal and extra-articular features

A variety of cutaneous, mucosal, serosal, and ocular manifestations may occur in IBD. These manifestations can be classified either by their association with the localization of the intestinal disease or by the correlation with the activity of the bowel disease (Table 9.1).

Skin lesions are most frequently associated and occur in 10–25% of the patients. Erythema nodosum (Fig. 9.6) parallels the activity of bowel disease, tends to occur in patients with active peripheral arthritis, and is probably a disease-related manifestation (Schorr-Lesnick and Brandt 1988). In the review by Greenstein *et al.* (1976), erythema nodosum occurred in 15% of patients with Crohn's colitis, 8% with ileocolitis, and 4% with isolated ileitis or ulcerative colitis. Lesions persisted for several weeks and recurrence was reported in 19% of cases. Patients with IBD who developed erythema nodosum had an increased frequency of arthritis (71%) (Mir-Madilessi *et al.* 1985).

Pyoderma gangrenosum is the most severe skin lesion in IBD and occurs in 1–5% of patients. Painful lesions tend to appear in the pretibial area, feet, trunk, or back, but can occur elsewhere (Fig. 9.7). They appear as discrete ulcers with a necrotic base. If lesions in the feet become deep then destruction of tendons may occur. They are present for weeks to months, and recurrence is

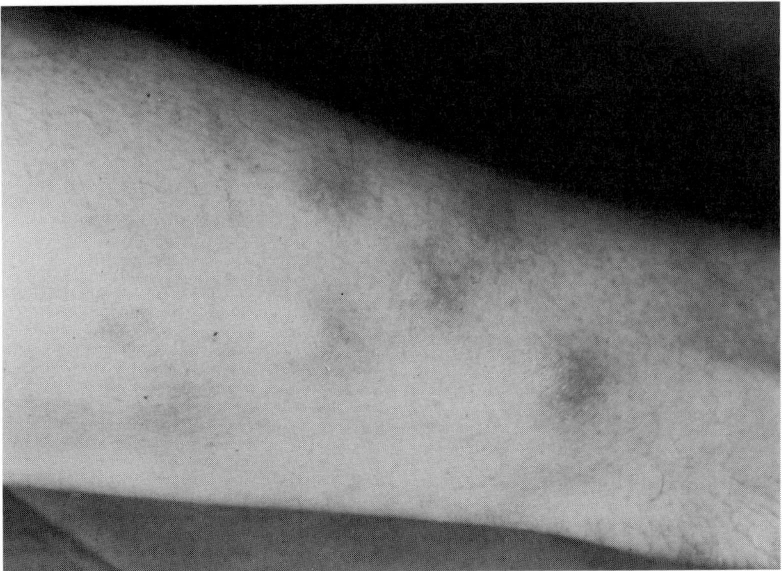

Fig. 9.6 Erythema nodosum of the leg: painful red subcutaneous nodules in a patient with Crohn's disease and AS.

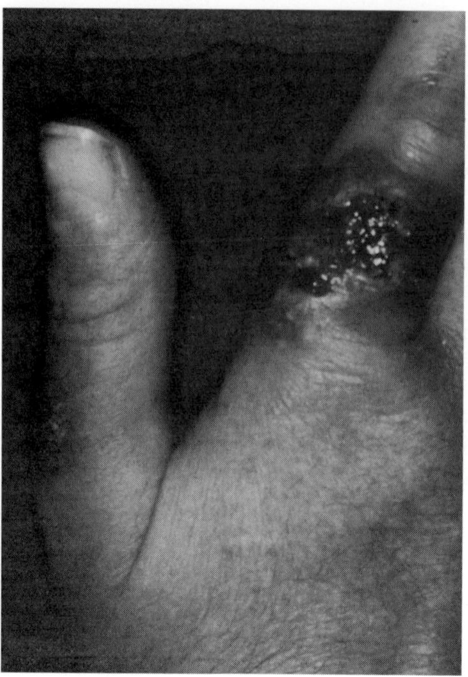

Fig. 9.7 Pyoderma gangrenosum in a patient with ulcerative colitis.

frequent. These lesions are not related to the activity of the bowel or joint disease (Mir-Madilessi *et al.* 1985) and have to be considered an independent associated disorder (Schorr-Lesnick and Brandt 1988). Leg ulcers and thrombophlebitis can also be seen. Psoriasis is increased in patients with IBD and their relatives (Lee *et al.* 1990). Aphthous ulcerations, mainly affecting the buccal mucosa and tongue, are more frequent in CD and can parallel disease activity.

The main ocular manifestation of IBD is acute anterior uveitis (AAU) and occurs in 3–11% of the cases. The uveitis is acute in onset, unilateral, and transient, but recurrences are common (Rosenbaum 1989*a*) (see Chapter 10). It generally spares the choroid and retina; however, a chronic course with lesions in the posterior part of the eye is possible in rare cases. A form of granulomatous uveitis has been described (Salmon *et al.* 1989; Bañares *et al.* 1997).

The relationship of AAU to intestinal manifestations of IBD is debatable. Most authors agree that uveitis will not parallel the acute inflammatory bowel activity and occurs independently of the bowel inflammation. Acute anterior uveitis is more closely related to the axial involvement and to HLA-B27. Some studies, however, reported that patients with IBD and arthritis had a greater incidence of eye lesions (Salmon *et al.* 1991) and that 70% of UC patients with iritis had associated arthritis (Mousen *et al.* 1990). Moreover, asymptomatic uveitis seems to be not infrequent in IBD (12% as reported by Strauss (1988)), whereas asymptomatic gut inflammation was found in 66% of patients with B27-positive AAU (Bañares *et al.* 1995). Intake of sulphasalazine was reported to prevent recurrent attacks of the eye disease (Dougados *et al.* 1991*b*). Conjunctivitis and episcleritis have also been described in IBD.

Clubbing of the fingers is described mostly in CD and seems to be related to proximal intestinal involvement and also to fibrotic lesions in resected gut specimens; it may regress after effective surgery (Kits *et al.* 1979).

At least 70% of patients with primary sclerosing cholangitis have IBD, most commonly UC, although patients with extensive Crohn's colitis are at risk as well (Lichtman and Sartor 1994). The patient may present with jaundice and pruritus, but more commonly only an asymptomatic elevated alkaline phosphatase is discovered (Fausa *et al.* 1991). About 25% of these patients develop gallstones.

Nephrolithiasis has been reported in 6% of patients with CD and 3% of patients with UC, but it is unrelated to the bowel involvement.

Anaemia is frequent in IBD and is related to the degree of disease activity.

Finally, amyloidosis is a well-recognized cause of death in CD. The incidence in clinical series is approximately 1%, but postmortem studies have revealed signs of amyloid in 25% of patients with CD (Greenstein *et al.* 1976). The prevalence of amyloidosis is indirectly related to the degree of gut inflammation, presumably via persistent elevation of acute-phase proteins.

Genetics and HLA

There is substantial evidence favouring a genetic cause for IBD. Familial aggregation for CD and UC has been amply documented. Both diseases are believed to be genetically linked because both occur within the same families (Kirsner 1973), but neither disease has been associated with HLA-antigens in family studies (Naom 1996). IBD, even when complicated by peripheral arthritis, is not associated with HLA-B27 (Mallas *et al.* 1976).

In IBD, sacroiliitis and spondylitis are associated with HLA-B27, but to a lesser degree than in uncomplicated AS (Woodrow and Eastmond 1978). The prevalence of HLA-B27 ranges between 50 and 70%, although it is lower when only sacroiliitis is present. AS patients not carrying the HLA-B27 antigen are at a higher risk of developing IBD than are B27-positive AS patients. On the other hand, a patient with IBD who is coincidentally HLA-B27 positive carries a compelling risk (increased by 200-fold) for developing spondylitis (Schorr-Lesnick and Brandt 1988; Weiner *et al.* 1991). The addition of HLA-B60 or -B44 further increases the risk for AS (Purrmann *et al.* 1988).

In a prospective study, B27-positive and -negative spondylarthropathy patients were compared (Mielants *et al.* 1993*a*): the B27-negative patients experienced more episodes of diarrhoea and had Crohn-like inflammatory gut lesions seen more frequently on ileocolonoscopy. Of 11 patients evolving to IBD, 5 were HLA-B27 positive. AS was the initial diagnosis in six patients, only two of whom were HLA-B27 positive (Mielants *et al.* 1995*b*). A follow-up study of AS patients after 12 years revealed that 6 out of 182 B27-positive patients had developed IBD (3%), versus 8 out of 24 B27-negative patients (33%) (Dekker-Saeys and Keat 1990).

HLA-B62 is present in a high proportion of spondylarthritic patients showing inflammatory and specifically CD-like lesions on gut biopsy (Mielants *et al.* 1995*b*), as well as in patients with proven CD (Mielants *et al.* 1995*a*). In the evolution of spondylarthropathy patients, HLA-B27 was found to be associated with persistent locomotor inflammation, whereas HLA-B62 was associated with clinical remission (Mielants *et al.* 1995*a*); this antigen could play a protective role in the evolution of locomotor inflammation, but is strongly associated with gut inflammation.

Although familial AS uncomplicated by IBD or psoriasis is almost always associated with B27, family studies of IBD patients have shown that axial involvement is often unrelated to HLA-B27 in relatives. The shared genetic predisposition to IBD and AS thus appears not to be HLA-linked. For example, familial aggregation for CD and AS was described in a B27-negative family (Czeizel 1992). Thus, whether IBD is familial or sporadic, B27 greatly increases the likelihood of axial inflammation in a given individual, but it is not a prerequisite (Enlow *et al.* 1980), whereas peripheral joint and tendon inflammation should be considered as a common disease manifestation of IBD completely unrelated to HLA.

Reactive arthritis (ReA)

Reactive arthritis can be defined as a joint inflammation initiated by infectious agents in which the causative microorganism cannot be cultured from the joint. The focus of the infection can be in the gut (enteric ReA) or in the urogenital tract (urogenital ReA). Immunofluorescence and molecular biopsy techniques have demonstrated microbial antigens (yersinia, salmonella, chlamydia) in the synovial fluid and membrane from patients with ReA (Granfors *et al.* 1989*a*, 1990). In contrast with urogenital ReA, in which chlamydia messenger-RNA was found in synovial tissue (Rahman *et al.* 1992*a*)—suggesting the presence of viable antigenic material in these cases—in enterogenic ReA no viable antigenic material could be demonstrated. This suggests a different pathogenic mechanism in enterogenic and in urogenital ReA. Reactive arthritis is included in the concept of spondylarthropathy because of the peripheral joint involvement, the possible occurrence of enthesopathies and sacroiliitis, and the increased prevalence of HLA-B27.

Different enterogenic bacteria are capable of initiating peripheral arthritis: *Shigella flexneri, Salmonella typhimurium, Yersinia enterocolitica* (especially serotype 1), *Yersinia pseudotuberculosis*, and *Campylobacter jejuni* are the most common species (Keat 1983), although arthritis has frequently been reported during outbreaks of diarrhoea in which no pathogens were identified.

Epidemiological aspects

There is a strong male preponderance in urogenital ReA, while in enterogenic ReA the sex ratio is only slightly in favour of males (1.5:1) (Keat 1983). The mean age of onset is 30 years, ranging from 20 to 60 years. The prevalence has been estimated at 5/100 000 individuals.

Intestinal symptoms

The intestinal symptoms associated with enterogenic ReA consist mainly of very profuse diarrhoea, accompanied by spiking fever, general ill-health, abdominal cramps, vomiting, and progressive dehydration. In some cases blood may be present in stools. The delay between infection and intestinal symptoms is very short. In salmonella epidemics the frequency of people reporting distress is between 1 and 10%, depending on the antimicrobial resistance pattern. Most patients recover within 1 month, although a fatal outcome is not uncommon. In urogenital ReA genital inflammation, balanitis, and urethritis are the major symptoms, but diarrhoea can be present (0.17%) (Keat 1983).

Peripheral arthritis

The peripheral arthritis resembles the clinical picture of spondylarthropathies: an asymmetrical pauciarticular pattern of joint involvement, predominantly of the lower limbs, accompanied by tendinitis (10%). Monoarthritis is a common finding as well as dactylitis (sausage fingers and toes). Synovial fluid analysis shows mild to marked inflammatory signs: the white blood cell count ranges from 4000 to 120 000 cells/mm^3 with predominantly polymorphonuclear cells. Enthesopathies usually involve the calcaneum (Fig. 9.8).

The duration of the joint symptoms is usually limited, and in more than 70% of the cases the patient is symptom-free after approximately 19 weeks (Keat 1983). Nevertheless, about 30% of the patients experience multiple episodes of flare-up of the joint disease and in 10–20% of cases (depending on the causative organism) the joint inflammation becomes chronic.

Radiographic lesions of the peripheral joints are seldom seen, and if they occur they are identical to those seen in association with IBD. In the course of the disease some patients complain of inflammatory buttock pain, and radiological evidence of sacroiliitis has been described in 6–9% of the patients, generally in those presenting a chronic or recurrent peripheral arthritis. In the majority of cases, short-term antibiotic treatment has no effect on the joint manifestations.

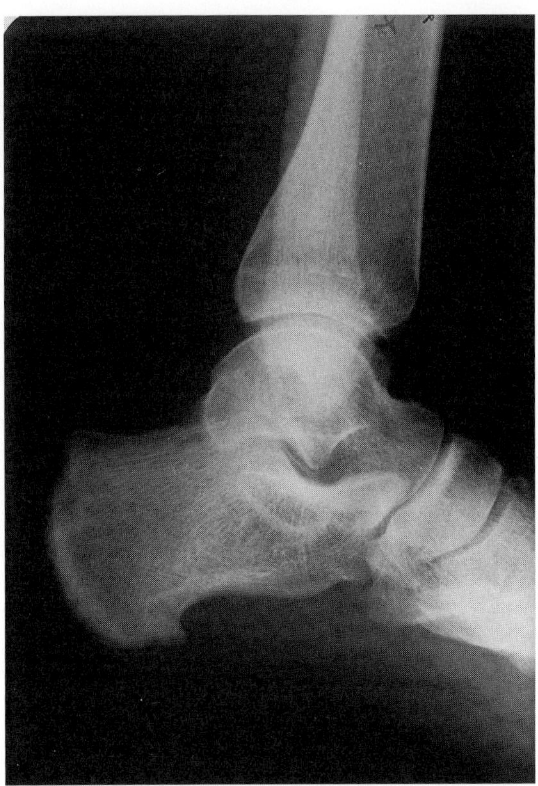

Fig. 9.8 Enthesopathy in spondylarthropathy: bone apposition at the insertion of the Achilles tendon and fascia plantaris.

Relationship between arthritis and gut inflammation (see Fig. 9.1)

The high frequency of infectious enteritis, especially of yersinia infections, and the fact that the gastrointestinal symptoms preceding the arthritis are often minimal and sometimes absent, make the definite diagnosis of enterogenic reactive arthritis difficult. A definite diagnosis of enterogenic infection can be made only by isolating the pathogen from the patient. However, by the time arthritic complications appear, the patient has usually recovered from the gastroenteritis and the pathogen may no longer be detectable in the faeces. In these cases, the diagnosis will be based on serological grounds (specific IgM antibody and/or increase of specific IgG and IgA antibody titres), or on antigen-specific synovial lymphocyte proliferation or by molecular biology techniques.

The arthritis generally develops 6–14 days after the diarrhoea. The interval is less than 30 days in 80% of the patients, although it may be as long as 3 months. The joint symptoms usually take longer to subside than the abdominal symptoms. In some cases, mainly of yersinia-induced ReA, diarrhoea and other intestinal symptoms can be absent (Keat 1983).

Table 9.2 Prevalence (%) of inflammatory gut lesions observed by ileocolonoscopy in spondylarthropathy patients

	Mielants *et al.* (1988)	**Grillet *et al.* (1987)**	**Simenon *et al.* (1990)**	**Leirisalo-Repo *et al.* (1994*b*)**	**Mielants *et al.* (1995*b*)**	**Schatteman *et al.* (1995)**	
Enterog. ReA	*n* = 12	*n* = 6		*n* = 18	*n* = 10		
Macro	50	33		50	ND		
Histol.	100	33		28	100		
Urog. ReA	*n* = 21	*n* = 2		*n* = 24	*n* = 10		
Macro	0	0		29	ND		
Histol.	14	0		36	30		
Undiff. SpA	*n* = 120	*n* = 17		*n* = 16	*n* = 51		
Macro	35	24		38	ND		
Histol.	72	24		31	65		
AS	*n* = 79	*n* = 28	*n* = 96	*n* = 37	*n* = 72		
Macro	29	29	37.5	49	ND		
Histol.	57	25	66.7	41	62		
Psoriatic Arthr.						non-SpA	SpA
						n = 26	*n* = 38
Macro						0	18
Histol.						0	26
Control Patients	*n* = 37	*n* = 24	*n* = 17	*n* = 33			*n* = 37
Arthritis					ND		
Macro	0	4	5.6	6			0
Histol.	3	4	12.5	36			3
Spastic Colon	*n* = 28	ND	*n* = 19	ND	ND		
Macro	0		0				
Histol	0		15.8				

Enterog. ReA, enterogenic reactive arthritis; Urog. ReA, urogenital reactive arthritis; Undiff. SpA, undifferentiated spondylarthropathy; AS, ankylosing spondylitis; Psoriatic Arthr., psoriatic arthritis; Macro, prevalence (%) of macroscopic signs of gut inflammation; Histol., prevalence (%) of histological signs of gut inflammation; non-SpA, psoriatic patients not belonging to the concept of spondylarthropathy; SpA, psoriatic patients belonging to the concept of spondylarthropathy.

There is no relationship between the severity of the bowel symptoms and either the development of articular symptoms or the severity of the joint symptoms.

A number of investigators have performed ileocolonoscopic studies in ReA (Table 9.2). In enterogenic ReA, most authors (Grillet *et al.* 1987; Leirisalo-Repo *et al.* 1994*b*; Mielants *et al.* 1988, 1995*b*) found macroscopic gut lesions in half of the cases. Histological abnormalities were seen in 28 to 100%. In urogenital ReA, macroscopic lesions in the gut are seldom seen, but histological gut inflammation was found in 14 to 36%. These lesions were mostly described as 'acute' lesions resembling the picture of acute bacterial enteritis (Cuvelier *et al.* 1987). This should be considered as a form of 'reactive' enteritis since the causative organism presumably does not infect the intestinal tract.

In follow-up studies of ReA an overall remission rate of 60–80% (Keat 1983; Mielants *et al.* 1995*a*) has been described. The prognosis seems to be better for enterogenic ReA (Bremell *et al.* 1991; Herrlinger and Asmussen 1992; Leirisalo-Repo and Suoranta 1988; Lindholm and Visakorpi 1991) than for urogenital ReA (Fox *et al.* 1979; Leirisalo-Repo *et al.* 1982).

Nevertheless, some ReA patients can develop AS: 10–25% of patients with enterogenic ReA (Bremell *et al.* 1991; Herrlinger and Asmussen 1992; Leirisalo-Repo and Suoranta 1988; Lindholm and Visakorpi 1991; Mielants *et al.* 1995*a*), depending on the triggering agent, and 14–60% of the patients with urogenital ReA (Fox *et al.* 1979; Leirisalo-Repo *et al.* 1982). The evolution of yersinia-ReA to IBD was reported in two studies (Leirisalo-Repo and Suoranta 1988; Mielants *et al.* 1995*a*), while the second study described one patient with urogenital arthritis developing UC. This confirms the place of ReA, as well as of IBD, in the concept of SpA.

Other extraintestinal and extra-articular features

The most common other extraintestinal features of ReA are ocular and dermatological manifestations, but these seem not to be related to the gut or joint disease. Acute anterior uveitis and conjunctivitis occur in about 5–30% of the cases and are usually self-remitting. Acute anterior uveitis occurs mainly in B27-positive patients, but appears to be independent and not related in time to the infectious episode which is actually considered to be the triggering agent of ReA. Mouth ulcers and erythema nodosum have been reported following yersinia infection. Keratoderma blenorrhagica, described in urogenital ReA, does not occur in enterogenic forms.

Genetics and HLA-B27

Predisposition to arthritis associated with gut infection is strongly linked with the HLA-B27 antigen, which is present in 60–80% of the patients. As in other diseases included in the SpA concept, there is a strong association of HLA-B27 with the presence of sacroiliitis, spondylitis, and acute anterior uveitis.

In epidemics of enteric bacterial infection, the relative risk of developing ReA in B27- positive patients is about 20%, while in B27-negative patients the risk is lower than 1%. Carriage of the HLA-B27 antigen influences not only the development of the disease but also the severity, extent, and duration of symptoms (Linssen and Feltkamp 1988; Mielants *et al.* 1991*a*, 1993*a*).

Undifferentiated SpA

At least 30% of patients presenting the clinical, biological, radiographic, and genetic features of SpA cannot be classified into one of the known clinical entities and are classified as having undifferentiated SpA.

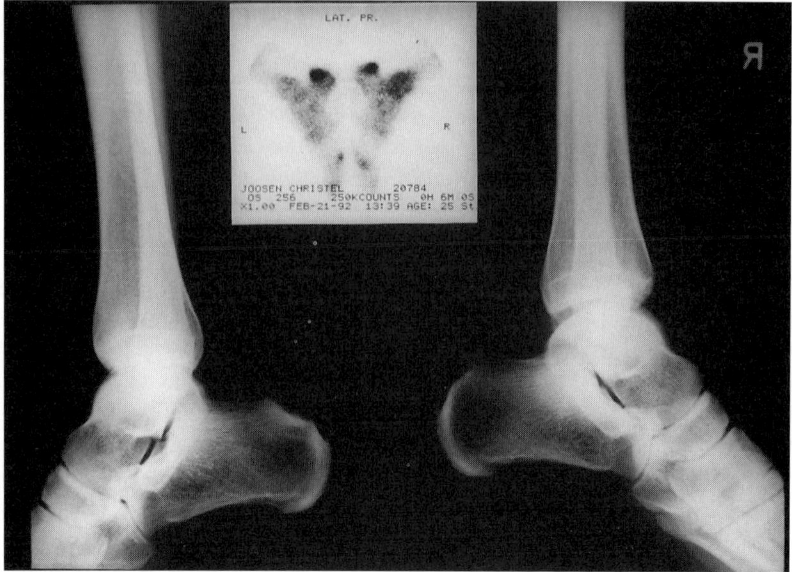

Fig. 9.9 Enthesopathy in undifferentiated spondylarthropathy: involvement of the insertion of the Achilles tendon described on a technetium scan, with an important erosion at the left calcaneum.

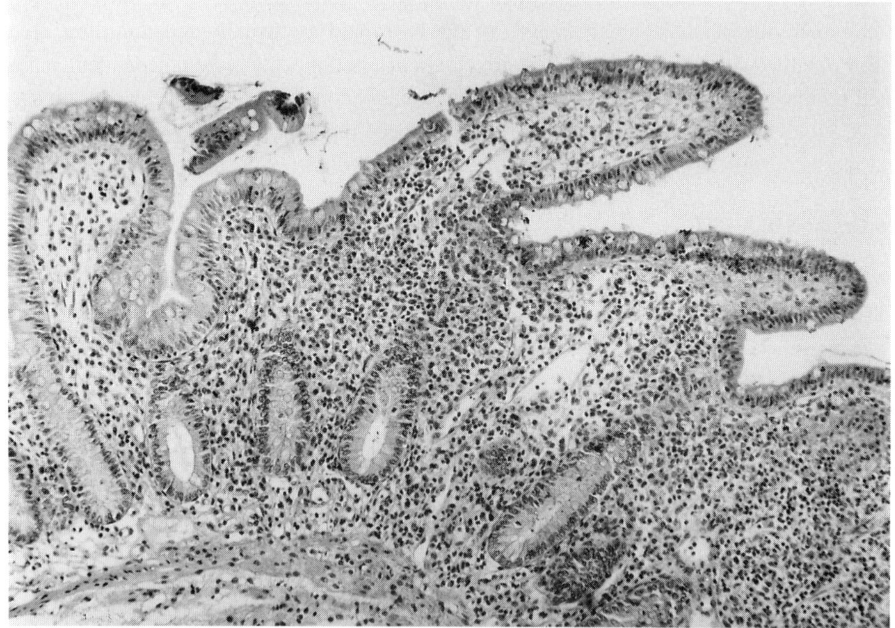

Fig. 9.10 Acute inflammatory gut lesion: the architecture of villi and crypts is intact. The epithelium of the lamina propria contains many polymorphonuclear cells (haematoxylin and eosin × 160).

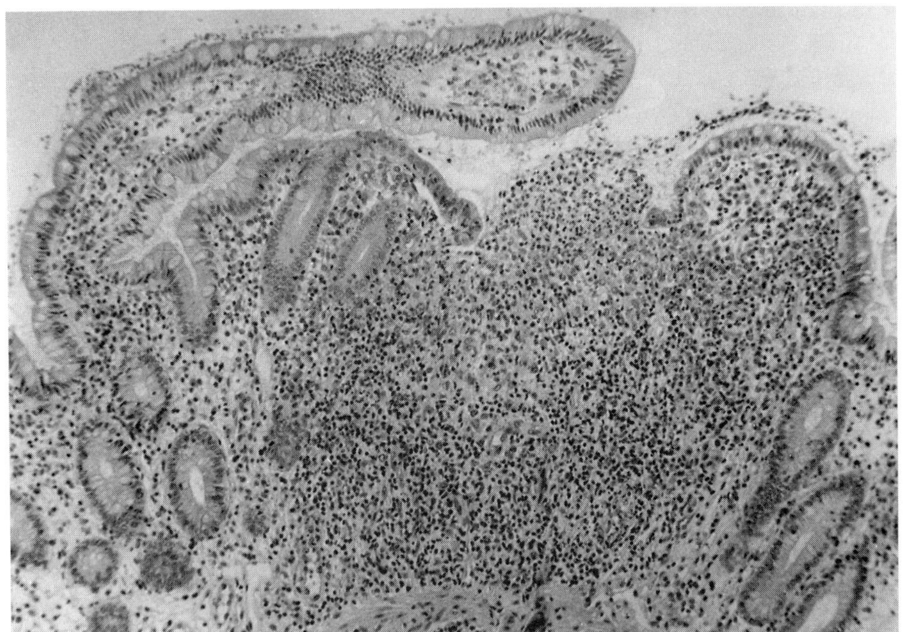

Fig. 9.11 Chronic inflammatory gut lesion: flattening and distortion of villi, aphthoid ulceration with streams of leucocytes localized above a lymphoid follicle, distortion of crypts, and an increased number of inflammatory cells in the lamina propria (haematoxylin and eosin × 160).

The musculoskeletal findings are similar to those seen in other forms of SpA, with an asymmetrical involvement of a restricted number of joints, predominantly of the lower limbs. Enthesopathies (Fig. 9.9), mainly of the feet, and dactylitis are frequently associated.

Erosive joint lesions, particularly of the small joints of the hands and feet are not uncommon; they resemble the lesions seen in RA, but differ in their asymmetrical and pauciarticular pattern. Acute anterior uveitis, erythema nodosum, and urogenital symptoms are the most frequent extra-articular features.

Relationship between arthritis and gut inflammation (See Fig. 9.1)

The majority of patients with undifferentiated SpA do not present with pronounced abdominal symptoms. However, about 20–30% regularly experience short episodes of diarrhoea or regularly have more than two stools per day (Mielants *et al.* 1991*a*).

Ileocolonoscopic studies have demonstrated a high prevalence of bowel inflammation in undifferentiated SpA (Table 9.2). Macroscopic abnormalities were found in 24–38% of the patients (Grillet *et al.* 1987; Mielants *et al.* 1988; 1995*b*; Leirisafo-Repo *et al.* 1994*b*), and histological features of inflammation were found in 24 to 72%. The histological gut lesions could be subdivided into two forms (Cuvelier *et al.* 1987): an 'acute' inflammation resembling acute bacterial enteritis, and the 'chronic' inflammation resembling the picture of IBD, especially CD. In acute lesions, the pattern of inflammation is similar to that seen in acute bacterial enterocolitis (Fig. 9.10). The normal architecture is well preserved. There is infiltration of the epithelium by neutrophils and eosinophils without a significant increase in lymphocytes. In the crypts as well, there is an infiltration of neutrophils and eosinophils, often causing crypt abscesses. Small superficial ulcers covered with fibrin and neutrophils overlying hyperplastic lymphoid follicles can occur. The lamina propria is oedematous and haemorrhagic, and contains mainly polymorphonuclear cells.

The principal features of chronic lesions (Fig. 9.11) are crypt distortion, atrophy of the villous surface of the colonic mucosa, villous blunting and fusion, increased mixed lamina propria cellularity, and basal lymphoid aggregates in the propria. In some of these patients the presence of some lesions, such as aphthoid ulcers, branching, pyloric metaplasia of the crypts, and sarcoid-like granulomas made them indistinguishable from patients with CD. Patients in whom acute lesions and chronic lesions were found in different biopsies were considered as having chronic inflammatory lesions. The classification of the inflammatory lesions into acute and chronic has been a convenient morphological concept, but it has not been shown to correlate clinically with either acute or chronic symptomatology (Cuvelier *et al.* 1987; Mielants *et al.* 1991*a*).

Whereas acute lesions are predominantly seen in ReA, in undifferentiated SpA the prevalence of both types of lesions is practically identical.

Repeat ileocolonoscopy (Mielants *et al.* 1987*a*) demonstrated a strong relationship between gut inflammation and peripheral arthritis in ReA and undifferentiated SpA; gut inflammation disappeared in almost all patients who were in articular clinical remission, whereas all the

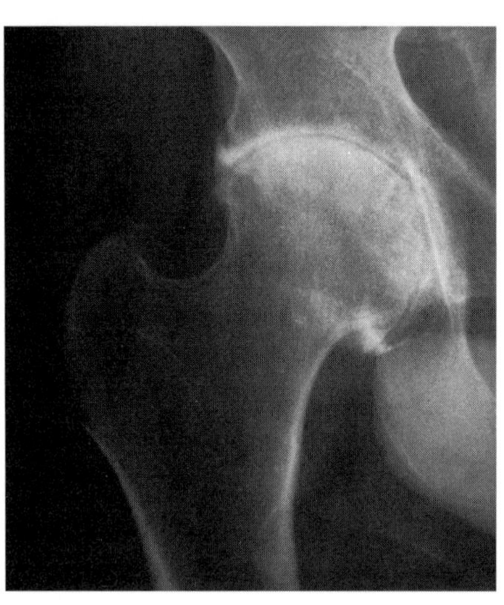

(a)

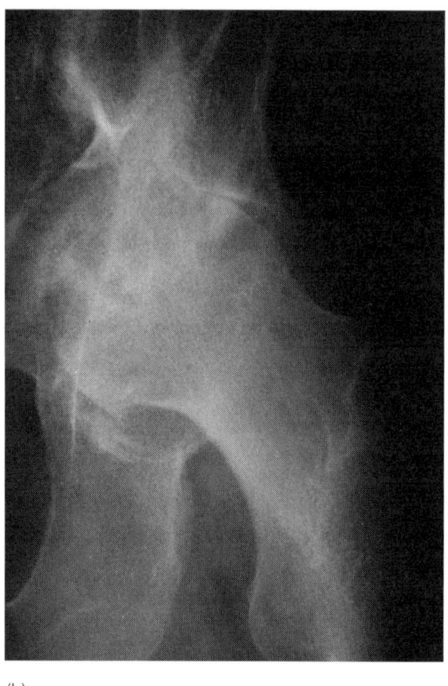

(b)

Fig. 9.12 Hip lesions in spondyloarthropathy. (a) Concentric hip involvement found mainly in AS and related to the spine involvement; (b) Destructive hip involvement resembling the hip involvement in rheumatoid arthritis, which tends to occur in patients with gut lesions suggestive of Crohn's disease (Mielants *et al.* 1990*a*)

patients with persistently active peripheral joint inflammation had persistent histologically evident bowel inflammation. In a recent study of 49 patients with different forms of SpA who underwent two consecutive ileocolonoscopies, 15 patients complained of having more than two stools per day. Of these 15 patients, 10 developed persistent diarrhoea, and 7 eventually developed IBD (De Vos *et al.* 1996).

Development of erosive joint lesions in undifferentiated SpA was found to be related to the presence of gut inflammation, especially the chronic lesions (Mielants *et al.* 1990*b*). Erosive and destructive lesions of the hip (Figs 9.12(a), (b)) have been reported and have been related to HLA-B62 and CD-like lesions on gut biopsy in undifferentiated SpA and in AS (Mielants *et al.* 1990*a*).

Genetics and HLA

HLA-B27 has been found in 40–60% of the patients with undifferentiated SpA. Within this population, B27 is not associated either positively or negatively with gut inflammation, since it was found in the same frequency in patients presenting a normal histology on gut biopsy as in those with acute and chronic inflammatory gut lesions (Mielants *et al.* 1993*a*). The presence of another HLA-antigen, HLA-B62, was found to be significantly elevated in patients with undifferentiated SpA (26%) compared with healthy blood donors (10%) (Mielants *et al.* 1987*b*). HLA-B62 was found to be significantly more prevalent in SpA patients presenting with chronic gut lesions (23%) compared with SpA patients with a normal gut histology (16%) or presenting with acute lesions (10%) (Mielants *et al.* 1993*a*).

In a family study, a son and daughter, both carrying HLA-B27 and B62, and both suffering from an undifferentiated SpA evolving to AS, were observed. Both had spondylarthropathy-related chronic lesions on ileocolonoscopy. Their father, who had no signs of musculoskeletal inflammation, carried HLA-B62 and was found to have chronic gut lesions on ileocolonoscopy, whereas the son, who also carried HLA-B62, had clinical Crohn's disease (Mielants *et al.* 1986*b*).

In a prospective study on the evolution of non-AS SpA (Mielants *et al.* 1995*a, b*), 71 patients with ReA or undifferentiated SpA, in whom IBD was initially excluded, were reviewed 2–9 years after a first ileocolonoscopy. Of these, joint disease had remitted in 60%, whereas 13% had persistent undifferentiated SpA. A total of 14 patients (20%) developed AS, 13 of whom had initially shown inflammatory gut lesions. Factors associated with the evolution of undifferentiated SpA to AS included episodes of inflammatory axial pain, elevated serum inflammatory markers, inflammatory gut lesions, and HLA-B27. IBD developed in 4 patients, (5.6%), all of whom also developed AS after presenting initially with gut inflammation. HLA-B27 was only present in one of these patients, while HLA-B62 was found in two.

Ankylosing spondylitis

Relationship between AS and gut inflammation (see Fig. 9.1)

The relationship between AS and IBD has largely been described above.

The majority of authors performing ileocolonoscopy on patients with SpA have found the highest prevalence of inflammatory gut lesions in the group with AS (Table 9.2). Macroscopic lesions are found in about 30–50% of the patients, and histological gut inflammation is described by most authors in more than 40%. The prevalence of gut lesions was higher in patients who had associated peripheral arthritis (67%) than in those presenting only axial involvement (42%) (Mielants *et al.* 1995*b*).

Histologically, AS patients present significantly more 'chronic' inflammatory gut lesions (52%) than 'acute' lesions (10%). The long-term evolution of AS gives a much lower remission rate of gut lesions (19%) than other forms of SpA (Mielants *et al.* 1995*a*). As described above, four patients who presented with AS eventually developed IBD (7.7% of the total AS patients followed). They all had inflammatory lesions at first ileocolonoscopy, but the spondylitis preceded symptomatic gut manifestations. In a recent Finnish study, IBD, mostly CD, developed in an extraordinary 35% of patients with AS (13/37). In this study too, the presence of chronic gut inflammation, especially in the colon, on initial examination was associated with evolution to IBD (Leirisalo-Repo *et al.* 1995). This high prevalence of evolution to IBD in AS patients supports the hypothesis that both disease entities bear common pathogenetic mechanisms and confirms the place of IBD in the concept of SpA, although it is unclear why there was a fivefold difference in the rate of IBD in the two follow-up studies of AS (Mielants 1995*a* vs Leirisalo-Repo *et al.* 1995).

Juvenile chronic arthritis (JCA)

Juvenile chronic arthritis has been defined as an inflammatory disease affecting one or more joints and beginning before the age of 16 years, with a minimum duration of 3 months. The disease is subdivided into three distinct types of disease onset: pauciarticular, polyarticular, and systemic (Ansell 1978). The first subgroup is subdivided into two groups: (1) a form with early onset, mostly affecting young girls before 8 years of age, who frequently carry antinuclear antibodies; and (2) a form with a late onset (over 9 years old), mainly occurring in boys, frequently presenting with tendinitis and sometimes sacroiliitis, accompanied by acute anterior uveitis, and associated with HLA-B27 (Schaller 1984). This subgroup, which also includes patients with juvenile-onset ankylosing spondylitis (JAS), Reiter's disease, ReA, and IBD, is part of the spondylarthropathy concept (Schaller 1984). Some investigators described these children as having the SEA syndrome (seronegativity, enthesopathy, and arthropathy) (Rosenberg and Petty 1982); many of them will later develop AS (Burgos-Vargas and Clark 1989).

Epidemiology

Data on the prevalence of JCA vary widely depending on the method used and the area in which the study is conducted. In studies from referral hospitals, prevalence rates range from 7 to 65/100 000 (Gewanter *et al.* 1983), whereas in population surveys the rates are much higher (56 to 220/100 000) (Gäre *et al.* 1987). By using a combination of both methods, even higher prevalence rates were obtained: 167/100 000 for definite JCA and 301/100 000 for possible JCA (Mielants *et al.* 1993*b*). Most studies agree that the late-onset form of pauciarticular JCA is the most frequently found and accounts for 75% of the JCA population (Kunnamo *et al.* 1983; Towner *et al.* 1983). Burgos-Vargas (1991) estimated the prevalence of this subgroup between 33 and 65/100 000.

The disease, mainly affecting males (3:1), predominantly manifests itself between the ages of 9 and 15 years, but there is no decrease in the frequency of onset at the end of the juvenile age. This suggests that the initial part of the frequency-distribution curve of SpA in adults, according to age of onset, overlaps with late-onset pauciarticular JCA cases, that is to say the two disorders are the same.

The bowel in late-onset pauciarticular JCA (see Fig. 9.1)

Mielants and co-workers have described two studies of ileocolonoscopy in late-onset pauciarticular JCA (Mielants *et al.* 1987*c*; 1993*c*). In the first, ileocolonoscopy was performed in a group of 32 adult SpA patients in whom the disease started before the age of 16 years as a form of late-onset pauciarticular JCA (Mielants *et al.* 1987*c*). Of these patients 80% had histological evidence of gut inflammation. The prevalence of gut inflammation was the same in patients who ultimately developed AS and in patients with only persistent peripheral arthritis and/or enthesopathy. All but one patient with AS had chronic gut lesions, while acute lesions were more frequent in patients with persistent peripheral arthritis. Out of the 32 patients, 2 developed IBD.

In the second study, ileocolonoscopy was performed in 12 juvenile patients with late-onset pauciarticular JCA who were then followed for 3–9 years (Mielants *et al.* 1993*c*). Histological signs of inflammation were found initially in 9 out of 12 patients, 4 of the acute type, 5 of the chronic type. At follow-up, four patients were in clinical remission, including the three patients with an initially normal gut histology. In all, five patients had developed AS, one with an associated CD, all of them initially showing chronic gut inflammation. The persistence of chronic gut inflammation was implicated in the pathogenesis of the disease and in the perpetuation of the musculoskeletal inflammation (Mielants *et al.* 1993*c*).

Genetics and HLA

As in other forms of SpA, late-onset pauciarticular JCA is strongly related to HLA-B27 (60–80%); this association is more pronounced if sacroiliitis, spondylitis, and uveitis are present or eventually develop. Furthermore, Burgos-Vargas (1991) found AS and sacroiliitis in 14 and 25%, respectively, of HLA-B27 first-degree relatives of probands with juvenile AS. HLA-B27, however, was not especially associated with subclinical bowel inflammation, since this antigen was present in the same frequency in patients with normal histology on gut biopsy as in those with acute or chronic inflammatory gut lesions (Mielants *et al.* 1987*c*). On the other hand, in this study HLA-B62 was absent in all patients with a normal histology or in those with acute gut lesions, but a striking 42% of JCA patients with chronic gut lesions carried this antigen. The five JCA patients who developed AS were B27 positive; one patient who developed both AS and CD carried both antigens, B62 and B27 (Mielants *et al.* 1993*c*).

Psoriatic arthritis (PsA)

Psoriatic arthritis was recognized as an articular disease distinct from RA in the middle of this century (Baker *et al.* 1963). Psoriatic arthritis was defined as the presence of arthritis in a patient with psoriasis in the absence of rheumatoid factor (Moll and Wright 1973). These authors proposed a classification of five subgroups:

(1) arthritis of the distal interphalangeal (DIP) joints;

(2) arthritis mutilans;

(3) polyarthritis with involvement of five or more joints;

(4) oligoarthritis with involvement of fewer than five joints;

(5) ankylosing spondylitis.

A recent classification was proposed in which only four clinical subgroups were recognized, the DIP subgroup no longer being considered a distinct clinical entity, since DIP-joint involvement is encountered in all subgroups and does not occur without characteristics of the other subgroups (Torre Alonso *et al.* 1991). The oligoarticular subgroup, occurring in 54–70% of the total group of PsA, presents features comparable to the other SpA patients: besides oligoarticular joint involvement, enthesitis may be found in up to 70% of cases and sacroiliitis in up to 40% (Schatteman *et al.* 1995). The associations between uveitis and HLA-B27 are discussed elsewhere.

The bowel in psoriatic arthritis (see Fig. 9.1)

Only one study reported ileocolonoscopic findings in psoriatic arthritis (Schatteman *et al.* 1995) (Table 9.2). None of the 26 PsA patients with polyarthritis showed lesions. In contrast, in the oligoarticular and in the axial subgroups, macroscopic lesions were found in 13 and 22%, and microscopic lesions in 20 and 30% of the cases, respectively. Chronic lesions were more frequently seen in the axial subgroup. The prevalence of these lesions is significantly higher than in the control groups, but significantly lower than in undifferentiated SpA or in AS. This suggests that the gut plays a role in the pathogenesis of musculoskeletal inflammation in the subgroups of PsA belonging to the SpA concept, but that other portals of entry for causative agents, for instance the skin and the nails, must be taken into consideration (Schatteman *et al.* 1995).

Acute anterior uveitis (AAU)

Acute anterior uveitis is a prominent manifestation of all forms of SpA; it is the most frequent extra-articular inflammatory site in AS (Linssen *et al.* 1991), ReA (Keat 1983), undifferentiated SpA (Keat 1983), PsA (Torre Alonso *et al.* 1991), late-onset pauciarticular JCA (Rosenberg 1987), and IBD (Mousen *et al.* 1990; Salmon *et al.* 1991; Strauss 1988) (see Chapter 10). The type of uveitis associated with the SpA is highly characteristic in its clinical manifestations: it is acute in onset, anterior, unilateral, transient, but recurrences are common (Rosenbaum 1989*a*). This recurrent unilateral AAU can also occur as an isolated disease without joint involvement, but with a strong association with HLA-B27 (50%) (Brewerton *et al.* 1973*b*).

The bowel in acute anterior uveitis (see Fig. 9.1)

The relationship between AAU and IBD is described in the section on extraintestinal manifestations of IBD, above. Although asymptomatic uveitis is frequent in IBD (Strauss 1988) and patients with both IBD and arthritis have a greater incidence of eye inflammation (Salmon *et al.* 1991), the uveitis does not parallel bowel activity.

Ileocolonoscopic studies have revealed the presence of gut inflammation in B27-positive AAU patients without any joint or gut symptoms (Bañares *et al.* 1995; Mielants *et al.* 1990*d*). Bañares *et al.* (1995) found histological signs of gut inflammation in 18 out of 27 patients with AAU (66%). IBD was found in three patients. The highest incidence of lesions was found in patients with uveitis and AS or sacroiliitis. Gut lesions were more prevalent in patients with frequently recurrent AAU, suggesting that bowel inflammation may trigger flares of AAU. On the other hand, a significantly higher incidence of gut lesions was found in B27-negative patients. This confirms the finding that HLA-B27 is not related to the gut inflammation (Mielants *et al.* 1991*a*), and that B27-negative SpA patients have a greater risk of developing IBD (Mielants *et al.* 1995*b*).

Risk factors for SpA patients to develop IBD

When different parameters at first investigation were compared between SpA and AS patients evolving or not to IBD, it was found that risk factors for IBD could be determined (Mielants *et al.* 1995*b*). Patients experiencing regular episodes of diarrhoea early in the disease, patients presenting persistently raised, inflammatory serum parameters, and patients demonstrating chronic inflammatory gut lesions are at highest risk of developing IBD. Another risk factor is HLA-B27 negativity in the presence of sacroiliitis and in AS. This confirms the hypothesis that B27-negative AS patients are at greater risk of developing IBD (Mielants *et al.* 1991*a*; 1995*b*). Spondylarthropathy may develop in B27-negative patients who carry genes associated with IBD, without showing clinical signs of IBD (Khan *et al.* 1980). It appears that HLA-B27 and gut inflammation are independent risk factors, but nevertheless show a complex set of interactions.

Repeat ileocolonoscopic studies demonstrated the strong relationship between joint and gut disease. This close relationship was confirmed in the animal model of the HLA-B27 transgenic rats (Hammer *et al.* 1990*b*) in which gut inflammation is mostly associated with joint inflammation, whereas in germfree conditions (Taurog *et al.* 1994) both forms of inflammation remain absent.

Therapeutic consequences

The demonstration of subclinical gut inflammation in SpA has had therapeutic consequences. Sulphasalazine is an effective drug in the treatment of UC, demonstrated both in the treatment of active disease (Dick *et al.* 1964) and in the prevention of relapses (Dissanayake and Truelove 1973). The efficacy of sulphasalazine in CD is more debatable, demonstrated in some double-blind controlled trials (Summers *et al.* 1979; Van Hees *et al.* 1981), but not confirmed in others (Malchow *et al.* 1984). The efficacy of sulphasazaline in preventing recurrences of CD is even more controversial (Wenckert *et al.* 1978).

Sulphasalazine is split in the colon into two components: a sulphonamide component which has been shown to be the active component in the treatment of the arthritis in RA (Pullar *et al.* 1985), and a 5-ASA (5-acetylsalicyclic acid) component which is the active moiety in the treatment of colonic inflammation in IBD (Azad Khan *et al.* 1977). Since arthritis is a major manifestation in SpA and since the gut evidently plays a crucial role in this disease, it seemed logical to use this drug in treating patients with the various SpA.

Sulphasalazine has been found to be effective in placebo-controlled double-blind studies in patients with AS, mainly for peripheral arthritis but in some studies also for axial disease

Table 9.3 Intake of sulphasalazine (SASP) in different gut histological subgroups in relation to the clinical evolution of the locomotor disease in spondylarthropathies

	n		n	SASP intake	SASP withdrawn for clinical remission > 2 years
Normal histology	39	Active disease	21	9 (43%)	
		Remission	18	12 (67%)	1 (5%)
Acute lesions	27	Active disease	15	10 (67%)	
		Remission	12	11 (92%)	10 (47%)
Chronic lesions	54	Active disease	31	24 (77%)	
		Remission	23	23 (100%)	13 (28%)

(Dougados *et al.* 1986; Feltelius and Hällgren 1986; Kirwan *et al.* 1993; Nissilä *et al.* 1988). Efficacy has also been found in other forms of SpA, including ReA (Trnavsky *et al.* 1990; Mielants *et al.* 1990*c*), PsA (Fraser *et al.* 1993), late-onset pauciarticular JCA (Gedalia *et al.* 1993; Joos *et al.* 1991) and AAU (Dougados *et al.* 1991*b*). Recently, a large double-blind multicentre study in AS, ReA, and PsA confirmed the overall beneficial effect of the drug, with improvement in both clinical and laboratory markers (Dougados *et al.* 1995*a*). The most pronounced effects were seen in patients with PsA. The prevalence of side-effects was relatively low: 10% of the patients dropped out and another 10% of patients experienced dose-dependent and/or transient side-effects. A second large double-blind multicenter study confirmed the beneficial effect of sulphasalazine in PsA and to a lesser extent in ReA in AS (Clegg *et al.* 1996*a,b,c*).

As noted above, the question remains whether sulphasalazine truly has beneficial effects on axial disease. Although the first trials (Dougados *et al.* 1986; Nissilä *et al.* 1988) and a meta-analysis of the available randomized, double-blind, placebo-controlled studies (Ferraz *et al.* 1990) showed benefit for both axial and peripheral joint inflammation, some authors (Kirwan *et al.* 1993) and the large multicentre study (Dougados *et al.* 1995*a*) described a more pronounced effect on the peripheral arthritis. This was confirmed in the recent studies of Clegg *et al.* 1996*a,b,c*), in which it was concluded that the efficacy of sulphasalazine in SpA is related to its effect on inflammatory peripheral arthritis.

In a recent follow-up study, 123 patients with SpA who underwent an ileocolonoscopy were regularly monitored and then re-evaluated clinically 2–9 years later (Mielants *et al.* 1996). In 49 patients a second ileocolonoscopy was performed. These patients were treated with NSAIDs, and if they still had active joint or axial disease after 3 months of treatment, enteric-coated sulphasalazine at a dosage of 2–3g/day was added and given continuously, being stopped only if there were major side-effects or if a sustained clinical remission was achieved after at least 2 years of administration.

Withdrawal of sulphasalazine for clinical remission was observed significantly more often in non-AS SpA patients (38%) than in AS patients (14%), further supporting the idea that sulphasalazine has a more pronounced effect on peripheral than on axial arthropathy.

In total, 89 of 120 SpA patients were treated with sulphasalazine. Of these 89 patients, 46 (52%) were in clinical remission upon re-evaluation. The remission rate in patients not treated with this drug (22.5%) was significantly lower. This provides further evidence of its efficacy in SpA and suggests that sulphasalazine can induce clinical remission in SpA. Moreover, sulphasalazine was withdrawn for a clinical remission of more than 2 years in only 1 of the 21 patients (5%) with a normal gut histology, vs. 23 of 68 (34%) in patients with inflammatory gut lesions on initial biopsy, a significant difference. Overall, in the group of patients with normal gut histology, 67% of those who went into clinical remission took sulphasalazine, whereas all except one with inflammatory gut lesions who went into remission were on this drug ($p < 0.01$). These findings indicate that sulphasalazine treatment could be more effective in SpA patients with gut inflammation than in those with a normal gut histology.

In the 49 patients who underwent a second ileocolonoscopy, a statistically significant correlation was found between treatment with sulphasalazine and resolution of inflammatory gut lesions. All 20 patients in whom these lesions resolved had taken sulfasalazine, compared with 8 out is with persistently normal histology and 5 out of 14 with persistent inflammatory gut lesions. One potential explanation for these findings is the possibility that the beneficial effect of this drug in SpA is due to its anti-inflammatory effect on gut inflammation. Consistent with this idea are recent case reports (Thomson *et al.* 1994*b*; Zwillich and Ritchlin 1991) in which treatment with 5-ASA components induced remission in SpA patients, together with a disappearance of inflammatory gut lesions. As noted above, the 5-ASA component is thought to play the major role in the treatment of the colonic inflammation in IBD (Azad Kanhan *et al.* 1977).

However, in contrast, another recent study suggested that the sulphapyridine component is the active moiety for AS, as for RA, although there was a trend toward a better outcome for the whole molecule (Taggart *et al.* 1996).

Moreover, sulphasalazine does not seem to prevent the emergence of IBD in patients with SpA (Mielants *et al.* 1996), although there are no data for the outcomes of treated and untreated SpA patients.

Role of non-steroidal anti-inflammatory drugs on the gut

Non-steroidal anti-inflammatory drugs (NSAIDs) are the agents of first choice in the treatment of most forms of SpA. However, these drugs do have adverse effects on different parts of the bowel.

Gut permeability

Non-steroidal anti-inflammatory drugs substantially increase gut permeability in normal subjects (Bjarnason *et al.* 1987, 1991; Mielants *et al.* 1991*b*) as well as in patients with RA (Bjarnason *et al.* 1984) and AS (Mielants *et al.* 1991*c*; Wendling *et al.* 1990). The increased permeability occurs predominantly in the small bowel (Bjarnason *et al.* 1991). Increased gut permeability has been observed in different forms of SpA, in some cases even when no NSAIDs have been taken before the investigation (Bjarnason *et al.* 1983; Mielants *et al.* 1991*c*; Serrander *et al.* 1986; Wendling *et al.* 1990). Moreover, altered gut permeability has been found in healthy relatives of patients with IBD (Hollander *et al.* 1986) or AS (Martinez-Gonzales *et al.* 1994). Significantly increased gut permeability has also been found in SpA patients with histological chronic gut inflammation. However, no study has yet investigated whether increased permeability induced by NSAIDs correlates with histological abnormalities. Moreover, one study of the stomach found no correlation between endoscopic appearances and permeability changes (Aabaikken *et al.* 1989).

Side-effects of NSAIDs on the bowel

Some NSAIDs may cause colitis. Histologically, this inflammation is mild and non-specific (Bjarnason *et al.* 1993). In the large intestine, NSAIDs may also provoke relapse of quiescent IBD (Kaufman and Taubin 1987), especially in UC, and those prone to relapse do so within a few days of receiving these drugs (Rampton *et al.* 1993; Riley *et al.* 1990). Nevertheless, most relapses in IBD patients are not caused by NSAIDs.

Perforation and bleeding of the small intestine attributable to NSAIDs have been described (Langman *et al.* 1985), and these agents can also induce subclinical intestinal abnormalities manifested by an increased intestinal loss of protein and blood (Bjarnason *et al.* 1993). Even bowel ulcerations have been described (Morris *et al.* 1991), and cases of intestinal strictures have been associated with the prolonged use of NSAIDs (Allison *et al.* 1992). NSAID-induced intestinal blood loss can be reduced by sulphasalazine treatment (Hayllar *et al.* 1994).

Gut inflammation in SpA and NSAIDs

Since most patients with SpA take NSAIDs at some point in the course of their disease, the possibility needs to be considered that the gut inflammation found in these patients may be largely attributable to their intake of NSAIDs. However, this appears not to be the case. Virtually all ileocolonoscopic studies (Altomonte *et al.* 1994; Leirisalo-Repo *et al.* 1994*b*; Mielants *et al.* 1988, 1995*c*, 1996; Simenon *et al.* 1990) in spondylarthropathic patients have demonstrated an absence of association between the inflammatory gut lesions found in these diseases and the use of NSAIDs. The proportion of SpA patients taking NSAIDs was comparable among those with normal gut histology and those with inflammatory gut lesions. Moreover, these lesions were found in a number of SpA patients who had never taken NSAIDs before the ileocolonoscopy.

NSAID-induced enteropathy is localized to the proximal-and mid-small intestine and is almost never evident in the terminal ileum (Bjarnason and Peters 1996), whereas the inflammatory gut lesions in SpA are found in the terminal ileum, ileocaecal valve, and colon. No histological evidence of subclinical gut inflammation localized in the terminal ileum and ileocaecal region caused by NSAIDs has been demonstrated.

Other enteropathic arthritides

Whipple's disease

Whipple's disease is a multisystem disorder primarily affecting Caucasian males between 35 and 60 years of age. Male patients outnumber female patients by more than 8:1 (Ludwig *et al.* 1981).

The clinical picture is dominated by steatorrhoea associated with abdominal pain, generalized lymphadenopathy, malaise, serositis, fever, weight loss, arthritis, dermal pigmentary changes, leucocytosis, and thrombocytosis. A variety of ophthalmological and neurological syndromes may occur, including anterior or posterior uveitis, vitritis, ocular palsies, and progressive encephalopathy (Fleming *et al.* 1988; Khan 1982).

The arthritis is a migratory symmetrical polyarthritis involving joints of both the upper and lower extremities. Joint pain without obvious synovitis is common. The arthritis tends not to be deforming and is rarely erosive or cystic. The arthritis frequently occurs in a remittent, intermittent pattern, lasting hours to days, and is rarely chronic. Synovial effusions contain between 4000 and 100 000 cells/mm^3, consisting mainly of polymorphonuclear cells. Joint symptoms may antedate the intestinal complaints by more than 5 years (Khan 1982). Arthritis flares are not related temporally to exacerbations of intestinal symptoms.

The incidence of sacroiliitis and spondylitis in Whipple's disease is controversial, as well as the relationship with HLA-B27. Dobbins *et al.* (1987) reported a prevalence of 28% (13/47) of B27 in patients with Whipple's disease, whereas Bai *et al.* (1991) found no increased prevalence (1/14 patients vs. 7/174 controls). Although originally considered one of the SpA (Moll and Wright 1973), in recent years most authorities have concluded that Whipple's is not related to these disorders, particularly since it has now been clearly established to be an infectious disease.

In Whipple's disease, characteristic periodic acid Schiff (PAS) staining deposits are found in the macrophages of the small intestine and in the mesenteric lymph nodes. These deposits contain rodshaped bacilli best seen by electron microscopy (Hawkins *et al.* 1976). These bacilliform bodies were long considered to be the aetiological agent, because they disappear when patients are successfully treated with antibiotics, despite a uniform lack of success in culturing the agent *in vitro* (Dobbins and Kawanishi 1981). Some synovial morphological studies suggest that the joint can also be directly invaded by this organism, and thus the arthritis of Whipple's disease may be infectious. Recently, a unique 1321-base bacterial 16S rRNA sequence was amplified from duodenal tissue of five patients with Whipple's disease, but not from duodenal tissue of ten patients without the disorder (Relman *et al.* 1992). Phylogenetic analysis showed the bacterium to be a Gram-positive actinomycete, which was designated *Tropheryma whipplii*. The polymerase chain reaction for this sequence now provides a specific test for the disease.

A correct diagnosis is important, since the condition responds very well to appropriate antibiotic therapy, usually tetracycline 1 g/day, which has to be continued for more than 1 year. However, functional abnormalities of the macrophages may persist after successful treatment, indicating a possible immunogenetic predisposition of the affected individual.

Coeliac disease

Coeliac disease is an illness caused by abnormalities in the small intestine that result from immunological sensitivity to dietary gluten. It is characterized by mucosal abnormalities of the small intestine, primarily villous flattening and atrophy, which result in malabsorption of nutrients by the involved section of the small intestine. Prompt clinical improvement follows dietary manipulation, specifically the avoidance of certain cereal grains in the diet.

Gastrointestinal symptoms

The most prominent gastrointestinal symptoms of coeliac disease result from the altered intestinal mucosal surface and malabsorption. Diarrhoea, weight loss, flatulence, and weakness are the dominant symptoms. The amount of diarrhoea is dependent upon the amount of mucosal surface altered.

Rheumatological symptoms

Arthritis has been reported in some patients with coeliac disease. It is described as a polyarticular symmetrical arthritis involving large joints, for example the hips, knees, and shoulders (Bourne *et al.* 1985; Chakravarty and Scott 1992; Pinals 1986). An increased frequency of HLA-B8, -DR3 has been described in these patients, but this haplotype is highly associated with coeliac disease itself. Some authors (Bourne *et al.* 1985; Chakravarty and Scott 1992) have observed a striking decrease in synovitis in those coeliac-disease patients prescribed a gluten-free diet, although rechallenge with gluten did not provoke a relapse of arthritis. No data are available on the synovial fluid or synovium of patients with arthritis associated with coeliac disease, and the pathogenesis of the joint disease is unknown.

Treatment

The prompt removal of dietary gluten, presumably after the diagnosis has been established by small-intestinal biopsy, nearly always results in significant improvement. So-called refractory cases typically improve with oral corticosteroids.

Intestinal bypass arthritis

Intestinal bypass surgery (jejunocolostomy or jejunoileostomy), most commonly performed as a treatment for morbid obesity, may give rise to an arthritis–dermatitis syndrome, sometimes associated with renal, hepatic, and haematological disorders. Polyarthritis has been reported in 20–80% of cases. Symptoms appear 2–30 months following surgery (Clegg *et al.* 1985; Wands *et al.* 1976). The arthritis is polyarticular, symmetrical, and migratory, affecting both the upper and lower limb joints. Chronic involvement occurs in up to 25% of the patients. The duration of the arthritis is unpredictable, and there is no relationship between the joint symptoms and abnormal bowel movements. Radiographic deformities or erosions are not seen. Sacroiliac or spinal involvement, although uncommon, has been described. In 66–80% of the patients, a variety of dermatological abnormalities are present. Erythema nodosum, macules progressing to papules and vesiculopustules, urticaria, and nodular dermatitis have been reported. Other associated features are Raynaud's phenomenon, paresthesia, pericarditis, pleuritis, glomerulonephritis, retinal vasculitis, and superficial thrombophlebitis.

The pathogenesis involves bacterial overgrowth and mucosal alterations in the blind loop. The disease seems to be immune-mediated: cryoprecipitates and other circulating complexes containing immunoglobulins, complement, antibodies to bacteria, and bacterial antigens are found in the serum (Clegg *et al.* 1985; Utsinger 1980). Bacterial overgrowth in the blind loop could be responsible for a substantial increase of antigenic stimulation.

Acute symmetrical polyarthritis involving the peripheral and axial skeleton has also been described 1–2 years after a restorative proctocolectomy with an ileal pouch-anastomosis for ulcerative colitis (Axon *et al.* 1993; Lohmuller *et al.* 1990). In these cases, bacterial overgrowth with increased absorption of bacteria leading to dissemination of immune complexes was considered pathogenic.

Non-steroidal anti-inflammatory drugs are usually sufficient to control the arthritis. Oral antibiotics such as tetracycline, clindamycin, or metronidazole, given intermittently or continuously, can reduce the symptoms through a reduction of bacterial overgrowth. However, only surgical reanastomosis of the bypassed segment of the intestine gives complete resolution of all symptoms and may be necessary in refractory cases.

10 The eye in spondyloarthritis

James T. Rosenbaum

Many internists tend to be intimidated by having to evaluate eye disease and, conversely, many ophthalmologists are daunted by the differential diagnosis of systemic illness. Consequently, a knowledge of the ocular manifestations of reactive arthritis and ankylosing spondylitis requires either an exceptional rheumatologist or an exceptional ophthalmologist. The eye is commonly involved in spondyloarthropathy and is vital with regard to both theoretical and therapeutic considerations. This chapter reviews the clinical manifestations of this eye disease, its treatment, and its possible aetiology.

Clinical manifestations

In general terms, inflammation can affect any portion of the eye or surrounding orbital tissue. Conjunctivitis, episcleritis, scleritis, keratitis, anterior uveitis, posterior uveitis, orbital myositis, and optic neuritis will have different clinical characteristics and different systemic disease associations.

During the course of either ankylosing spondylitis or Reiter's syndrome, 20–40% of patients will develop anterior uveitis (see Table 10.1), a term which is synonymous with iritis. The largest series surveyed 1331 patients with AS; 40% had a history of iritis which was usually recurrent (Edmunds *et al.* 1991*b*).

The vast majority of patients with spondyloarthritis who develop iritis are HLA-B27 positive. In many series of patients with uveitis, it is the most frequently identified systemic disease. For example, in one North American study in a uveitis clinic, spondyloarthropathy accounted for approximately 13% of all patients (Rosenbaum 1989*b*). In a Swiss study,

Table 10.1 Representative studies on the likelihood of iritis in association with spondyloarthritis[a]

Author	Disease	With iritis (%)
Birkbeck *et al.* 1951	Ankylosing spondylitis	9
Edmunds *et al.* 1991*b*	Ankylosing spondylitis	40
Feltkamp 1985	Ankylosing spondylitis	29
Haarr 1960	Ankylosing spondylitis	33
Romanus 1953	Ankylosing spondylitis	28
Wilkinson and Bywaters 1958	Ankylosing spondylitis	25
Ansell 1980	Juvenile ankylosing spondylitis	27
Hancock 1960	Reiter's syndrome	37

[a] Modified from Rosenbaum 1992.

Table 10.2 Frequency of Reiter's syndrome, ankylosing spondylitis, or B27-associated iritis among patients with uveitis[a]

Location of patient population	B27-associated	Ankylosing spondylitis	Reiter's syndrome
Oregon (Rosenbaum 1989*a*)	1.7	5.5	7.2
Iowa (Perkins and Folk 1984)	ND	5.8	5.2
Southern California (Henderley *et al.* 1987)	3	1.5	1
England (Perkins and Folk 1984)	ND	10.5	17.2
Holland (Rothova *et al.* 1992)	12.1	5.5[d]	ND
Israel[b] (Weiner and BenEzra 1991)	3	3.3	1
Turkey (Soylu *et al.* 1993)	0.6	1.9	0
China (Chung *et al.* 1988)	10.8[c]	22.1	4.2

ND, not determined; data expressed as the per cent of patients relative to the total series.
[a] Modified from Rosenbaum (Pepose *et al.* 1996).
[b] Includes only patients with chronic uveitis.
[c] Includes patients with psoriatic arthropathy.
[d] Reiter's syndrome and ankylosing spondylitis are classified together as seronegative spondyloarthropathy.

HLA-B27 accounted for 15.4% of all patients with uveitis (Tran *et al.* 1994). A Dutch uveitis study found that 17% of patients had B27-associated disease; 6% of the patients in this series were found to have spondyloarthropathy (Rothova *et al.* 1992). In a Yugoslavian study, 50% of the uveitis patients who were HLA typed were HLA-B27 positive (Karaman-Kraljevic *et al.* 1990). Additional studies that indicate the worldwide association of HLA-B27 with uveitis are shown in Table 10.2.

Many of these surveys are biased by originating from university clinics that tend to provide tertiary care to patients with more severe or atypical disease. Most of these studies use uveitis as the denominator rather than anterior uveitis or iritis. Most referral centres encounter a disproportionate percentage of patients with posterior uveitis because this is more difficult to treat than anterior uveitis. Spondyloarthropathy, of course, is rarely associated with posterior uveitis. A recent community-based study in Los Angeles found that 17% of patients with anterior uveitis were either HLA-B27 positive or had B27-associated joint disease (McCannel *et al.* 1996). In an additional 41.5% of patients with a sudden onset of anterior uveitis, as evaluated in ophthalmological practices, HLA-B27 status was not determined. If one assumes that half of these patients are HLA-B27 positive (see below), about 40% of all patients with uveitis in a community study will have B27-related disease. In a recent large series from a university-based uveitis clinic in Spain (Bañares *et al.* 1997), in which the patterns of uveitis were classified, of 247 patients with anterior uveitis, of those whose disease was acute, recurrent, and unilateral 60% had either a spondyloarthropathy (48%) and/or HLA-B27 (12%). The corresponding percentage for those with acute nonrecurrent unilateral anterior uveitis was 39%, for acute bilateral disease 9%, and for chronic disease 5%. Of 181 patients with posterior uveitis or panuveitis, only 2% had a spondyloarthropathy.

Iritis, like arthritis, has many different aetiologies (Rosenbaum 1991). Iritis is a common manifestation of the pauciarticular, antinuclear antibody (ANA)-positive, female subset of juvenile rheumatoid arthritis. It may be seen in Behçet's disease, sarcoidosis, relapsing polychondritis, Kawasaki's disease, or inflammatory bowel disease.

HLA-B27-associated iritis can usually be distinguished clinically from these other subsets of iritis because it has a characteristic course (Rosenbaum 1989*a*; Rosenbaum 1992; Rothova *et al.* 1987; Santin *et al.* 1990; Tay-Kearney *et al.* 1996). It usually begins with a prodromal period lasting from 12 to 48 hours, during which one eye will feel irritated or uncomfortable. The full-blown iritis is typified by unilateral pain and redness. Vessels around the limbus (the junction between the cornea and sclera) are especially prominent, in contrast to the diffuse redness of conjunctivitis or the sectorial redness that often characterizes scleritis. The diagnosis of iritis is established by a slit-lamp examination which can document that leuckocytes are present in the anterior chamber of the eye and that the blood–aqueous barrier is disrupted. In some patients with iritis in association with spondyloarthritis, white cells are also seen just posterior to the lens, indicating that the ciliary body is also inflamed. This is termed an iridocyclitis. Inflammation throughout the vitreous humour, that is to say a posterior uveitis, occurs in a minority of patients (Rodriguez *et al.* 1996). The presence of a retinal vasculitis, a chorioretinitis, or simultaneous onset in both eyes should raise concern that the uveitis is not a manifestation of spondyloarthropathy. B27-associated iritis has a sudden onset and is unilateral, but it tends to recur and may recur in the contralateral eye. In one uveitis clinic series, for example, 66% of all episodes of iritis had a sudden onset, but 100% of episodes of iritis in association with spondyloarthritis had a sudden onset (Rosenbaum 1989*a*). In the same report, 66% of patients with iritis had unilateral disease, but 96% of patients with spondyloarthropathy had iritis with the first attack in a single eye. The iritis generally resolves completely between attacks. Typical episodes last no more than 2 months. The inflammation is often intense. For example, hypopyon describes the presence of pus in the anterior chamber of the eye. Hypopyon in the absence of infection in patients from North America is usually associated with HLA-B27 (D'Alessandro *et al.* 1991). Fibrin can be observed using a slit lamp, and a fibrinous or plastic iritis usually indicates the presence of HLA-B27 (Feltkamp 1985). A frequent concomitant of anterior uveitis is the deposition of clumps of leucocytes against the corneal endothelium. These cell clusters are known as keratic precipitates. When the clumps are large, the patient is likely to have a granulomatous disease such as sarcoidosis. In B27-associated iritis, the keratic precipitates are consistently of a small enough size to be appropriately labelled non-granulomatous.

The complications of iritis include band keratopathy (the deposition of calcium in the corneal endothelium), cataract, glaucoma, posterior synechiae (the adherence of the iris to the surface of the lens), and cystoid macular oedema. Synechiae and macular oedema are common components of B27-associated eye inflammation, whereas cataract, glaucoma, and band keratopathy are rare (Feltkamp 1985; Rosenbaum 1989*a*). Occasionally, the synechiae extend for 360 degrees. This impedes the flow of aqueous humour and causes a dramatic rise in intraocular pressure. This phenomenon, known as an iris bombe, is a medical emergency. The degree of lost visual acuity with B27-associated iritis usually correlates with the extent of cystoid macular oedema. Visual acuity is usually normal between attacks. Chronic, posterior inflammation or scarring that leads to permanent visual loss can occur, but this is the exception rather than the rule. Seasonal factors have been implicated in some but not all studies (Edmunds *et al.* 1991*b*). Some patients ascribe the onset of iritis to non-penetrating ocular trauma (Rosenbaum *et al.* 1991). Pregnancy might be a risk factor for female patients who are HLA-B27 positive (Rosenbaum 1989*a*). The characteristics of the uveitis associated with HLA-B27 are summarized in Table 10.3. The eye disease in association with spondyloarthropathy is obviously very distinct from the iritis of the pauciarticular, juvenile rheumatoid arthritis subset, which is characterized by an insidious onset, is bilateral, and of chronic

Table 10.3 Typical features of B27-associated uveitis

Most frequent findings
Anterior
Sudden onset
Unilateral
Recurrent, with many recurrences affecting the opposite eye from that initially affected
Non-granulomatous
Additional clues to diagnosis
Usually male
Often with associated enthesopathy
Intraocular pressure reduced relative to unaffected eye
Posterior synechiae
Rare findings which suggest B27-associated disease
Hypopyon
Iris bombe
Fibrin in the anterior chamber

Table 10.4 Representative studies on the likelihood of rheumatic disease with iritis[a]

Author	Conclusion
Beckingsale *et al.* 1984	60% of patients with B27-associated iritis had significant back pain
Feltkamp 1985	80% of patients with B27-associated acute anterior uveitis had definite or possible AS
Haarr 1960	34% of patients with acute iritis had AS
Linssen and Meenken 1995	66% of HLA-B27 uveitis patients had rheumatological disease; males were more likely than females to have systemic disease
Lynch *et al.* 1979	37% of B27-associated iritis patients had spondyloarthropathy
Pedersen 1980	33% of patients with acute anterior uveitis had rheumatic disease
Rosenbaum 1989*b*	84% of patients with B27-associated acute anterior uveitis had AS, RS, or incomplete RS
Russell *et al.* 1976	63% of patients with acute anterior uveitis had sacroiliitis
Saari *et al.* 1982	51% of B27-associated acute anterior uveitis had rheumatic disease
Stanworth and Sharp 1956	42% of patients with non-granulomatous anterior uveitis had AS or RS
Tay-Kearney *et al.* 1996	58% of 129 patients with B27-associated uveitis had spondyloarthropathy (colitis or psoriatic arthritis are included)
Vinje *et al.* 1983	35% with acute anterior uveitis had radiographic sacroiliitis
Wakefield *et al.* 1984	56% of B27-associated iritis patients had spondyloarthropathy

[a] Modified from Rosenbaum 1992.

duration. The iritis associated with HLA-B27 is also very different from the bilateral, recurrent disease which typifies Behçet's syndrome. The latter condition often includes a retinal vasculitis, has much more posterior involvement, and generally does not resolve completely between attacks.

Of all patients with anterior uveitis, approximately half are HLA-B27 positive (Brewerton *et al.* 1973*b*). If one restricts the analysis to more particular subsets of anterior uveitis such as recurrent or unilateral, or sudden in onset, the role of HLA-B27 increases (Ehlers *et al.* 1974). About two-thirds of patients with B27-associated iritis are male. The frequency of joint disease among uveitis patients who are HLA-B27 positive has been addressed in several series. These observations are summarized in Table 10.4. The estimates range from 33 to 84%. The eye disease can alert the astute clinician to the diagnosis of B27-related joint disease. The iritis is often the clue that helps to identify the cause of the chronic back pain or recurrent, migratory pauciarticular joint disease (Rosenbaum 1989*a*).

What is the likelihood of developing uveitis if one is HLA-B27 positive? The most comprehensive study found that the risk was 1% (Linssen *et al.* 1991). My own more limited study, which considered residual changes such as keratic precipitates or anterior lens capsule debris as evidence for prior uveitis, suggested that as many as 50% of 'healthy' B27-positive individuals may have had a previous iritis, often without the inflammation being diagnosed. However, this definition of iritis resulted in 2 out of 15 matched controls also demonstrating evidence for prior anterior uveitis. A 30% cumulative incidence has been suggested by another study involving only 20 male subjects (Cohen *et al.* 1976). This study noted iritis in 7% of controls. Other factors in addition to HLA-B27 appear to contribute to the predisposition to iritis. A family study found that first-degree relatives of B27-positive iritis patients who are also HLA-B27 positive are 13-fold more likely to develop iritis, compared with B27-positive individuals without a family history of iritis (Derhaag *et al.* 1988*b*). Several subtypes of HLA-B27 have been shown to be no more associated with iritis risk than HLA-B27 itself (Derhaag *et al.* 1988*a*). A recent Japanese study implicated HLA-DR8 in uveitis in association with ankylosing spondylitis (Islam *et al.* 1995). A Canadian study, using an isotope method to diagnose sacroiliitis, concluded that sacroiliac inflammation was a greater risk factor for iritis than HLA-B27 (Russell *et al.* 1976). Another Canadian study found that peripheral arthritis in a patient with ankylosing spondylitis enhanced the likelihood that iritis would develop (Maksymowych *et al.* 1995*b*). The complement allotype, C4B2, has been linked to iritis susceptibility, especially in males who are HLA-B27 positive (Wakefield *et al.* 1988). Other genetic factors which have been implicated include alpha-1 antitrypsin deficiency (Wakefield *et al.* 1991) and certain immunoglobulin Gm allotypes (Kijlstra *et al.* 1984), although the alpha-antitrypsin association has been disputed (Brewerton *et al.* 1985). More recently allelic differences in genes related to protein-antigen processing have been related to the predisposition to develop acute anterior uveitis. Among patients with B27-positive ankylosing spondylitis, the TAP 1B allele appears to increase the likelihood of developing extraspinal disease (Maksymowych *et al.* 1995*c*), and these investigators (Maksymowych and Russell 1995) have also reported that the LMP2 (low molecular weight polypeptide) arginine variant increases the risk among ankylosing spondylitis patients for developing anterior uveitis by a factor of three.

Other portions of the eye can also be involved in the spondyloarthropathies. Classic Reiter's syndrome is, of course, associated with conjunctivitis (Hancock 1960; Popert *et al.* 1964). This process is generally bilateral. In contrast to sudden-onset iritis, conjunctivitis is not painful, although patients may complain of discomfort, irritation, or itching. Conjunctivitis is usually a self-limiting problem in Reiter's syndrome and is only rarely associated with visual loss. Conjunctivitis must be distinguished from other causes of a red eye such as iritis, and other aetiologies, such as allergy or chemical irritants, must be excluded.

Several case reports document that corneal inflammation or keratitis can be a manifestation of Reiter's syndrome (Mark and McCulley 1982; Rowson and Dart 1992). Scleritis has also been ascribed to spondyloarthropathy (Foster and Sainz de la Maza, 1994; Watson and Hezleman 1976). Scleritis is a painful vasculitis of scleral vessels most commonly seen in patients with rheumatoid arthritis in association with active joint disease, a high titre of rheumatoid factor, and often vasculitis elsewhere. In one university referral centre study that included 172 patients with scleritis, one patient had AS, three had Reiter's syndrome, seven had inflammatory bowel disease, and two patients had psoriatic arthritis (Foster and Sainz de la Maza 1994). Episcleritis is a vascular inflammation of vessels that are more superficial than those in the sclera, and is typically less painful than scleritis. It is also more transient, normally does not have severe visual consequences, and is usually not a manifestation of a systemic illness. In this same series (Foster and Sainz de la Maza 1994), 1% of patients with episcleritis had Reiter's syndrome and none had AS.

Iritis also occurs in the other forms of seronegative spondyloarthropathies. About 7% of patients with psoriatic arthritis experience iritis (Lambert and Wright 1976; Møller *et al.* 1981; Vinje *et al.* 1983), but the likelihood of developing iritis increases to 15% in those with sacroiliitis in addition (Lambert and Wright 1976). The role of HLA-B27 or the hallmarks of the eye inflammation are incompletely characterized in psoriatic arthritis. An estimated 2–9% of patients with inflammatory bowel disease will develop episcleritis, scleritis, or uveitis (Billison *et al.* 1967; Greenstein *et al.* 1976). In our own referral clinic, approximately 80% of patients with eye disease and bowel inflammation have Crohn's colitis (Lyons and Rosenbaum 1995). This may reflect a referral bias, as it is conceivable that the eye involvement with Crohn's disease is more severe or more persistent compared to eye disease associated with ulcerative colitis. In contrast to the uveitis which is seen in association with ankylosing spondylitis or Reiter's syndrome, the uveitis in association with colitis is more likely to be bilateral, to have an insidious onset, to follow a chronic course, to be associated with cataract or glaucoma, and to have a significant posterior component (Lyons and Rosenbaum 1995). Only about 45% of patients with uveitis in association with inflammatory bowel disease are HLA-B27 positive.

Aetiology

The mechanism underlying iritis in association with spondyloarthritis is unknown. The pathogenesis of iritis may resemble the pathogenesis of peripheral arthritis in spondyloarthropathy, but this hypothesis is largely untested.

In addition to the critical genetic factors discussed above, several other immunological changes have been detected in patients with iritis in association with spondyloarthropathy. As is true for both Reiter's syndrome and ankylosing spondylitis, occult bowel pathology has frequently been found to be present (Banares *et al.* 1995). The likelihood of finding occult bowel pathology with biopsy obtained by ileocolonoscopy appears to correlate with a history of iritis rather than with the presence of HLA-B27 (Banares *et al.* 1995). A serological study strongly implicated a recent yersinia infection as a trigger in a subset of patients with anterior uveitis (Wakefield *et al.* 1990). Ankylosing spondylitis patients with iritis tend to have increased IgA antibodies against either *Klebsiella pneumoniae* or *Escherichia coli* lipopolysaccharide compared with patients with AS and no history of iritis (Maki-Ikola *et al.* 1995*a*). Some have proposed that antibodies to klebsiella may cross-react with antigens present in vitreous humour (Kijlstra *et al.* 1984). These investigators also found that klebsiella is more likely to be present in the stool of AS patients who are experiencing a flare of anterior uveitis (Ebringer *et al.* 1979). B27-positive patients with uveitis reportedly demonstrate more lymphoproliferation in response to chlamydia compared with patients with uveitis who are HLA-B27 negative (Wakefield and Penny 1983). Paradoxically, the phagocytic response to *Chlamydia trachomatis* is reduced when B27-positive uveitis patients are compared with uveitis patients who are HLA-B27 negative (Wakefield *et al.* 1985). Immune complexes are occasionally present in the sera of patients with B27-associated uveitis, but apparently complexes are more commonly present in uveitis patients who are HLA-B27 negative (Andrews *et al.* 1979). A T-cell lymphopenia has been detected in patients with ankylosing spondylitis; the lymphopenia is also present in household contacts when the spondyloarthritis patients experience a flare of uveitis (Byron *et al.* 1979).

Animal models may help to clarify the pathogenesis of B27-associated eye disease. Endotoxin-induced uveitis is a widely used model for acute onset anterior uveitis (Rosenbaum *et al.* 1980). In most rat strains, the subcutaneous, intraperitoneal, or intravenous injection of modest doses of Gram-negative bacterial endotoxin will induce a bilateral anterior uveitis. The disease begins within 12–24 hours and usually resolves completely within a few days. Recurrent challenges with endotoxin produce progressively less eye inflammation as the rat rapidly develops pharmacological tolerance (Rosenbaum *et al.* 1980). The dose of endotoxin required to induce eye inflammation leaves other organ systems normal at the light microscopic level. The many possible relationships between HLA-B27 and Gram-negative bacteria, as discussed elsewhere in this volume, suggest that this model is very relevant to human disease. However, the model shows consistent differences from the inflammation seen in patients. First, as noted above, anterior uveitis in B27-positive patients is consistently unilateral. Second, the rat disease appears to be independent of the major histocompatibility complex, although a few strains such as the Buffalo rat are relatively resistant to the ocular effects of endotoxin. Mice also develop a similar uveitis which is strain-dependent (Li *et al.* 1995). The disease in mice is milder than that which develops in rats, but it also appears to be independent of MHC class I antigen allotype. Third, in patients, arthritis and sometimes iritis typically develop 1–4 weeks after a precipitating Gram-negative infection; in contrast, the iritis in rats develops within 12–24 hours of exposure to the endotoxin. Finally, the human disease is typically recurrent, whereas recurrent disease is difficult to establish in rats.

The creation of B27-positive rats and mice which develop spontaneous bowel and joint disease may also facilitate an understanding of the eye disease (Hammer *et al.* 1990*b*; Khare *et al.* 1995*a*). Lewis rats that express a low copy number of the B27 transgene and do not develop spontaneous disease (Hammer *et al.* 1990*b*) are no more predisposed than non-transgenic Lewis rats to the development of endotoxin-induced uveitis (Baggia *et al.* 1997), nor do they seem any more susceptible to a recently observed model of 'reactive' iritis that develops 7–9 days after oral or intravenous challenge with live *Salmonella enteritidis* (Baggia *et al.* 1997).

Retinal S antigen, or arrestin, can be used as an autoantigen to induce an autoimmune uveitis in rodents that has many analogies to the model of experimental autoimmune encephalomyelitis. The S antigen model is primarily a chorioretinitis, so its relevance to HLA-B27 disease is questionable. However, a uveitogenic peptide from S antigen shares sequence homology with a segment of HLA-B27, and the B27-derived amino-acid sequence is uveitogenic if injected into Lewis rats (Wildner and Thurau 1994). Since posterior uveitis is clinically quite distinct from anterior uveitis, the clinical implication of this observation requires additional clarification.

Laboratory testing and therapy

The differential ophthalmic diagnosis of the red eye relies primarily on the findings from the slit-lamp examination. If a diagnosis of iritis is established, an important issue is the role of HLA-B27 typing or sacroiliac joint radiographs. A recent study found that the prognosis for sudden-onset anterior uveitis did not differ between B27-positive and negative patients (Linssen and Meenken 1995). However, 66% of B27-positive patients had spondyloarthritis at the time of eye-disease presentation or after 9 years follow-up. In contrast only 6% of B27-negative patients with iritis had spondyloarthritis. The presence of HLA-B27, of course, does not establish a diagnosis *per se* since it may be unrelated to the disease, but it helps to suggest a diagnostic category and may alert an ophthalmologist to be more vigilant in evaluating rheumatic symptoms.

The author's practice is to obtain sacroiliac-joint imaging primarily for those patients with back pain if the patient's history does not permit a clear distinction between a mechanical versus an inflammatory cause.

The therapy of iritis in association with spondyloarthropathy can be divided into treatment of the acute attacks and prophylactic therapy. Most attacks of iritis can be managed with topical corticosteroids and a mydriatic agent to dilate the pupil. The latter approach reduces pain resulting from spasm of the muscles controlling the iris and helps to prevent synechiae from forming. The intensity of topical steroid usage should be monitored by an ophthalmologist to minimize such complications as cataract and glaucoma. Although topical steroids are not indicated to prevent attacks of iritis, topical steroids should be instituted during the prodrome of the iritis even if a minimal cellular response is present on slit-lamp examination. Several different topical non-steroidal preparations are available for ophthalmic use. Their relative utility in iritis has not been demonstrated.

Very severe episodes of iritis can benefit from a periocular injection of corticosteroid. Occasionally a 10–21-day course of oral prednisone with a rapid tapering of the dosage can also be an adjunct in therapy. The role of oral non-steroidal anti-inflammatory drugs has not been studied, but these may be effective in reducing pain. The author has anecdotal experience that chronic oral non-steroidal intake may reduce the frequency or intensity of attacks of iritis, but this too has not been rigorously tested.

Sulphasalazine is emerging as a potential promising adjunct to therapy. Two well-designed studies have now reported that sulphasalazine may reduce the frequency and duration of recurrent attacks of iritis (Breitbart *et al.* 1993; Dougados *et al.* 1991*b*). The patient and clinician need to weigh the risks and costs of taking a medication continuously against the potential benefit of limiting future attacks that evolve with an unpredictable pattern.

11 Enteric infections and arthritis: bacteriological aspects

Jaakko Uksila, Paavo Toivanen, and Kaisa Granfors

Introduction

Reactive arthritis (ReA) was initially described as a sterile joint inflammation after *Yersinia enterocolitica* enteric infection (Ahvonen *et al.* 1969). Subsequently, enteric infections caused by salmonella, shigella, campylobacter, and *Yersinia pseudotuberculosis* have also been found to be followed by this complication. In other forms of spondylarthropathies such as ankylosing spondylitis (AS) and arthritis or sacroiliitis associated with inflammatory bowel disease, an association with infection has been suggested, but not established.

ReA has provided investigators with an opportunity to focus on the properties of the triggering organisms, and recent studies have indicated that microorganisms are intimately involved not only in the pathogenesis during the intestinal phase of disease, but also in the target organ, the joint. It is anticipated that a continued study of microorganisms and the immune reactions directed against them will reveal how synovial inflammation is initiated, how the immune system maintains the reactivity, and what dictates the final outcome of the disease—either recovery or chronicity.

Triggering pathogens

Several bacteria are known to be associated with the development of arthritis. Among these, the most common triggers of ReA are bacteria causing enteric infections together with

Table 11.1 Bacteria triggering reactive arthritis

HLA-B27 association **Established**	**Not established**
Campylobacter	Borrelia
Chlamydia	Brucella
Salmonella	Clostridium
Shigella	Haemophilus
Yersinia	Hafnia
	Leptospira
	Mycobacterium
	Neisseria
	Staphylococcus
	Streptococcus
	Ureaplasma
	Vibrio

Chlamydia trachomatis, a urogenital pathogen (Toivanen and Toivanen 1994). In addition to these, numerous other bacteria have been implicated in the induction of ReA (Table 11.1). However, the difference between the first group of pathogens and this last one is relatively clear-cut: classical ReA, triggered by yersinia, salmonella, shigella, campylobacter, and chlamydia, is highly associated with HLA-B27 (Aho *et al.* 1975; Calin and Fries 1975*b*; Keat 1983) and these bacteria cause mucosal infections, whereas no association with HLA-B27 has been established for the other organisms and the infections are primarily localized to tissues other than mucosa. Furthermore, the enteric bacteria causing B27-associated arthritis, unlike most of the others, are Gram-negative, invasive, lipopolysaccharide-containing microbes which can adapt themselves to live intracellularly (Granfors 1992).

Host–microbe interactions

Normally, the intestinal mucosa functions as a barrier to prevent bacteria that colonize the gut from invading systemic tissues: entry into host cells is a critical step in the initiation of infection triggering ReA. Invasion and intracellular replication by salmonella, shigella, and yersinia have been widely studied *in vitro*. These bacteria are able to invade non-professional phagocytes and replicate intracellularly. *In vivo*, salmonella and yersinia pass through the intestinal epithelial layer and enter reticuloendothelial compartments of the intestine, such as lamina propria and lymphoid follicles, where they multiply within mononuclear cells. Different stages of host–organism interaction considered to be important in the development of ReA are shown in Table 11.2. These will now be considered in turn.

Adherence and invasion

Microbial adherence to cell surfaces is a prerequisite to invasion. This occurs with the aid of specific cell-surface structures of the microorganism and the host cells. The next step, invasion, may take place with the aid of the same structures involved in adherence, or with the aid of other structures. Invasin, Ail, and YadA proteins are known to be important in the uptake of yersinia into mammalian cells (Pierson 1994). YadA was also found to be important in the yersinia-induced rat arthritis model, since a mutated strain of *Yersinia enterocolitica* O:8 not expressing YadA was found to be less arthritogenic than the wild-type strain

Table 11.2 Stages of host–microbe interaction possibly important in the pathogenesis of reactive arthritis

Entry of bacteria into body
Adherence and invasion/uptake of bacteria into cells
Intracellular survival
Killing of bacteria
Degradation of bacteria
Persistence of bacteria
Transport and deposition of bacterial components into joints
Antigen presentation and recognition

(Gripenberg-Lerche *et al.* 1994). Invasion by salmonella is evidently more complicated. Findings suggesting that expression of HLA-B27 on the host-cell surface modulates the invasion of ReA-triggering microbes into transfected mouse fibroblasts have been reported (Kapasi and Inman 1992; 1994). If this is true, then persistence of ReA-triggering bacteria in B27-positive positive patients could be due to decreased invasion and, consequently, decreased intracellular killing. In this case, yersinia would evade host-killing mechanisms by remaining extracellular. However, in other studies, no such effect of B27 was found on bacterial invasion into the same mouse fibroblasts (Virtala *et al.* 1997) or on bacterial uptake by monocytic cells (Laitio *et al.* 1997).

Intracellular survival and killing

Experiments looking at the intracellular survival, as opposed to uptake, of arthritogenic bacteria have suggested an effect of HLA-B27. In these experiments, fibroblasts and monocytic cells that had been transfected with HLA-B27 showed a prolonged intracellular survival time for salmonella, compared with cells transfected with HLA-A2 (Laitio *et al.* 1997; Virtala *et al.* 1997). This could be explained either by the more rapid replication of salmonella in the B27-positive cells, compared with the control cells, or by less efficient bactericidal mechanisms in B27-positive cells. That the same phenomenon was seen in two different cell types, which preferentially use different bactericidal mechanisms, suggests that HLA-B27 may interfere with several killing mechanisms.

Degradation of bacteria

With regard to ReA triggered by enteric organisms, only degraded bacterial material, not live bacteria, have been detected in peripheral blood and synovial fluid cells and tissue in patients with ReA (Granfors *et al.* 1989*a*, 1990, 1992*a*,*b*). This suggests the possibility that ReA may result from a defect in the degradation of causative bacteria, even if bactericidal activity is not impaired. However, there is no evidence for this so far. When peripheral blood monocytes from healthy people were allowed to ingest killed *Yersinia enterocolitica* O:3 bacteria, no difference in the degradation of bacterial components was seen between B27-positive and B27-negative cells, when followed with immunocytochemical techniques (Wuorela *et al.* 1993).

Persistence of bacterial antigens

The clinical picture of bacterial enteritis is highly variable, ranging from asymptomatic subclinical illness to profound diarrhoea. However, most cases are self-limiting and subside without antibiotic treatment. Stool cultures usually reveal the pathogenic organism during the acute phase of the disease, but only seldom does a patient remain a manifest carrier of an enteric pathogen. The pathogenic bacteria are normally so rapidly cleared from the intestine that by the time joint symptoms develop, usually 1–3 weeks after enteric infection, stool cultures may already be negative and only serum antibody responses against enteric bacteria can reveal the triggering organism. If the infection remains uncomplicated, antibody titres diminish gradually and reach the normal range within a few months (Granfors and Toivanen 1986; Toivanen *et al.* 1987*b*). In ReA, serum antibody levels against the causative agent can remain high even for years, suggesting persistence of occult bacteria somewhere in the body in an immunogenic but non-culturable form. In the best studied example, yersinia-triggered ReA, different isotypes of yersinia-specific antibodies can persist for prolonged periods. Particularly characteristic of yersinia ReA is the persistence of IgA antibodies. This indicates that the bacteria are continuously stimulating mucosal immunity, because the biological half life of serum IgA is only 5–6 days. The persistence of microbe-specific IgA responses has also been found in other reactive arthritides of intestinal origin, including those triggered by *Yersinia pseudotuberculosis* (Ståhlberg *et al.* 1987*c*), *Shigella flexneri* (van Bohemen *et al.* 1986*a*) and Salmonella spp. (Mäki-Ikola, *et al.* 1992). Another piece of evidence favouring persistence is the presence of circulating immune complexes in yersinia-ReA (Lahesmaa-Rantala, *et al.* 1987*b*). More directly, the persistence of bacteria has been shown by immunofluorescence studies in gut mucosal biopsies (Hoogkamp-Korstanje *et al.* 1988). Thus, it is believed that, in spite of negative results in stool cultures, bacteria are still present and are closely associated with the mucosa in those patients who develop ReA. The mechanisms behind bacterial persistence are not known. At present, we have no solid evidence for or against aberrant immunity of ReA-prone individuals. Still, antimicrobial defence mechanisms involved in the elimination of intracellular bacteria must play a critical role and, in this context, the role of HLA-B27 deserves closer attention (Kapasi and Inman 1994; Laitio *et al.* 1997; Virtala *et al.* 1997).

Antibodies to enteric pathogens are produced both during the acute infection and later during the reactive joint disease. Studies on humoral immunity in ReA have shown that antibody responses to enteric pathogens develop against multiple bacterial epitopes. Sera from ReA patients recognize a variety of outer-membrane proteins as well as lipopolysaccharide (Granfors *et al.* 1989*b*; Ståhlberg *et al.* 1987*b*). Some authors have reported antibody specificities that are found to be more prevalent in ReA patients, compared with patients with uncomplicated bacterial enteritis (Grönberg *et al.* 1989; Ståhlberg *et al.* 1987*b*). In general, however, serological studies have revealed no prominent arthritogenic antigen (Ståhlberg *et al.* 1987*a*). Antibodies in the synovial fluid seem to reflect the antibody response in the serum with regard to concentration, specificity, and isotype distribution (Mäki-Ikola *et al.* 1994), suggesting that local synovial antibody production may not be very strong in ReA. Antibody responses against epitopes homologous to HLA-B27 will be discussed under the topic dealing with molecular mimicry.

Transport and deposition of bacterial antigens in to joints

ReA was originally described as a sterile inflammation of the joint following a microbial infection elsewhere in the body (Ahvonen *et al.* 1969). Subsequent studies have not changed this basic concept: bacterial culture of joint tissue and fluid has consistently given negative results in patients with arthritis following enteric infection (Granfors *et al.* 1989*a*; Merilahti-Palo *et al.* 1991). Yersinia immune complexes detected in synovial fluid (Lahesmaa-Rantala 1987*a*) have suggested, however, that bacterial antigens present in the inflamed joint may stimulate local antibody production. This finding, along with persistently elevated antibody titres, prompted a number of studies that have now firmly established the presence of different enteric bacterial antigens in synovial fluid cells and tissues from yersinia-ReA patients (Table 11.3). The same holds true for chlamydia-triggered reactive arthritis (Keat *et al.* 1987; Mascia *et al.* 1992; Taylor-Robinson *et al.* 1992). Monocytic and polymorphonuclear cells in the synovial fluid were shown to contain bacterial lipopolysaccharide (LPS) in both yersinia and

Table 11.3 Enteric bacteria in ReA joint[a]

Detection method[b]				Reference
Bacteria	**Culture**	**Antigen detection**	**DNA detection**	
Salmonella				
	9/9 patients negative	9/9 patients positive (IF or IP)		(Granfors *et al.* 1990)
Shigella				
		1 patient positive (IF)		(Granfors *et al.* 1992)
Yersinia				
		1 patient positive (IF)		(Toivanen *et al.* 1987*a*)
	12/12 patients negative	3/12 patients positive (IC)		(Lahesmaa-Rantala *et al.* 1987*a*)
	3/13 patients negative	12/15 patients positive (IF)		(Granfors *et al.* 1989*a*)
		4/7 patients positive (IF)		(Hammer *et al.* 1990*a*)
	9/9 patients negative	8/10 patients positive (IP)		(Merilahti-Palo *et al.* 1991)
	5/5 patients negative	4/4 patients positive (IF)	5/5 patients negative (PCR)	(Viitanen *et al.* 1991)
	13/13 patients negative	13/13 patients positive (IF or IP)	13/13 patients negative (PCR)	(Nikkari *et al.* 1992)

[a] Adapted from (Nikkari 1994).

[b] IF, immunofluorescence staining; IP, immunoperoxidase staining; IC, immune complex determination; PCR, polymerase chain reaction.

salmonella-triggered ReA. Bacterial heat-shock protein has also been found in peripheral blood cells of yersinia-infected individuals (Granfors *et al.* submitted). On the other hand, attempts to detect bacterial DNA in the inflamed joint have not given positive results in the case of yersinia-ReA (Nikkari *et al* 1992; Viitanen *et al.* 1991), suggesting that live bacteria are not present in the inflamed joints of patients with enteroarthritis. In chlamydia-triggered reactive arthritis, *Chlamydia trachomatis* DNA has been identified in the joint tissue of at least some patients (Hammer *et al.* 1992; Mascia *et al.* 1992; Nanagara *et al* 1995; Rahman *et al* 1992; Taylor-Robinson *et al.* 1992). There is one such report for *Chlamydia pneumoniae* as well (Gérard *et al.* 1995*b*).

Other bacterial components have also been searched for in acute inflammatory arthritis. Analysis for muramic acid, a bacterial cell-wall component, by gas chromatography–mass spectrometry revealed that 4 out of 14 patients with culture-negative arthritis, but with a history of recent bacterial (non-enteric) disease, had traces of muramic acid in the synovial fluid (Lehtonen *et al.* 1994). This suggests that a proportion of undefined acute inflammatory arthritides are of bacterial origin and that similar mechanisms may underly the development of arthritis following both enteric and non-enteric infections.

In conclusion, antigenic structures derived from enteric pathogens are deposited in the joint in ReA. How this deposition occurs is not known in detail. It is evident that cells which are exposed to local infection in the intestine and take part in the process of degradation of intracellular bacteria recirculate, probably for long periods of time. Due to specific adhesion properties that favour the localization of mucosa-derived cells not only to mucosal but also to joint tissues (Salmi *et al.* 1995), these cells may home to the synovium and there start a T-cell mediated inflammatory process. The inflammation might then be expected to enter a chronic phase when autoreactive T lymphocytes come into play.

Role of bacteria in ankylosing spondylitis

Of all enteric bacteria, *Klebsiella pneumoniae* has gained perhaps the strongest attention in studies on AS, although no definite role for this bacteria has been identified after two decades of investigation. Based on early reports of an increased occurrence of klebsiella in stool cultures from patients with active ankylosing spondylitis (AS) (Ebringer *et al.* 1977, 1978), as well as of elevated serum antibody levels (Trull *et al.* 1983, 1984), klebsiella has been suggested to play an aetiopathogenetic role in AS. Further evidence was obtained from studies on immunological cross-reactivity between klebsiella and HLA-B27 (Avakian *et al.* 1980; Welsh *et al.* 1980). However, many negative results on the faecal carriage of klebsiella have also been reported (Eastmond *et al.* 1980; Hunter *et al.* 1981; van Kregten*et al.* 1991; Warren and Brewerton 1980). Serological findings have shown elevated anti-klebsiella antibodies in some studies but not in others (Collado *et al.* 1994; Russell and Suarez-Almazor 1992; Shodjai-Moradi *et al.* 1992). It has also been suggested that some serotypes of klebsiella are more strongly associated with AS than others (Sahly *et al.* 1994*a,b*), suggesting that certain capsular polysaccharides could be involved in triggering the disease.

Not all investigators have found increased bacterial antibodies in AS to be a klebsiella-specific phenomenon. For example, van Bohemen *et al.* (1986*b*) reported increased antibody levels also against other species of Enterobacteriaceae. Similar results were reported by Mäki-Ikola (Mäki-Ikola *et al.* 1995*c*), who observed that AS patients with exclusively axial disease had increased antibody levels not only against klebsiella but to some extent also against

Escherichia coli and proteus. On the other hand, in patients with AS and peripheral arthritis, antibodies were elevated against klebsiella alone, suggesting a parameter of clinical heterogeneity in AS. High IgA antibody levels against klebsiella in patients with inflammatory bowel disease (Cooper *et al.* 1988; O'Mahony *et al.* 1992) indicate that the association between klebsiella and AS may be at the level of intestinal mucosal lesions, thus leaving the aetiological role of klebsiella in AS open. Of interest in this respect are reports of sulphasalazine treatment for AS. Total IgA and secretory IgA and IgM contents of jejunal fluid were reduced to normal by this treatment (Feltelius *et al.* 1994), and the concentrations of serum IgA antibodies against klebsiella, *E. coli* and proteus were decreased (Nissilä *et al.* 1994). These findings further emphasize the role of gut lymphoid tissue and intestinal bacteria in the pathogenesis of AS. It still remains to be seen whether discrepant findings of antibody responses in AS can be explained by technical differences, including the use of different bacterial strains and/or antigen preparations.

Bacteria as triggers of autoreactivity: role of molecular mimicry

Taken as a fact that degradation products of bacteria (for example cell-wall components such as LPS or muramic acid), or bacteria in a more complete but non-culturable form, are present in the inflamed joint, it remains to be explained how the destructive process in the joint is turned on. The association with HLA-B27, although incomplete, has suggested that antigenic determinants shared by arthritis-causing enterobacteria and HLA-B27 might trigger immunological self-reactivity. As noted above, such an association, based on serological cross-reactivity, was first observed between klebsiella and HLA-B27 (Avakian *et al.* 1980; Welsh *et al.* 1980). In recent years, molecular biology has brought us to a new level in the study of antigenic determinants and molecular mimicry.

The search for epitopes shared by MHC molecules and bacteria has revealed a number of enterobacterial proteins with linear and non-linear amino-acid homologies to HLA-B27 (Table 11.4). Klebsiella nitrogenase contains a hexapeptide which is homologous to the α_1-helix of HLA-B* 2705 (Schwimmbeck *et al.* 1987). A plasmid carried by *Shigella flexneri* encodes a potential pentapeptide with homology to the same polymorphic region of HLA-B27. This plasmid has shown close association with arthritogenicity in shigella (Stieglitz *et al.* 1989, 1993), but to date there is scant evidence that the peptide is produced. Two other ReA-associated bacterial species, *Yersinia enterocolitica* and *Salmonella typhimurium* also share amino-acid homology with HLA-B27. YadA of *Y. enterocolitica* is a plasmid-encoded, high molecular weight, outer-membrane protein with virulence properties due to its ability to mediate adhesion (Heesemann and Gruter 1987; Kapperud *et al.* 1987; Skurnik and Wolf-Watz 1989). It has also proven to be arthritogenic in a rat model (Gripenberg-Lerche *et al.* 1994, 1995). OmpH is an outer-membrane protein present in salmonella, *E. coli*, and *Y. enterocolitica (Koski et al.* 1989). A non-linear sequence of five amino acids homologous to HLA-B27 has been observed in OmpH of *S. typhimurium* and *E. coli,* but not in that of *Y. enterocolitica.* In addition, amino-acid sequences shared by a number of other Gram-negative enteric organisms and HLA-B27 have been found (Scofield *et al.* 1993), and it is of interest that some of these peptides are capable of binding to HLA-B27 molecules (Scofield *et al.* 1995).

Table 11.4 Peptide sequences containing linear/non-linear amino-acid homology to HLA-B27

Bacterium	Protein	Sequence[a]	Binding HLA-B27	Reference
Bacillus megaterium	26.2K protein	ARVTARRYL	yes	(Scofield *et al.* 1995)
E. coli	Protein 168	RRYLEWGAT	no	"
	26K protein	VRTLLRRVK	no	"
	FeaD	YRYSDDNGK	no	"
Kl. pneumoniae	Nitrogenase	LRRCVEAFGL	yes	"
	Nitrogenase	QTDRED	nd[b]	(Schwimmbeck *et al.* 1987)
	PulD secretion protein	DRDE	nd	(Fielder *et al.* 1995)
Ps. aeruginosa	Methyltransferase	LRRYLEARR	yes	(Scofield *et al.* 1995)
S. typhimurium	Aminotransferase	LRTLLELTR	yes	"
	OmpH	KAGSDRTKL	nd	(Lahesmaa *et al.* 1991)
Sh. flexneri	2mD plasmid encoded protein[c]	AQTDRHSL	nd	(Stieglitz *et al.* 1989)
Y. enterocolitica	YadA	TDRE	nd	(Lahesmaa *et al.* 1991)

[a] The amino acids shared by HLA-B27 and any of the microbial antigens are underlined.

[b] nd, not done.

[c] predicted only

In spite of the observed peptide homologies, immunological reactivity of arthritic patients towards these epitopes appears not to be extensive. In one study, one-third of AS patients and one-half of patients with Reiter's syndrome had antibodies against synthetic peptides containing the homologous sequence to Klebsiella nitrogenase (Schwimmbeck 1987). Similarly, one-third of patients with B27-associated diseases had antibodies against YadA-and OmpH-derived peptides, but further analysis demonstrated the responses were directed against a flanking peptide sequence and not against the area of peptide homology (Lahesmaa *et al.* 1991). Furthermore, peripheral blood and synovial fluid T-cell responses of ReA patients have given negative results, and most workers in the field have concluded that the existing data do not support the idea of molecular mimicry being the primary driving force in the pathogenesis of reactive enteroarthritis (Lahesmaa *et al.* 1993). To prove such a possibility, studies with T-cell stimulation and peptide binding are needed, similar to those carried out to find antigenic peptides decisive in the pathogenesis of multiple sclerosis (Wucherpfennig and Strominger 1995). In this light, the newly reported homology between *Klebsiella pneumoniae* and type II collagen (Fielder *et al.* 1995) awaits further clarification.

Role of other bacterial components; lessons from animal models

Susceptibility of certain rat strains to joint inflammation provides another way of addressing the question of bacteria and arthritis. Although these models do not simulate human diseases in all aspects, they have made it possible to dissect further the arthritogenic properties of arthritis-inducing bacteria by studying isolated bacterial components and genetically modified strains.

Mertz *et al.* (1991) found a cationic 19 kDa yersinia protein which was capable of inducing experimental antigen-induced arthritis. This protein turned out to be the β subunit of yersinia urease (Skurnik *et al.* 1993), which Probst *et al.* (1993*a*) in turn observed to be a prominent stimulator of synovial T cells in human reactive arthritis. It was also shown to contain peptides with predicted binding affinity for HLA-B27 (Mertz *et al.* 1994). As already predicted on the basis of the amino-acid sequence (Skurnik *et al.* 1993) however, it is hard to believe that the urease β subunit would be a crucially decisive arthritogenic molecule in yersinia. We are currently exploring this question using another experimental model of arthritis (Gripenberg-Lerche *et al.* 1994, 1995).

Peptidoglycan–polysaccharide (PG–PS) has been found to be an important component in arthritis induced by bacterial cell walls. Streptococcal PG–PS (Stimpson *et al.* 1986) and PG–PS isolated from *Eubacterium* species (Severijnen *et al.* 1990) both trigger chronic joint inflammation in susceptible Lewis rats. Components of intestinal bacteria are also thought to play a role in the reactivation of arthritis where the inciting stimulation is induced by intra-articular injection of streptococcal PG–PS. Reactivation was obtained when self-filling, small-bowel blind loops were constructed surgically (Lichtman *et al.* 1995), allowing overgrowth of intestinal bacteria. Anaerobes seemed to be more important than aerobic bacteria in the reactivation of arthritis, since treatment with metronidazole prevented arthritis but gentamicin had no effect. A similar type of arthritis has been noted in humans subjected to jejunoileal bypass surgery. The overgrowth of intestinal bacteria may result in deposition of bacterial antigens in the joint in the form of immune complexes (Clegg *et al.* 1985), and possibly also by other mechanisms. As such, this condition resembles ReA, in spite of the fact that HLA-B27 is not associated with this type of arthritis. This could be explained by an abnormally high bacterial antigen load associated with intestinal blind loops.

In another animal model, yersinia-triggered arthritis of Lewis rats, the role of the YadA protein of *Yersinia enterocolitica* has been further evaluated. As mentioned above, this outer-membrane protein has amino-acid homology to HLA-B27 and virulence properties associated with binding to extracellular matrix molecules. A mutated strain of *Y. enterocolitica* O:8 not expressing YadA was found to be less arthritogenic (arthritis incidence only 6%) than the wild-type strain (arthritis incidence 51%) (Gripenberg-Lerche *et al.* 1994). The decrease in arthritis incidence by this YadA null mutant may partly be due to impaired binding to extracellular matrix, since another YadA mutant unable to bind collagen also showed significantly decreased arthritogenicity (Gripenberg-Lerche *et al.* 1995).

Animal models of the spondylarthritides are discussed further in Chapter 15 in this volume.

T cell responses to bacterial antigens

The elimination of microbes is without doubt one of the major functions of the immune system. With a skin-surface of close to 2 m^2 and an internal mucosa estimated to cover some 400 m^2, a person is continuously exposed to a huge load of environmental antigens, a large part of which is of microbial origin. This antigenic load may be even higher in patients with spondylarthropathies, in whom intestinal inflammation as well as increased gut permeability are frequently observed. As a consequence, the task of the immune system in eliminating foreign material would also be expected to be increased.

Antibodies can act directly against bacteria by neutralizing harmful products, such as toxins, by preventing the mucosal binding of bacteria by blocking adhesion molecules, and by opsonizing bacteria together with the complement system. Phagocytosis, enhanced by opsonins, completes the work of antibodies and provides material for T cells to enhance more specific, secondary-type antibody responses and memory functions. All of this is well suited to dealing with pathogens that live extracellularly. However, for eliminating intracellular microbes, including those capable of triggering HLA-B27 associated ReA, T lymphocytes dominate the antibacterial action. As noted above, it has been hypothesized, but remains unresolved experimentally, whether individuals carrying HLA-B27 possess a defect in antimicrobial activity and, if so, by what mechanism. The persistence of bacterial antigens, as indicated by continued antibody production, supports this hypothesis. Alternatively, such microbial persistence may be common, but only those with a susceptible genetic background develop the disease, presumably on an immune-mediated basis.

In ReA, T cells specific for the triggering microbe are observed at the site of inflammation (Burmeister 1995; Hermann 1993). In yersinia-triggered ReA, T cell lines and clones have been found to respond to distinct bacterial antigens (Probst *et al.* 1993*b*) but having a somewhat restricted T cell receptor Vβ gene usage (Lahesmaa *et al.* 1995). Among this seemingly polyclonal response, antigens such as YopH (Lahesmaa *et al.* 1995), a 19 kDa urease β subunit (Probst *et al.* 1993*a*), and an evolutionally conserved 50S ribosomal protein (Mertz *et al.* 1994), have been identified to elicit specific responses. The urease β subunit of yersinia contains a peptide sequence with an HLA-B27 binding motif and homology to several human proteins. However, other bacteria not implicated in ReA, such as *Helicobacter pylori, Streptomyces albus,* and *Mycobacterium leprae,* possess highly similar epitopes as candidates for T cell reactivity (Mertz *et al.* 1994). This suggests that the presence of a single antigenic epitope capable of triggering T cell responses is not decisive for arthritogenicity, but requires other contributing bacterial properties as well. The experience gained from studies with YadA yersinia mutants points in the same direction (Gripenberg-Lerche *et al.* 1994, 1995).

MHC class I restricted CD8+ synovial fluid T cells isolated from patients with HLA-B27 associated diseases have been reported (Hermann *et al.* 1993), but the great majority of T cells from ReA are CD4+ and TH1 in type (Lahesmaa *et al.* 1992*b*; Schlaak *et al.* 1992), similar to T cells in Lyme arthritis (Yssel *et al.* 1991). Methods to propagate synovial T cells from inflamed joints *in vitro* may affect their subclass distribution. It is also possible that antigenic responses of T cells may change as the disease progresses; such an evolution has been noted in a case of persistent arthritis (Southwood and Gaston 1993), and it will be of interest to see how HLA-B27 is associated with such a process. T cell responses are discussed further in Chapter 13.

Concluding remarks

ReA induced by enteric infections has been useful for studying the relationship of bacteria to arthritis. Enterogenic ReA is evidently a multifactorial disease. The triggering microbe comprises one cornerstone of this condition. HLA-B27 is another important, although by no means essential, component. What additional mechanisms are involved remains to be established. Likewise, the exact mechanisms of disease initiation, maintenance, and resolution are not yet known. However, recent data allow one to propose the following sequence of events:

1. HLA-B27 originally influences the fate of enteric pathogens by allowing, through a so far unknown mechanism, bacterial persistence (this function may be borne by other risk factors in B27-negative cases).
2. Bacterial antigens are conveyed within circulating leucocytes and deposited in healthy and/or previously traumatized joints.
3. Components of intestinal bacteria leaking from an inflamed gut, and later from other hidden reservoirs, maintain the inflammatory process within the joint tissue.
4. Antigenic similarities between arthritogenic bacteria and host components lead to the development of either autoreactive and/or pathogen-reactive T cells and chronic disease.

The evidence for all these events has been discussed above. Nevertheless, it is possible that we are not yet playing this game of scientific dominoes correctly, and it is more than likely that some pieces are still missing.

Acknowledgements

Our original studies were supported by the Academy of Finland and the Sigrid Jusélius Foundation.

12 HLA-B27, ankylosing spondylitis, and the spondyloarthropathies

Paul Wordsworth and Matthew Brown

Ankylosing spondylitis is one of a group of conditions thought to have an autoimmune pathogenesis, which also includes several other rheumatic disorders, such as rheumatoid arthritis and juvenile chronic arthritis. They are characterized by disordered immunological responses, causing tissue-specific inflammation and damage, and by their striking immunogenetic associations (Wordsworth 1995). In 1973 the description of a very strong association between HLA-B27, one of the immune response genes, and ankylosing spondylitis (Brewerton *et al.* 1973*a*; Schlosstein *et al.* 1973) prompted enormous interest in the immunogenetics of this condition. The odds ratio for HLA-B27 in ankylosing spondylitis is in excess of 100, and is fairly constant across ethnic groups. Much has now been learned about the structural biology and function of HLA-B27 and the other immune response genes. It is known, for example, that these genes encode transmembrane glycoproteins which lie at the very heart of specific immune responses. They form an integral part of a trimolecular complex (HLA molecule, its peptide antigen ligand, and the T-lymphocyte antigen receptor), the formation of which can lead to T-cell activation. However, the precise mechanisms by which HLA-B27 is involved in ankylosing spondylitis and related disorders still remain conjectural.

Structure and function of HLA molecules

The HLA molecules are encoded within the major histocompatibility complex (MHC) on the short arm of Chromosome 6, a segment of DNA approximately four megabases in length which contains in excess of 110 genes (Fig. 12.1) (Albertella and Campbell 1994). The HLA genes encode several isotypes, the most important of which are the class I molecules (HLA-A, HLA-B, and HLA-Cw series) (Spencer Wells and Parham 1996) and the HLA class II molecules (HLA-DR, HLA-DQ, and HLA-DP) (Apple and Erlich 1996). These are all involved in the binding and presentation of antigenic peptide fragments for recognition by the immune system, but there are important differences in structure and function between them. The HLA class I molecules are expressed on virtually all nucleated cells and are particularly involved in cytotoxic responses to virus-infected cells and tumours. HLA class II molecules are expressed on a relatively limited range of cell types, often referred to as 'professional antigen-presenting cells' (dendritic cells, macrophages/monocytes, B lymphocytes, and activated T lymphocytes) which can also present exogenous antigens and are involved in both cellular and humoral responses. In addition to the HLA loci the MHC contains a number of other well-characterized genes, some of which have potentially important immunological functions. These include molecular chaperones (the heat-shock protein HSP-70, HLA-DM), cytokines (tumour necrosis factor-α, lymphotoxin), and complement components (C2, C4, factor B). Of interest, many of these genes are upregulated by interferon-γ, which is typically present at sites of inflammation, suggesting a mechanism by which these products may function synergistically.

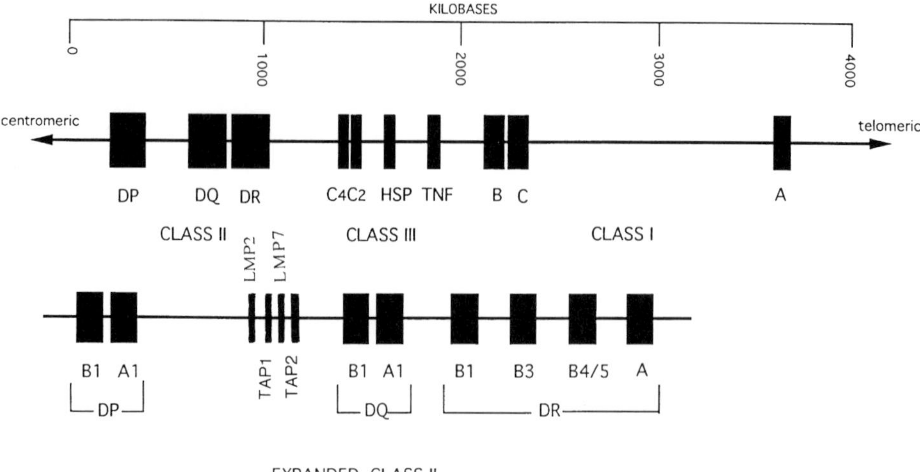

Fig. 12.1 Representation of the organization of the major histocompatability complex on Chromosome 6.

HLA class I

HLA class I molecules bind peptides derived from endogenously synthesized proteins, which may include tumour antigens and viral products. Soon after virus-specific cytotoxic T cells were first described it was noted that they only lysed their targets, derived from various inbred strains of mice, if they shared the same HLA class I alleles (Zinkernagel and Doherty 1979). This was the first description of MHC restriction, and subsequently it was also shown that cytotoxic T cells actually recognize antigens as peptide fragments derived from viral proteins (Townsend *et al.* 1985). The majority of antigens presented by HLA class II molecules are also self-peptides, but exogenous antigens derived from the endosomal breakdown of ingested pathogens are also presented.

HLA class I molecules are members of the immunoglobulin superfamily. They are heterodimers, consisting of a polymorphic heavy chain (45 kDa) including three globular domains ($\alpha1$, $\alpha2$, and $\alpha3$) stabilized by intrachain disulphide bonds, non-covalently bound through the $\alpha3$ domain to a non-polymorphic light chain $\beta2$-microglobulin (12 kDa). A high degree of homology is found among all HLA class I molecules in the framework regions, and their polymorphism is concentrated in those amino-acid residues adjacent to the antigen-binding site. The crystal structure of several class I antigens, including HLA-B27, has now been solved. This clearly reveals a groove-like antigen-binding site which contains electron-dense material indicating the presence of bound peptide fragments (Fig. 12.2). This groove is bounded by two antiparallel α-helices, about 10–18 Å apart, derived from the $\alpha1$ and $\alpha2$ domains of the heavy chain. The floor of the binding site is formed by eight strands of β-pleated sheet (Bjorkman *et al.* 1987; Garrett *et al.* 1989; Madden *et al.* 1992). Typically, the peptide ligands consist of nonamer fragments, usually in an extended conformation, although larger or shorter peptides may also bind. The interactions between the HLA molecules and specific peptide ligands have been studied at high resolution in some instances by the co-crystallization of HLA molecules with a variety of peptides (Matsumura *et al.* 1992). Slightly longer peptides may be accommodated in the groove by the formation of a small kink, while

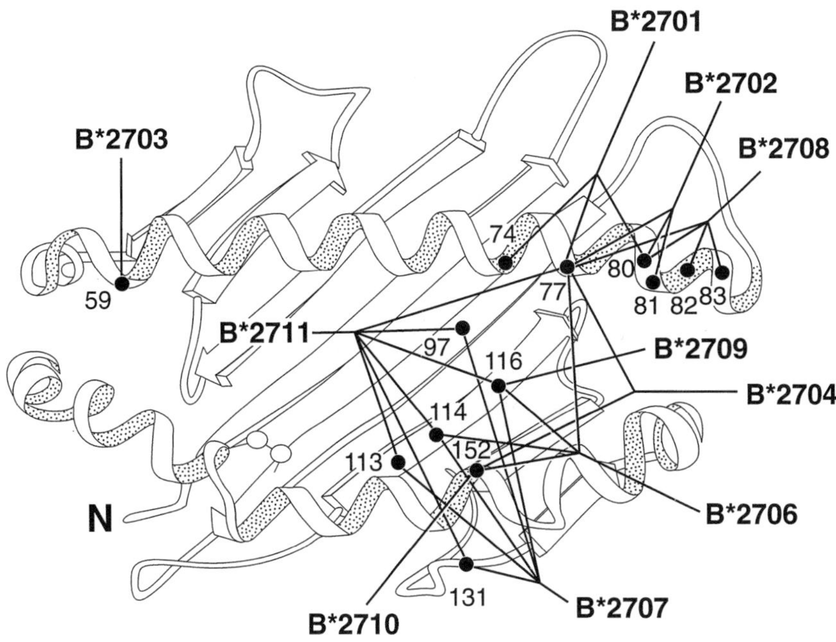

Fig. 12.2 Ribbon diagram of HLA-B27 indicating the position of allelic diversity relative to HLA-B*2705 for subtypes 01 through 11.

Table 12.1 The amino acids that distinguish the twelve known HLA-B27 subtypes

Subtype	Amino acid residue															
	59	69	70	71	74	77	80	81	82	83	97	113	114	116	131	152
B*2705	Y	A	K	A	D	D	T	L	L	R	N	Y	H	D	S	V
B*2701	—	—	—	—	Y	N	—	A	—	—	—	—	—	—	—	—
B*2702	—	—	—	—	—	N	I	A	—	—	—	—	—	—	—	—
B*2703	H	—	—	—	—	—	—	—	—	—	—	—	—	—	—	—
B*2704	—	—	—	—	—	S	—	—	—	—	—	—	—	—	—	E
B*2706	—	—	—	—	—	S	—	—	—	—	—	—	D	Y	—	E
B*2707	—	—	—	—	—	—	—	—	—	—	S	H	N	Y	R	—
B*2708	—	—	—	—	—	S	N	—	R	G	—	—	—	—	—	—
B*2709	—	—	—	—	—	—	—	—	—	—	—	—	—	H	—	—
B*2710	—	—	—	—	—	—	—	—	—	—	—	—	—	—	—	E
B*2711	—	—	—	—	—	S	—	—	—	—	S	H	N	Y	R	—
B*2712	—	T	N	T	—	S	N	—	R	G	—	—	—	—	—	—
Pocket	*A*	—	*B*	—	*C*	*F*	*F*	*F*	—	—	*C*	*D*	*E*	*F*	—	*E*

A dash indicates identity at that position with the B*2705 sequence. Residues 59-83 are in the $\alpha1$ domain, 97-152 are in the $\alpha2$ domain. B*2708 and B*2712 are homologous with HLA-B7 at positions 77-83, and B*2712 is homologous with many other HLA-B alleles at positions 69-71. B*2707 and B*2711 are homologous with HLA-B8 at positions 97-131. One letter amino acid code: A, alinine; D, aspartic acid; E, glutamic acid; G, glycine; H, histidine; I, isoleucine; K, lysine; L, leucine; N, aparagine; R, arginine; S, serine; T, threonine; V, valine; Y, tyrosine. From Hildebrand *et al.* 1994; Fiorello *et al.* 1995; Marcos *et al.* 1996; Hasegawa *et al.* 1997; Marsh 1997.

occasionally much longer peptides may be bound, probably by overlapping the ends of the binding site (Urban *et al.* 1994; Collins *et al.* 1994).

HLA class II

These molecules are similar in structure to the HLA class I molecules but the binding site is open ended with the consequence that longer peptides are usually bound, overlapping the binding site at both ends. Most of the peptides which are bound are derived from self-proteins, but exogenous peptides can also be presented. The HLA class II molecules are heterodimers of α and β polypeptides, the amino-terminal ends of which constitute a similar binding site to the class I molecule (Stern *et al.* 1994). In contrast to class I molecules, the class II molecules bind invariant chain (including the CLIP peptide that occupies the binding site) which prevents peptide binding initially. This complex passes through the Golgi apparatus and is targeted to the early endosome, which subsequently fuses with endocytic vacuoles containing complex exogenous antigens, to form the late endosome. Here the pH falls, leading to dissociation of the CLIP peptide from the binding site of the HLA class II molecule, which can then bind self or foreign peptides. The class II molecule is expressed on the cell surface, whence it may be recycled periodically by endocytosis.

Peptide antigen processing

Antigen fragments presented by HLA class I molecules are generated in the cytosol and actively transported to the endoplasmic reticulum (Cerundolo and Braud 1996; Elliott *et al.* 1993). Here the peptides (usually nonamers) associate with nascent class I molecules, inducing a conformational change in the heavy chain which enhances its stability. After associating with β2-microglobulin the HLA molecule is expressed on the cell surface where it can interact with the antigen receptors of specific T lymphocytes.

Generation of peptides for presentation

The generation of peptide fragments for presentation by HLA class I molecules is dependent on the activity of a large multicatalytic protease complex in the cytosol known as the proteasome (Hilt and Wolf 1996). This enzyme complex acts largely on proteins marked by ubiquitination. Following the attachment of a chain of multiple units of the 76 amino-acid polypeptide ubiquitin to the protein, it is then unfolded and transported to the centre of the proteasome where it undergoes catalytic degradation in an ATP-dependent manner. The central core of the proteasome is a 700 kDa (20S) cylinder composed of low molecular weight subunits arranged in a stack of four rings each composed of seven subunits. At either end of the central 20S cylinder are 19S caps which are thought to be involved in the unfolding of the protein and their transport into the proteolytic central core (Hilt and Wolf 1996). Experiments in yeast demonstrate that 'gene knockout' of any of the 14 known yeast 20S proteasome genes are lethal, as are deletions of any of the 19S cap genes.

In humans two genes (LMP2 and LMP7), which lie in the MHC class II region (telomeric to HLA-DP), as well as a third non-MHC gene, encode non-essential β subunits of the 20S proteasome (Fig. 12.1) which can be induced by interferon-γ. These can replace three of the constitutive subunits, which are suppressed by interferon-γ (Aki *et al.* 1994). This alters the peptide-cleaving activities of the proteasome. In particular, peptides with basic amino acids at the carboxyl terminus are preferentially generated, which are more likely to bind to HLA class I molecules in general, and HLA-B*2705 in particular.

Peptide transporters

Before the peptide products of proteolysis can be presented by the immune system they must be transported into the endoplasmic reticulum where they bind to the nascent HLA class I heavy chain as it comes off the ribosome. The binding of peptide stabilizes the heavy chain which also associates through its $\alpha 3$ domain with $\beta 2$-microglobulin and then passes to the cell surface where it is available for interaction with T lymphocytes through the T-cell antigen receptor. The importance of the peptide transport mechanism, encoded adjacent to the LMP2 and LMP7 genes within the MHC class II, can be clearly seen in mutant cell lines or mice lacking these genes. These genes encode the two components of a peptide transporter known as Transporters Associated with antigen Processing (TAP1 and TAP2). They are members of an ATP-dependent superfamily of membrane transporters which also includes the multidrug resistance and cystic fibrosis chloride-transport genes. Mutants with substantial deletions in the HLA class II region, including these loci, may fail entirely to express HLA class I at the cell surface, or more usually express markedly reduced amounts. This defect can partially be reversed by incubating the cells with peptide which can bind to the empty class I molecules on the cell surface thereby increasing their stability. In the rat, polymorphism of the TAP genes influences the nature of the peptides transported to the endoplasmic reticulum (Powis *et al.* 1993). However, in humans only very limited polymorphism exists, and its role in determining the range of peptide available for expression at the cell surface seems limited (Obst *et al.* 1995). One Moroccan family has been reported in which inheritance of a non-functional TAP2 gene resulted in non-expression of HLA class I molecules and a propensity to recurrent bacterial infection (de la Salle *et al.* 1994). Cell lines derived from a small-cell lung cancer with a defective TAP1 gene similarly do not express HLA class I molecules, and this may be one mechanism by which tumours avoid detection by immune surveillance (Chen *et al.* 1996). In ankylosing spondylitis, polymorphism of the LMP2 gene and the TAP genes appear to be of little relevance (Burney *et al.* 1994; Westman *et al.* 1995), although it has been tentatively suggested that iritis and peripheral arthritis may be more common in those with both a particular LMP polymorphism (Maksymowych *et al.* 1994, 1995*a*) and TAP1 polymorphism (Maksymowych *et al.* 1995*c*).

Peptide interactions with HLA class I molecules

The side chains of the constituent peptide amino acids intimately interact with the HLA molecule through hydrogen bonds. Typically there are six pockets (A–F) around the binding site, each potentially with the capacity to accommodate side chains of individual amino acids in the peptide. The A and F pockets, which bind the amino and carboxyl terminus of the peptide, respectively, play a particularly important role and are highly conserved across the range of HLA molecules. There are also additional important binding pockets which differ between individual HLA molecules, providing allele-specific anchor sites for the binding of particular amino acids. The binding of peptides to individual HLA molecules has been extensively studied by sequencing peptides eluted from purified class I molecules. This reveals allele-specific peptide-binding motifs for many HLA class I molecules, conferring a high degree of specificity to peptide binding. The amino acid at position 2 of the peptide is frequently crucial to the binding affinity, as discussed below (Falk *et al.* 1991; Jardetsky *et al.* 1991; Tanigaki *et al.* 1994).

In the A pocket, tyrosine residues at positions 7, 59, 159, and 171 of the heavy chain are highly conserved across all HLA-B molecules and contribute to hydrogen bonding with the amino-terminal residue of the peptide. However, in one HLA-B27 variant (HLA-B*2703) there is a tyrosine to histidine substitution at position 59 (Fig. 12.2), which could conceivably influence peptide binding (Table 12.1). Likewise, in the F pocket, tyrosine at position 143 and tyrosine at position 84 are highly conserved, interacting with the carboxyl-terminal peptide residue while the tryptophan at position 147 is also conserved and interacts with the carbonyl group of the penultimate residue of the peptide. The high degree of conservation of the F pocket also explains why the carboxyl-terminal peptide residue is also restricted, since this side chain points straight into the F pocket (Rötzschke *et al.* 1994). Of peptides binding to class I molecules, 95% have isoleucine, leucine, valine, arginine, lysine, threonine, or phenylalanine at the carboxyl terminus. Furthermore, the amino acids at position 77 and 116 also influence peptide binding: class I molecules with aspartic acid at position 77 and 116 select for peptides with a positively charged carboxyl-terminal residue; of those with serine at position 77 and 116, two-thirds of the bound peptides have tyrosine at the carboxyl terminus; and in those class I molecules with phenylalanine/tyrosine at position 116, 8 out of 10 bound peptides have a hydrophobic residue at the carboxyl terminus. In general, for the three common groups of class I molecules, tyrosine^{116} correlates with leucine/isoleucine or valine at the peptide carboxyl terminus, aspartic acid^{116} correlates with arginine or lysine, and serine^{116} correlates with tyrosine at the carboxyl terminus. The commonest HLA-B27 variant in Caucasians (HLA-B*2705) has aspartic acid^{77}, leucine^{81}, leucine^{95}, aspartic acid^{116}, and the peptide carboxyl terminus is typically arginine or lysine (Elliott *et al.* 1993). Other important peptide anchor residues can be found within the binding site and these vary between HLA molecules.

The B pocket

The B pocket is an important peptide anchor site in many HLA class I molecules, including HLA-B27 which predominantly binds peptides with arginine at position 2. In some other class I molecules the importance of the B pocket is reduced or abolished because of the limited access permitted by the tertiary structure. For example, the presence of phenylalanine or threonine at position 67 which lies at its mouth can completely block access to the B pocket. More commonly, access is partially occluded by substitutions at position 45, halfway down the pocket, for example tyrosine^{45} found in HLA-B8. In this case, peptide specificity is derived from pocket 3 instead (Sutton *et al.* 1993). However, this is not the case for all class I molecules having this tyrosine^{45} substitution since proline at position 2 is preferentially accepted by the B pockets of HLA-B35, -B7, -B51, and -B53 (Hill *et al.* 1992). The importance of the B pocket in determining binding specificity is further illustrated by experiments using site-directed mutagenesis to effect a 'B pocket transplant' from HLA-A2 to HLA-B*2705. The resulting hybrid HLA molecule binds peptides with leucine rather than the expected arginine at position 2 (Colbert *et al.* 1993).

The relative importance of the A, F, and other anchor pockets in HLA-B27 and other class I molecules has been investigated by assessing the binding affinities of specific peptides and their derivatives. In general, the peptide binding affinities can be reduced 100-fold by substituting the carboxyl-terminal residue with alanine or by amidation of the carboxyl-terminal residue. These modifications impair interactions with the F pocket. Even more strikingly, blocking binding to the A pocket by acetylation of the amino-terminal peptide residue can reduce binding by a factor of 10^4. By comparison, substitutions to other anchor sites, such as the B pocket of HLA-B27, can reduce binding 500-fold (Parker *et al.* 1994).

HLA-B27 and antigen presentation

The mechanisms by which HLA-B27 presents antigen to the immune system are identical to those for other HLA class I molecules. However, the nature of the associated peptide ligands and their stability at the cell surface may be different from other class I molecules. There are also differences among the twelve HLA-B27 subtypes (allotypes) currently recognized. These variants can be distinguished by their amino-acid or DNA sequences, but all are recognized by serological reagents for HLA-B27, with the exception of HLA-B*2708 which was originally detected as a serological variant of HLA-B7, and B*2712, which has only been identified at the DNA level and does not react with most anti-B27 alloantisera. The differences in amino-acid sequence among the HLA-B27 allotypes is shown in Table 12.1 and the prevalence in different ethnic groups is shown in Table 12.2. These allotypes are thought to have arisen from B*2705 by three different mechanisms: point mutation (B*2703), gene conversion (B*2701, B*2702, B*2704, B*2706, and B*2708) and reciprocal recombination (B*2707, B*2709) (Lopez de Castro 1989). The polymorphic residues around the B pocket are conserved throughout the B27 allotypes, so that peptides with arginine at position 2 are required for binding. B27 differs from many other class I molecules in having a relatively large pocket to interact with the carboxyl terminus of the peptide, formed by a coalescence of the C and F pockets. In contrast to the B pocket, which is identical throughout the B27 subtypes, the C/F pocket may be influenced by amino-acid substitutions at position 74, 77, 80, 81, 97, and 116 in several of these allotypes. Likewise, the

Table 12.2 HLA-B27 subtype distribution in different ethnic groups

Population	B27 subtype	
	Common	Rare
European	B*2705,2	B*2701,8,9,10
Jews	B*2702,5	B*2704
Asian Indians	B*2705,4	B*2702,7
Thai	B*2704,6	
Chinese	B*2704,5	B*2706
Japanese	B*2704,5	B*2711
Amerindians	B*2705	
Eskimo	B*2705	
West Africans	B*2705,3	

tyrosine → histidine[59] substitution in B*2703 could influence binding to the A pocket. However, experiments to date have shown relatively minor differences in the repertoire of peptides bound to B*2703 compared to B*2705 (Colbert *et al.* 1994).

Peptide binding to HLA-B27 subtypes

Potentially significant differences exist in the peptide-binding motifs of the different HLA-B27 subtypes (Fuzakawa *et al.* 1994; Tanigaki *et al.* 1994) (also, see Chapter 18). HLA-B*2701 binds only a minority of peptides which will bind to B*2705, almost certainly because of the loss of acidic charges at position 74 and 77 in the C/F pocket. In B*2705 the aspartic acid[77] stabilizes basic amino-acid side chains in the C/F pocket, whereas in B*2701 the bound peptides have either histidine or an aliphatic residue at the carboxyl terminus. In addition to substitutions at positions 77, 114, 116, and 152 relative to B*2705, there is a point mutation resulting in a glycine for alanine[211] substitution in B*2704/B*2706. This probably occurred shortly before or after the divergence of B*2704/6 from B*2705, but is unlikely to be of significance in antigen binding (Rudwaleit *et al.* 1996). The change to aspartic acid[74] in B*2706 produces a lower binding affinity for peptides with basic residues at the carboxyl terminus, but although B*2704 shares the same serine with B*2706 it is otherwise more similar to B*2705 and has greater similarity with B*2705 in the peptides which it binds. B*2709 differs from B*2705 only by the substitution of histidine for aspartic acid[116]. This affects pocket F, making B*2709 unable to bind peptides with arginine or tyrosine carboxyl-terminus residues (Damato *et al.* 1995).

Mechanisms of involvement of HLA-B27 in disease

Not only was the association between ankylosing spondylitis and HLA-B27 in 1973 (Brewerton *et al.* 1973*a*; Schlosstein *et al.* 1973) one of the first to be described, but it is still one of the strongest with an odds ratio between 100 and 200 (Brown *et al.* 1996*a*). Although a great deal has since been learned about the molecular biology of HLA-B27 and its role in antigen presentation, there is still a considerable debate about the mechanism of this association: it could represent the function of B27 as a restriction element; peptides derived from B27 could be relevant in the initiation or perpetuation of the disease; or B27 could provide a target for cross-reactive serological responses by molecular mimicry with cell-surface antigens from bacteria.

The reactive thiol hypothesis

The unique position of the reactive thiol cysteine[67] opposite the basic lysine[70] at the mouth of the B pocket led to the theory that altered oxidation of cysteine[67] may lead either to changes in peptide recognition and presentation by HLA-B27, or altered antigenicity of B27 itself (the 'reactive thiol hypothesis') (Whelan and Archer 1993).

It has been reported that humoral recognition of B27 is altered by increased oxidation of cysteine[67] (Archer *et al.* 1990), but other studies have found no effect of exposure of B27-positive cells to free radicals on the binding of anti-B27 monoclonal antibodies (MacLean *et al.* 1992). Recently, homocysteine-treated cells were shown to be specifically lysed by CTL from patients with spondyloarthropathy, but other antigens in addition to B27 were implicated (Gao *et al.* 1996). Whether the oxidation of cysteine[67] has any direct effect on T-cell recognition of B27 or disease pathogenesis is still not known.

The 'promiscuous peptide' theory

HLA-B27 and fragments of other class I molecules are frequently found in elution products from class II molecules (Chicz *et al.* 1993). This led to the suggestion that fragments of B27 may be presented by class II molecules, thereby inducing autoimmunity. This could explain the predominance of CD4-positive cells at sites of inflammation in the spondyloarthropathies. The lack of a strong class II association may simply reflect the relatively promiscuous binding of peptides by class II molecules (the 'promiscuous peptide' theory) (Davenport 1995). Mouse and animal models of spondyloarthritis support this theory. In B27 transgenic rats, the development of arthritis is closely linked to the number of copies of the B27 transgene (Taurog *et al.* 1993), as would be predicted by this theory. In humans, however, B27 acts as a dominant susceptibility allele and no 'dose effect' occurs (Rubin *et al.* 1994; Suarez and Russell 1987). In mice transgenic for B27 but lacking β_2-microglobulin, B27 is present at very low levels on the cell surface, and yet arthritis has been described in such mice when conventionally housed (Khare *et al.* 1995*b*). These mice have very low CD8 lymphocyte counts, and it has been suggested that B27 fragments may be being presented by mouse class II molecules to CD4 lymphocytes thereby inducing arthritis. Class II knockout experiments in either mice or rats may determine the veracity of this theory.

Molecular mimicry

Some form of molecular mimicry is central to many of the theories explaining the association of HLA-B27 and ankylosing spondylitis. In its original form, molecular mimicry between bacterial organisms and B27 was postulated to result in a cross-reaction between a humoral reaction to bacteria and B27 (Benjamin and Parham 1990). Other possibilities include cross-reactivity between bacterial and B27-presented endogenous antigens. The theory has been modified by some to explain disease models where cellular rather than humoral immunity plays a central role, as in the arthritogenic peptide theory.

Potential targets for molecular mimicry exist, with evidence of homology between numerous bacteria and B27 (Schwimmbeck and Oldstone 1988; Scofield *et al.* 1993). However, whether this plays any role in the pathenogenesis of ankylosing spondylitis remains conjectural. That B27 is capable of presenting such peptides has been demonstrated (Scofield *et al.* 1995), but evidence of cytotoxic T lymphocytes recognizing such peptides has not. Further, HLA class I-derived peptides are not commonly found amongst elution products from class I molecules (Rammensee *et al.* 1995).

Numerous studies have investigated evidence of humoral immunity to HLA-B27 cross-reactive sequences with a range of bacteria although with conflicting results (Inman and Scofield 1994). The most commonly studied of these is a hexapeptide QTDRED, derived from *Klebsiella pneumoniae* nitrogenase and homologous with part of the first hypervariable region of B*2705. The aspartate[77] is not shared by other subtypes known to be associated with ankylosing spondylitis (B*2702 or B*2704), nor is the sequence included in a B27 peptide-binding motif, so it is unlikely to be a target for cross-reactive T-cell recognition. Chance occurrence of homology in short peptide sequence like this is quite likely, and of its own accord provides no evidence of an aetiological role. Klebsiella is not a recognized trigger of reactive arthritis either, which would seem likely if it has a causal role in ankylosing spondylitis. Patients with ankylosing spondylitis have repeatedly been demonstrated to have increased antibody levels against a variety of klebsiella components (Ebringer 1992), but again this may merely reflect increased carriage rather than a causal role. Considerable evidence of humoral cross-reaction between B27 and klebsiella has been documented (Avakian *et al.* 1980; Welsh *et al.* 1980). However, attempts to demonstrate that anti-klebsiella sera could differentiate ankylosing spondylitis-affected and -unaffected B27-positive individuals have largely been unsuccessful (Beukelman *et al.* 1990).

An interesting hypothetical homologous pentapeptide (amino-acid sequence deduced from DNA code) (AQTDR) coded for by a shigella plasmid pHS-2 may have a role in some forms of reactive arthritis. This plasmid has been found in three arthritogenic shigella strains, but not in two strains unassociated with reactive arthritis (Stieglitz and Lipsky 1993). Humoral cross-reactivity between this peptide and B27 is stronger than with *K. pneumoniae* nitrogenase and B27. However, the majority of ankylosing spondylitis and reactive arthritis samples studied had no antibody to a synthetic peptide from which the homologous sequence is derived, suggesting that it may have a role in a minor subset of patients only (Tsuchiya *et al.* 1990).

'Linked gene' hypothesis

It is now widely accepted that HLA-B27 itself is directly involved in the pathogenesis of ankylosing spondylitis. However, it is conceivable that HLA-B27 itself is merely a marker for another tightly linked gene which has the primary association with ankylosing spondylitis. More likely, it is possible that additional genes on some HLA-B27 haplotypes may also affect the penetrance of B27 or the expression of the disease, as has been suggested by evidence from association studies of TAP, LMP, and DR genes as discussed below. A causal link with B27 is strongly suggested by the fact that in numerous population studies worldwide the prevalence of ankylosing spondylitis reflects the underlying frequency of B27 in the corresponding ethnic group (Table 12.3). In Caucasians, over 90% of patients with ankylosing spondylitis are B27- positive, and if patients with associated disorders such as inflammatory bowel disease or psoriasis are excluded, 98% of patients with the 'pure' form of the disease are B27 positive. It has been suggested that since a small minority of patients with the disease are B27 negative this gene may, in fact, be a marker for another nearby gene in even stronger association with the condition, but attempts to define such a gene using restriction fragment length polymorphisms of DNA in the region of the HLA-B locus have generally been unsuccessful in defining stronger associations (Reveille *et al.* 1994). The minor shortfall in the proportion of patients who are B27 positive can almost certainly be explained on the basis of

Table 12.3 HLA-B27 subtype distribution in UK Caucasian patients with ankylosing spondylitis and healthy controls (antigen frequencies)

	B*2705	B*2702	B*2708
AS patients	169	3	0
Healthy controls	147	5	2

genetic heterogeneity. This is common in even monogenic disorders and is likely to be important in complex traits such as ankylosing spondylitis. Other HLA genes, and very likely non-HLA genes, may be involved (Brown *et al.* 1995*b*; Rubin *et al.* 1994).

Arthritogenic peptide theory

In the 'arthritogenic peptide' theory, cross-reactive responsiveness is invoked at the level of the T cell directed at a peptide presented by HLA-B27. Such responses could be directed against either endogenous or exogenous antigens, or both. Possible examples of each have been described: B27-restricted CD8 responses against type II collagen peptides have been found in isolated patients with reactive arthritis (Gao *et al.* 1994); similar responses to arthritogenic bacteria have also been observed in patients with ankylosing spondylitis and reactive arthritis (Hermann *et al.* 1993).

There has been considerable interest in the possibility that the twelve distinct HLA-B27 allotypes currently defined may not be associated equally with ankylosing spondylitis, not least because this might be explicable on the basis of their different binding affinities to peptide antigens (Lopez de Castro 1995). This might give clues as to the nature of the 'arthritogenic peptide' putatively incriminated in the disease. Some of these subtypes are much commoner that others, allowing conclusions to be drawn from rigorous population studies, while with the rarer variants much of the evidence is relatively anecdotal. Thus, in Caucasian, Amerindian, and Eskimo populations B*2705 predominates, B*2704 is common in many Asian groups, and B*2702 is the commonest variant in Jews with ankylosing spondylitis. In contrast, the other variants are rare, and their status in relation to ankylosing spondylitis susceptibility is unclear, since population studies have proved either impossible or limited in their power. Patients with B*2701, B*2706, and B*2707 have been described, but it is not known whether the strength of the association mirrors that observed with the commoner subtypes. Recently, it has indeed been suggested that B*2706 may not be strongly associated with ankylosing spondylitis since a study in Thailand showed that the allotype was markedly under-represented in patients compared with ethnically matched controls (Lopez-Larrea *et al.* 1995). This finding has been supported by a smaller study in Indonesians, which none the less reported two cases of ankylosing spondylitis associated with B*2706 (Nasution *et al.* 1996) HLA-B*2709 is found in 3% of B27-positive Italians and 25% of B27-positive Sardinians. One epidemiological study of Sardinians has recently suggested that it may not be associated with susceptibility to ankylosing spondylitis (Damato *et al.* 1995). A similar argument has been made for B*2703 which is relatively common in West Africa and where ankylosing spondylitis is reputedly a rare condition (Hill *et al.* 1991). Our recent epidemiological survey in The Gambia indicated that the frequency of B27 amongst the Fula was 6% consisting of both B*2703 (32%) and B*2705 (68%). However, in this population no cases of ankylosing spondylitis were found, and in this particular geographical location the disease did not appear to be associated with either B*2703 or B*2705, suggesting that there were other protective factors (environmental or genetic) (Brown *et al.* 1997). Recently, ankylosing spondylitis and B*2703 have been reported in African-American patients (Reveille *et al.* 1996).

In Northern Europe, HLA-B*2705 is by far the dominant allotype associated with ankylosing spondylitis and numerous studies have now confirmed this fact (Breur-Vriesendorp *et al.* 1987; Brown *et al.* 1996; MacLean *et al.* 1993). Recently, we undertook a large study in the United Kingdom which showed that both B*2705 and B*2702 were positively associated with the

Table 12.4 HLA haplotype-sharing in ankylosing spondylitis

	Share 0	Share 1	Share 2
Observed	6	54	43
Expected	26	51	26

$\chi^2 = 28.1$, $p = 7.8 \times 10^{-7}$

disease, and also that there did not appear to be any preferential association with either of these allotypes (Table 12.4). Of interest, 1.3% of the controls but none of the patients had B*2708.

MHC/non-MHC genes in ankylosing spondylitis

Although the HLA association with ankylosing spondylitis is the strongest of any autoimmune disease, it is likely that non-MHC genes play a significant role in an individual's susceptibility to disease. A small minority of patients develop ankylosing spondylitis in the absence of B27, indicating that B27 is not absolutely essential for the development of ankylosing spondylitis. The proportion of B27-negative cases increases if one considers related conditions such as reactive arthritis and colitic and psoriatic spondyloarthritis, in which as many as 40–50% of patients may not carry B27. B27-positive first-degree relatives of patients with ankylosing spondylitis are 5.6–15 times more likely to develop ankylosing spondylitis themselves than B27-positive individuals with no such family history, suggesting the presence of other shared susceptibility factors (Calin *et al.* 1983; van der Linden *et al.* 1984*b*). The rate of decline of recurrence risk for ankylosing spondylitis in successively more distant-degrees of relatives is more rapid than occurs in monogenic diseases, and is most consistent with polygenic disease models where there is multiplicative genetic interaction determining disease susceptibility (Lawrence 1977). B27 transgenic strains of mice and rats show different penetrances for spondyloarthritis, dependent on the non-transgenic genetic background of the animal (Taurog *et al.* 1996; Weinreich *et al.* 1995). Recently, it has been shown that backcrossing the HLA-B27 transgene locus of arthritis-prone F344 rat strains into inbred Dark Agouti rats resulted in suppression of the disease phenotype (Taurog *et al.* 1996). This finding suggests the presence of either added non-B27 susceptibility genes in F344 rats (and other arthritis-prone rat strains) or protective genes in the Dark Agouti strain. Identification of these genes may well have relevance to human spondyloarthritis.

Other HLA class I molecules and ankylosing spondylitis

Complex genetic interactions between HLA haplotypes are recognized in other autoimmune diseases, including rheumatoid arthritis (Wordsworth *et al.* 1992) where the compound heterozygote HLA-DRB1*0401/*0404 genotype is particularly associated with susceptibility to disease. In ankylosing spondylitis a similar situation exists where the presence of HLA-B60 on the non-B27 haplotype increases the risk threefold (Robinson *et al.* 1989; Rubin *et al.* 1994). These results have been confirmed in the United Kingdom and extended to individuals who are B27 negative (Brown *et al.* 1996*c*). This result may not be consistent across all ethnic groups, and negative reports regarding the association have been published (Reveille *et al.* 1994; Sanmarti *et al.* 1991; Yamaguchi *et al.* 1995). This could possibly indicate that B60 is a marker for a further susceptibility allele, and that a differential strength of linkage exists between this allele and B60 in the different populations studied. Similarly, HLA-B39 has been reported to be associated with B27-negative ankylosing spondylitis in Japanese (Yamaguchi *et al.* 1995) and Caucasian populations (Khan *et al.* 1980). It has also been associated with psoriatic arthritis (Gladman *et al.* 1986). In our own study of 25 B27-negative Caucasian patients with ankylosing spondylitis and 5398 B27-negative controls, no such association was seen (Brown *et al.* 1996*c*).

Varying differences in the structure and peptide-binding characteristics exist between B27 and the other HLA class I molecules for which associations with ankylosing spondylitis have been described (HLA-B39 and HLA-B60). HLA-B39 shares the important B pocket amino acids glutamic acid^{45}, cysteine^{67}, and also tyrosine^{99} with B27, but not lysine^{70} which is characteristic of all B27 allotypes (Yamaguchi *et al.* 1995). In common with B27 it preferentially binds positively charged amino acids at position 2, including arginine. HLA-B60 shares residues threonine^{24} and tyrosine^{99} with B27, but preferentially binds glutamine not arginine at position 2 (Kawaguchi *et al.* 1993; Rammensee *et al.* 1995). This suggests that HLA-B60 either presents different 'arthritogenic peptides', or acts in a different manner to B27 in increasing susceptibility to ankylosing spondylitis.

Other MHC genes

Weak associations with a range of class II genes have been reported, including DR1, DR2, DR7, and DR8. Ethnic differences in linkage disequilibrium with HLA-B27 and the small scale of most of these studies probably explains the lack of agreement. We have found an association between DR1 and ankylosing spondylitis in 112 familial and 172 sporadic cases compared with 675 B27-positive controls. Only 31.4% of B27-positive controls carry DR1, compared with 50% of familial ankylosing spondylitis cases ($\chi^2 = 7.6$, $p = 0.006$, $OR = 1.8$), 41% of sporadic cases ($\chi^2 = 5.3$, $p = 0.02$, $OR = 1.5$), and 39% of B27-negative cases ($\chi^2 = 5.4$, $p = 0.02$, $OR = 2.9$ compared with general population controls). No other DR association was found (Brown *et al.* 1995*a*).

Population studies of tumour necrosis factor (TNFα) polymorphisms have shown no specific associations with disease (Verjans *et al.* 1994). An association with a complotype and susceptibility to ankylosing spondylitis in Mexicans has been reported but not replicated in any other population (Vargas-Alarcon *et al.* 1994). Given the large number of candidate 'linked genes' in the MHC, the prior probability of positive findings in population-association studies in this area is small, and future efforts at linkage disequilibrium mapping may be more fruitful.

Non-MHC component

In 15 multicase Canadian ankylosing spondylitis families, Rubin *et al.* found a maximum LOD score for HLA-B27 and ankylosing spondylitis of 7.5 with a penetrance of 20% (Rubin *et al.* 1994). Segregation analysis suggested an autosomal dominant model of genetic action, consistent with previous evidence that homozygosity for B27 does not further increase disease susceptibility (Arnett *et al.* 1997). Rubin also calculated the attributable risk of B27 to be

50%, consistent with our own findings for HLA-linked genes. In a study of 103 affected sibling pairs we have also confirmed linkage to HLA (LOD score 6.9). However, a significant proportion of sibling pairs did not share HLA haplotypes identical by descent from their parents (Table 12.3), indicating a significant role for non-MHC genes. We estimate that no more than 36% of the genetic variance in ankylosing spondylitis is due to HLA (Brown *et al.* 1995*b*, 1997).

A small number of non-MHC candidate genes have been investigated. An association between the secretor status locus and ankylosing spondylitis has been found, with non-secretors of ABO antigens having a relative risk for disease of 2.6 (Shinebaum *et al.* 1987). Non-secretors have lower immunity to mucosal infections, suggesting a possible mechanism for this potential association. Two subsequent studies, however, have reported no association between secretor status and ankylosing spondylitis (Møller 1990; Pal *et al.* 1997).

Recently, an association between inactive alleles of a cytochrome P450 enzyme, CYP2D6, and ankylosing spondylitis was reported (Beyeler *et al.* 1996) with a relative risk for disease of 2.7. A weak association of α1-antitrypsin has been reported with B27-related acute anterior uveitis (Brewerton *et al.* 1978) and ankylosing spondylitis (Buisseret *et al.* 1977). Each of these associations awaits confirmation.

Other spondyloarthropathies

Spondyloarthritis may occur in association with psoriasis, inflammatory bowel disease, and urogenital or enteric infections (reactive arthritis). The strength of association of HLA-B27 with each of these diseases is significantly lower than in ankylosing spondylitis, suggesting a role for non-B27 genetic susceptibility factors.

Uncomplicated psoriasis is associated with HLA-B13, B16 (and its splits B38 and B39), B17, Cw6, and DR7 (Armstrong *et al.* 1983; Gladman *et al.* 1986; O'Donnell *et al.* 1993). B27 is associated with the development of sacroiliitis (Suarez and Russell 1990) and DR4 has been linked with peripheral arthritis (McHugh *et al.* 1987), but this has not been a universal finding (Gladman *et al.* 1986). The B7 cross-reactive group of HLA antigens is increased in some groups with 'undifferentiated spondyloarthritis', and in B27-negative spondyloarthritis in American-Africans (Khan *et al.* 1978; Stein *et al.* 1990). The psoriasis-associated HLA-B antigens belong to this group, consistent with the finding that much B27-negative spondyloarthritis is associated with psoriasis or inflammatory bowel disease. Chronicity of joint disease is associated with B27, B39, and DQw3 (Gladman and Farewell 1995). The reported association with B39 is of particular interest in view of the suggestion that this antigen is also increased in B27-negative patients with ankylosing spondylitis (Yamaguchi *et al.* 1995).

Reactive arthritis is associated with HLA-B27 in up to 70% of cases, and this association is strongest with more persistent forms of the disease. There is an overall male predominance in this disease of approximately 3:1, but in outbreaks of enteric arthritogenic infection the gender ratio is equal. This probably reflects greater environmental exposure of males to triggering urogenital infections. No other HLA associations have been consistently found with this disease (Laivoranta *et al.* 1995), although associations with the B7 cross-reactive group HLA antigens have been reported (Khan 1983). Only approximately 10% of B27-positive individuals develop arthritis following infections with known triggering bacteria, suggesting a role for susceptibility factors other than B27 (Mattila *et al.* 1994).

Approximately 20% of patients with inflammatory bowel disease (either ulcerative colitis or Crohn's disease) develop spondyloarthritis (Scarpa *et al.* 1992*a*). Inflammatory bowel disease itself is not associated with B27, but approximately 50% of patients with associated spondylitis are B27 positive. A recent association with DR1*0103 and colitic arthritis is consistent with findings of a DR1 association and ankylosing spondylitis (Roussomoustakakai *et al.* submitted). Terminal ileal inflammation has been found in ankylosing spondylitis patients (Leirisalo-Repo *et al.* 1994*b*), as has evidence of increased intestinal permeability (Smith *et al.* 1985). It has been postulated that increased intestinal permeability results in absorption of some arthritogenic factor in these diseases (Mielants and Veys 1995). Surprisingly, although B27 has not been associated with inflammatory bowel disease, B27 transgenic rats develop autoimmune colitis. When raised in a germfree environment they develop neither arthritis or colitis, although they do develop other diseases such as psoriasis and genital inflammation (also B27-related human diseases). This supports a role for gut flora in the development of gut inflammation and B27-associated arthritis (Taurog *et al.* 1994). Given this finding, it is surprising that colitic spondyloarthritis does not resolve following surgical removal of all inflamed intestinal segments in patients with either Crohn's disease or ulcerative colitis.

Clearly a considerable amount has been learnt about the structure and function of HLA class I molecules in general, and B27 in particular, and how it may induce arthritis. However, persuasive evidence for a mechanism to explain the association is still awaited. There is also a dearth of published research regarding other interacting genes, although there is strong evidence to suggest that they do exist and do play a significant role in this disease, as they have been shown to do in other autoimmune diseases such as type 1 diabetes (Davies *et al.* 1994). Better understanding of the genetic mechanisms for this disease, and, in turn, the disease pathogenesis, is the best hope for the development of effective prevention or treatment for ankylosing spondylitis and the other spondyloarthropathies.

13 Triggering mechanisms and T-cell responses in the spondylarthropathies

Joachim Sieper and Jürgen Braun

Introduction

The term spondylarthropathy (SpA) applies to a group of different, although closely related, diseases: ankylosing spondylitis (AS); reactive arthritis (ReA); a subset of psoriatic arthritis (PsA); arthritis/sacroiliitis in inflammatory bowel disease; and undifferentiated SpA. All these diseases have an HLA-B27 association, sacroiliitis, a characteristic type of peripheral joint involvement, enthesitis, and some extra-articular manifestations in common (Dougados *et al.* 1991*a*). Their pathogenesis is not clear, but the interaction of bacteria, T cells, and the HLA-B27 molecule seems to be important (Kingsley and Sieper 1993).

The detection of bacterial antigen in synovial fluid and synovial membrane in ReA (Granfors *et al.* 1989*a*; Schumacher *et al.* 1988), a specific T-cell response in synovial fluid to the triggering bacterium in ReA (Ford *et al.* 1981*a*; Gaston *et al.* 1989; Sieper *et al.* 1991), a better definition of the role of the MHC class I molecule in the immune response (Germain 1994), and results indicating that HLA-B27 might behave not simply as a restriction element (Chicz *et al.* 1993; Taurog *et al.* 1993) make the SpA group uniquely interesting among the immune-mediated diseases. They offer a special opportunity for evaluating the interaction between bacterial antigen, MHC molecule, and T cells which leads either to hypersensitivity (damage from the immune response rather than direct damage to cells by microbes) or to autoimmunity.

Although bacteria have been hypothesized to play a role in the aetiology of all subtypes of SpA (see discussion below), causative bacteria have only been identified in ReA. *Chlamydia trachomatis*, *Yersinia enterocolitica*, *Salmonella typhimurium*, *Campylobacter jejuni*, and *Shigella flexneri* are those most likely to induce ReA after a preceding urogenital or gastroenteral infection. Recently, ReA has also been described after a preceding infection of the respiratory tract with *Chlamydia pneumomiae*, but it does not seem to be a frequent cause of ReA (Braun *et al.* 1994*d*). The following discussion will concentrate on the urogenital/enteric bacteria because most information is available for them.

Triggering bacteria in reactive arthritis: common features and differences

In the past, the common features of these bacteria have been stressed, namely that these bacteria are either obligate (*Chlamydia* spp.) or facultative (enterobacteria) intracellular bacteria. However, attention should also be paid to the differences in the biology of these pathogens, since these may better explain the pathogenesis of ReA.

Biology of reactive arthritis-associated bacteria

The mucosal surface is the port of entry of all ReA-associated bacteria. This is true not only for the enterobacteria in the gut but also for *Chlamydia trachomatis* in the reproductive system, and for *Chlamydia pneumoniae* in the airways. The mucosal immune system of the gut is the best investigated, but the others may not be so different (Kaufmann 1993; Service 1994). The M cells in Peyer's patches of the gut are the major window for invasion. They are specialized cells that are free of the mucous layer that covers other intestinal epithelial cells. They pass antigen and microbes to underlying antigen-presenting cells (mainly macrophages) and lymphocytes. The macrophages serve not only as antigen-presenting cells but also as distributors of intracellular bacteria to distant sites, probably including joints. Many intracellular bacteria exploit this permeable window to penetrate the body.

Although entry through M cells seems to be common to Yersinia, Salmonella, and Shigella spp. they behave differently afterwards. Yersinia have been found on or inside M cells and phagocytes in Peyer's patches, but intracellular replication is not a major feature of their infection; they mainly multiply and persist extracellularly. Although macrophages are easily infected *in vitro* by Yersinia, the extent to which this organism resides within cells *in vivo* is less clear (Bliska *et al.* 1993; Heesemann *et al.* 1993). In contrast, Salmonellae are believed to be transported to other tissues from the gut only via intracellular traffic (Bliska *et al.* 1993). The same seems to be likely for *Chlamydia trachomatis*—an obligate intracellular bacterium which resides comfortably inside macrophages, fibroblasts, and epithelial cells. Shigellae also enter the body via the M cells, and subsequently they are found mainly inside resident macrophages (Perdomo *et al.* 1994). However, these infected macrophages are rapidly killed by apoptosis, making it unlikely that shigellae can persist intracellularly (Zychlinsky *et al.* 1992). In acute enteritis, mainly non-professional phagocytes are infected. Inside the cell the bacteria gain easy access to the cytoplasm where they multiply, destroy the host cell, and spread to other cells. After infection the shigellae are cleared from the body; chronic persistence is only rarely observed. Therefore it is likely that salmonella- and chlamydia-infected macrophages can reach the joint, while this is less likely although possible for yersinia, and unlikely for shigella.

HLA-B27 association for different bacteria in reactive arthritis

Although the HLA-B27 frequency in ReA is generally reported to lie between 60 and 80%, recent studies in epidemics reveal that there is considerable variation among different bacteria. It is striking that the HLA-B27 association in acute salmonella-induced ReA can be as low as 0% (Thomson *et al.* 1992), 22% (Thomson *et al.* 1995), and 33% (Mattila *et al.* 1994). In chlamydia-induced ReA a relative low HLA-B27 frequency of between 40 and 50% has also been reported (Kvien *et al.* 1994; Wollenhaupt and Zeidler 1990*b*). Furthermore, when Chlamydia trachomatis DNA was defected by PCR in the synovial fluid from patients with oligoarthritis, HLA-B27 was only found in 20% of cases (Bas 1995). In yersinia-induced ReA, HLA-B27 is found in 70–80% of patients (Herrlinger and Asmussen 1992; Leirisalo-Repo and Suoranta 1988). This may reflect ascertainment base: yersinia-induced ReA does not normally result from outbreaks, so only the more severe cases may be seen by rheumatologists. The highest HLA-B27 association of 80–90% is found in shigella-induced ReA, both during epidemics (Calin and Fries 1976; Finch *et al.* 1986; Sairanen and Tiilikainen 1975;

Simon *et al.* 1981; Stieglitz *et al.* 1989; van Bohemen *et al.* 1985) and in sporadic cases (Sieper *et al.* 1993*a*).

While the extent of the HLA-B27 association in acute ReA seems to depend on the initiating organism, HLA-B27 is a severity marker for all bacteria. This is especially true for sacroilitis, enthesitis, iritis, and to a lesser degree for chronic arthritis. On long-term follow-up studies of patients with ReA, radiologically determined sacroiliitis (15–35%), recurrent arthritis (10 to 20%) and acute iritis (about 8%) were found nearly exclusively in B27-positive patients with salmonella- and yersinia-induced ReA (Leirisalo-Repo 1994*a*; Leirisalo-Repo and Suoranta 1988; Leirisalo-Repo 1994; Thomson *et al.* 1995), and with an even higher frequency in patients with chlamydia-induced ReA (Leirisalo-Repo 1994*a*). In a small sample, 80% of individuals with shigella-induced B27-positive ReA had chronic symptoms after 10 years postinfection (Calin and Fries, 1976).

Bacteria in the joint: alive or dead?

If live bacteria persist in the joint, they might drive the inflammation independently from HLA-B27, and this arthritis might therefore be associated with a low HLA-B27 frequency. Although live persistence seems to be true for chlamydia (Bas *et al.* 1995; Nanagara *et al.* 1995; Taylor-Robinson *et al.* 1992), no bacteria-specific DNA or mRNA was detected in yersinia-induced ReA even when yersinia were found by immunocytochemical staining in synovial fluid (Nikkari *et al.* 1992). Continuing elevation of the yersinia-specific IgA levels in ReA argues for the persistence of Yersinia in the gut mucosa (De Koning *et al.* 1989), resulting in dead bacteria or bacterial protein possibly reaching the joint. At present, no data are available concerning the presence of salmonella- or shigella- DNA or-mRNA in the joint. As pointed out above, persistence seems to be unlikely for shigella.

T-cell responses to bacteria in spondylarthropathies

How do these considerations fit with the known facts about antigen-specific T-cell responses to these bacteria, in general, and especially in ReA? Although surprisingly little is known about the immune response to infection by these pathogens in humans, there is growing evidence that T cells play an important role in fighting these bacteria (Autenrieth 1992; Burmester *et al.* 1995; Kaufmann 1993; Kingsley and Panayi 1992; Kingsley and Sieper 1993). In general the immune system recognizes foreign antigen in a way dependent on its cellular location. The MHC class II antigen-processing pathway presents peptides, from proteins that are either extracellular or have access to the endosomal pathway to CD4 T cells. In contrast, the MHC class I processing pathway presents peptides, from proteins that are either cytosolic or nuclear (but able to enter the cytosol), to CD8 T cells (Germain 1994). However, it is becoming increasingly clear that such a strict dichotomy in the antigen-presenting pathway does not exist. It has been shown that a subset of antigen-presenting cells can also acquire and present exogenous antigens in MHC class I molecules (Rock 1996).

Proteins from extracellular pathogens or intracellular pathogens residing in vacuoles (like chlamydia, salmonella, and yersinia) are normally presented by pathway II, and pathogens with access to the cytoplasm (such as shigella) by pathway I. The ReA-triggering bacteria, salmonella (Pfeifer *et al.* 1993; Pope *et al.* 1994), yersinia (Hermann *et al.* 1993) and *Chlamydia trachomatis* (Beatty *et al.* 1994; Starnbach *et al.* 1994*b*) can also induce a CD8+ T-cell response. The possible mechanisms by which they might do so have been discussed (Rock 1996), but the relevance of CD8+ T cells to an effective immune response against these bacteria is unknown. One might speculate that the CD8 response will turn out to be as important for shigella (Sansonetti 1992) as it is for listeria (Brunt 1990) because of the similarity in the intracellular behaviour of these organisms. Therefore, in the context of the HLA-B27 association, the question arises whether an arthritogenic bacterial peptide presented by the MHC class I molecule HLA B27 to CD8+ T cells drives the pathogenesis.

CD4+ T-cell response

So far there is more evidence for a dominant role for CD4+ T cells than for CD8+ T cells in SpA. About twice as many CD4 T cells than CD8 T cells are present in the synovial fluid of ReA-patients (Braun *et al.* 1994*b*) and in the synovial membrane of the sacroiliac joint in AS (Braun *et al.* 1995*a*); the synovial T-cell proliferative response to bacteria is predominantly a CD4 one (Gaston *et al.* 1989). The antigen-specific, proliferative T-cell response to all the triggering bacteria is clearly higher in synovial fluid than in peripheral blood. This seems to result from a local T-cell expansion, probably driven by bacterial antigens residing in the joint. Limiting dilution analysis has shown that the frequency of antigen-specific T cells in synovial fluid lies between 1/600 and 1/5000, and is clearly greater than in peripheral blood (Sieper *et al.* 1993*b*). Although some authors found that the increased synovial fluid T-cell response was, at least in part, due to more effective presentation of bacterial antigens by synovial antigen-presenting cells (APCs), we were unable to detect any difference between APCs from peripheral blood and synovial fluid, suggesting that the origin of the APCs was not a critical feature (Sieper *et al.* 1993*b*). Another possible explanation for the increased T-cell proliferation response to bacteria seen in synovial fluid could be the greater number of CD45RO (memory) cells at that site than in blood. However, depletion of the CD45RA (naive) cells did not change the clear difference between synovial fluid and peripheral blood (Braun *et al.* 1994*c*). Therefore the most likely explanation for the high antigen-specific T-cell proliferation in synovial fluid is a higher antigen-specific T-cell frequency compared to peripheral blood, although a non-specific part (highly activated cells in synovial fluid) might also contribute to a minor extent.

Not only is the proliferative T-cell response to triggering bacteria in peripheral blood in ReA patients clearly lower compared with synovial fluid, but this response has also been reported to be even lower than in the peripheral blood of healthy controls (Hassell *et al.* 1994; Hermann *et al.* 1995; Inman *et al.* 1989). This has led to the assumption that an effective systemic response against these bacteria is somehow hampered in patients with SpA that should normally alleviate the spread of bacteria to the joint.

CD8+ T-cell response

It is much more difficult to find a CD8+ T-cell response to triggering bacteria in synovial fluid. None the less, a CD8+, B27-restricted T-cell response to yersinia (Hermann *et al.* 1993; Ugrinovic *et al.* 1997) and salmonella (Hermann *et al.* 1993) has been found with cloned T-cells or T-cell lines derived from the synovial fluid of ReA-patients. Oligoclonal T-cell receptor usage in these T-cell clones has been described, but its relevance to pathogenesis is not clear (Duchmann *et al.* 1996). A B27-restricted cytotoxic T-cell response to *Chlamydia trachomatis* has been demonstrated in the HLA-B27 transgenic mice (Kuon *et al.* 1997). Thus, although a CD8 response can be detected, it is not known whether it is of importance for mounting an effective immune response.

Immunodominant antigens

If the immune response is driven by a persistent bacterial antigen, this antigen could be one shared among all the pathogens which are implicated in the aetiology.

In many cases of ReA the triggering bacterium can be identified (and differentiated from other bacteria) by means of an antigen-specific proliferative response of synovial fluid T cells (Braun *et al.* 1994*d*; Ford *et al.* 1981*a*; Gaston *et al.* 1989; Sieper *et al.* 1991, 1992*a*, *b*, 1993*a*). Each bacterium possess several intracellular antigens that are recognized by CD4+ T cells. The membrane proteins important for the humoral response are usually not recognized by the synovial T cells of chlamydia- or yersinia-induced ReA patients (Deane *et al.* 1994; Hassell *et al.* 1993; Mertz *et al.* 1994). This correlates nicely with the downregulation of bacterial membrane proteins and the upregulation of the 60 kDa heat-shock protein (hsp) observed during persistent infection of cells with *Chlamydia trachomatis in vitro* (Beatty *et al.* 1993), a situation similar to that in arthritis. It has recently been shown that the intracellular protein concentration correlates directly with antigenicity in listeria infection, thus emphasizing the importance of the amount of protein expressed for immunodominance (Villanueva *et al.* 1994). As yet, no data regarding this question are available for ReA.

Among the immunodominant proteins of yersinia and chlamydia are the highly conserved ribosomal proteins L2 and L23, the 60 kDa heat shock protein, and the urease 19 kDa subunit of yersinia (Mertz *et al.* 1994, 1997; Probst *et al.* 1993*a*); the conserved 18 kDa histone-like protein and the 60 kDa heat-shock protein of *Chlamydia trachomatis* are also immunodominant in ReA (Deane *et al.* 1994). Thus the specificity of the CD4 response for each bacterium and the presence of different immunodominant antigens for chlamydia and yersinia argues against CD4 T cells recognizing a common bacterial antigen.

However, as with other bacteria such as listeria, the CD8 response is narrowly confined to a few proteins and often to only one epitope on each (Villanueva *et al.* 1994). This makes it more likely that CD8+ T cells would recognize a common epitope shared by different bacteria. It is less clear how frequently such an epitope is located on a protein that is also immunodominant for CD4 T cells. Several groups have recently reported on the CD8-responses to immunodominant peptides derived from the 13 kDa and 60 kDa hsp of yersinia (Sieper and Kingsley 1996; Ugrinovic *et al.* 1997), the yersinia 19 kDa hsp (Ackermann *et al.* 1995), and the 75 kDa hsp of *Chlamydia trachomatis* (Bowness *et al.* 1995). However, it is too early to judge the relevance of these findings, but it should be noted that all these peptides (except the 19 kDa one) are derived from conserved proteins.

Chlamydia and yersinia immunodominant proteins are not only highly conserved among different bacterial species but also between prokaryotes and eukaryotes. The L23 ribosomal protein has a 32% identity and an overall homology of 56% between yersinia and humans (Mertz *et al.* 1994). The B27-binding peptides derived from such proteins might be highly cross-reactive or even identical between man and bacteria, and presentation of such peptides by B27 could thus lead to autoimmunity via the presentation of 'mimetopes'. All the known immunodominant proteins of chlamydia and yersinia are nuclear and/or cytosolic. The hypothetical self-peptide might therefore be derived from a self-protein with a similar distribution, in which case it would be presented preferentially to CD8 T cells via the class I pathway.

T-cell cytokines

Undoubtedly cytokines are of crucial importance for mounting an effective immune response against intracellular bacteria. T_{H1} cells, mainly secreting IFN-γ, help to eliminate these bacteria, while T_{H2} cells, mainly secreting IL-4 and IL-10, prevent this (Paul 1994). Initially, T cells cloned from the synovial fluid of patients with ReA yielded a predominantly T_{H1} pattern (Schlaak *et al.* 1992; Simon *et al.* 1993). However, this may have resulted from bias introduced by the cloning procedure or from a less-sensitive method for detecting IL-4. More recently, synovial membranes from 9 patients with ReA and 12 patients with rheumatoid arthritis (RA) were analysed for IL-2, IFN-γ, IL-4, and IL-10 mRNAs using the polymerase chain reaction technique (PCR) and *in-situ* hybridization (ISH) (Simon *et al.* 1994). The crucial finding was that IFN-γ was found in both ReA and RA synovial membranes, while IL-4 was more often present in ReA compared with RA. This raises the possibility that IL-4 may mediate bacterial persistence in the joint by inhibiting the effects of IFN-γ. ISH revealed that only 1/1000 T cells were positive for IL-4 mRNA and 1/300 for IFN-γ, suggesting that quite a small number of T cells can orchestrate an immune response. The importance of an optimal IFN-γ concentration for the effective elimination of chlamydia and yersinia has recently been demonstrated *in vitro* (Beatty *et al.* 1993), and in mice (Autenrieth *et al.* 1994; Bohn *et al.* 1994). Therefore, in those cases of ReA and SpA where bacterial antigens are present in the joint, the appearance of IL-4 may indicate an ineffective immune response (Yin *et al.* 1997). The situation regarding T_{H1} and T_{H2} in autoimmunity is less clear, although here IL-4 might act beneficially by suppressing the inflammation (Liblau *et al.* 1995).

Hypotheses concerning the interaction of bacteria, T cells, and HLA-B27 in the pathogenesis of spondylarthropathies

(Table 13.1)

The strong association of HLA-B27 in SpA is the most challenging aspect from an immunological point of view. Despite considerable efforts, the riddle has not yet been solved. While older hypotheses, such as molecular mimicry for cross-reacting antibodies, are now less attractive (Lahesmaa *et al.* 1992*a*), five interesting new hypotheses based on new findings have emerged. These will be considered in the following discussion. While in the first three hypotheses HLA-B27 plays a crucial role as a restriction element for the stimulation of CD8 T cells, alternatives are discussed in the other two hypotheses.

Hypothesis I

The first possibility, the so-called arthritogenic-peptide theory, is that bacterial antigen persists in the joint and is presented by HLA-B27 to CD8 T cells which then mediate immunopathology (Hermann *et al.* 1993). This mechanism is known to be operative in chronic

Table 13.1 Role of HLA-B27 in the pathogenesis of spondyloarthropathies

Hypothesis	Possible mechanisms
I. B27 presents persistent bacterial antigen to CD8 cells	One or a few arthritogenic epitopes expressed by triggering bacteria
II. B27 presents self-antigens to CD8 T cells	Cross-reactivity with a conserved bacterial epitope
III. B27 inhibits the protective antibacterial CD8+ immune response: dominant CD4 response causes disease	a. B27 molecule is not directly involved. Rather, a molecule encoded by a B27-linked gene interferes with the normal processing of bacterial antigen b. B27 captures the protective epitope(s) from other potentially more effective class I MHC molecules c. B27-restricted CD8 repertoire is biased towards inhibitory (TH2) cytokines
IV. B27-derived peptides presented by MHC class II molecules become the target of autoimmune attack by CD4 T cells	A cross-reacting bacterial peptide induces a response to a B27 peptide not normally recognized by CD4 T cells
V. B27 inhibits or otherwise alters bacterial entry into cells and/or clearance *in vivo*	B27 competes with a surface integrin molecule for binding bacteria (yersinia)

Modified, with permission, from Sieper and Braun (1995)

immune responses to some low cytopathic viruses, such as hepatitis B and lymphocytic choriomeningitis virus (LCMV), with consequent tissue destruction (Zinkernagel 1993).

Hypothesis II

This is another version of the arthritogenic-peptide theory. It assumes that autoimmunity is evoked by bacteria cross-reacting in the joint with self-antigens which are presented by HLA-B27 to CD8 T cells. Although cross-reactivity between bacterial peptides and self-peptides at the humoral level is unlikely (Lahesmaa *et al.* 1992*a*), such cross-reactivity could occur at the T-cell level and could result in the breakage of tolerance (or 'termination of ignorance') leading to autoimmunity. Under certain circumstances peptides from different proteins can cross-react even if they share only two or three critical positions in the peptide nonamer (Selin *et al.* 1994). How tolerance can be broken has been shown nicely with mice transgenic for the LCMV-glycoprotein gene linked to an insulin promoter, which is expressed exclusively in the insulin-producing cells of the pancreatic islets (Oldstone *et al.* 1991). Autoimmune diabetes occured only when these animals were infected with live LCMV, in which case the T cells invading the islets were mainly anti-LCMV CD8+. Additional proteins of the virus were evidently needed to break tolerance, presumably by generating inflammation, and possibly via intermolecular help (Zinkernagel *et al.* 1990). Recently, a possible instance of such a cross-reactivity in a human disease has been presented: DR2-restricted T-cell clones, derived from patients with multiple sclerosis, that are responsive to the immunodominant epitope of myelin basic protein cross-react with viral peptides from common viruses such as the Epstein–Barr virus (Wucherpfennig and Strominger 1995). These viruses may have driven the initial expansion of the T cell and, because of long-term viral persistence, might continuously or repeatedly activate these autoreactive T cells. Interestingly, a cytotoxic T-cell response to collagen type II derived self-peptides has been reported in a SpA patient (Gao *et al.* 1994).

Hypothesis III

A third possibility, although less likely, is that the CD8 response is crucial for eliminating the bacterial antigen, and is somehow inhibited in B27-positive individuals, failure of which might permit an ongoing stimulation of CD4 T cells, which, in turn, could mediate immunopathology in the joint. It has been shown in one family that B27-positive members could not present certain peptides which are normally presented by B27 molecules to T cells (Pazmany *et al.* 1992; Rowland-Jones *et al.* 1993). As this was not due to a defect in the B27 molecule itself, an alteration in antigen processing or transportation genetically linked to the B27 gene, or coincidentally inherited, has been suggested. Differences between disease and healthy controls in the proteasome genes, which are responsible for protein degradation in the cytoplasm, or in the TAP (transporter associated proteins) genes, responsible for the transport of peptides through the endoplasmic reticulum, have not yet been found. However, such a difference is not excluded and, furthermore, other as yet ill-defined mechanisms might lead to qualitatively or quantitatively different epitope presentation (Villanueva *et al.* 1994).

Another version of this hypothesis is that B27 itself does not present an arthritogenic antigen effectively to CD8 T cells. This could act either through competition for an epitope with the other MHC class I molecules present, or through competition of different epitopes for HLA-B27 (Sercarz *et al.* 1993). Regarding the first possibility, a hierarchy of peptide affinities for different MHC class II molecules has been suggested to explain the complex MHC class II genetics of insulin-dependent diabetes mellitus (Nepom 1990). This hypothesis could also apply to MHC class I molecules. Protection against a microorganism would fail if a dominant peptide has a higher affinity for B27, but it could induce an effective immune response if presented by another MHC class I molecule. In this case, the immune response would depend on which other MHC class I molecules were present besides B27. It has been reported recently that competition among class I MHC molecules for the same peptide can alter the immune response. Co-expression of HLA-B8 and HLA-B*2702 prevented the presentation of influenza-derived immunodominant peptides by HLA-B8 to CD8 T cells, by competition for the peptide occuring between the two HLA class I molecules (Tussey *et al.* 1995). A higher susceptibility to AS in B27-positive individuals has indeed been reported provided that HLA-Bw60 is also present (Robinson *et al.* 1989).

A further version of this hypothesis is that the B27-restricted CD8 response is somehow biased towards inhibitory (in this context presumably TH2) cytokines (Erard and LeGros 1994).

Does HLA-B27 as a restriction element play a role in the pathogenesis of SpA?

Taken together, the presence of bacterial antigen in the joint and an antigen-specific CD4 T-cell response argues for locally persistent bacterial antigen driving the immune response in ReA. Although a CD8 response against these bacteria remains possible, the failure to detect live yersinia in the joint and the improbability of chronic shigella persistence cast doubt on the hypothesis of a bacterium-derived arthritogenic peptide presented by HLA-B27 being responsible for a chronic immune response. Rather an acute CD8 T-cell response to a bacterial peptide could trigger a B27-restricted chronic cytotoxic T-cell response to a cross-reacting self-peptide.

Why is the presence or absence of live organisms in the joint so informative? In general, only proteins (and not, for example, lipopolysaccharide (LPS)) can induce such specific T-cell responses as seen in ReA, and it is highly improbable that proteins could remain undegraded inside cells for months or years. Although there is some debate about how long the immune system can maintain memory without being restimulated by antigen (Matzinger 1994), the higher bacteria-specific T-cell frequency in synovial fluid compared to peripheral blood argues for a local persistence of bacterial antigen (Sieper *et al.* 1993).

In addition to the different biologies of the ReA-associated bacteria, we also have to take into account the pathogenesis of the other SpAs. Recent evidence indicates that AS occurs in 20–30% of patients 20 years after the first manifestation of ReA (Leirisalo-Repo, personal communication). Considering that many, if not most, of the preceding infections in ReA can be asymptomatic, ReA-associated bacteria could also play an important role in the pathogenesis of AS. Other bacteria discussed are gut bacteria such as *Klebsiella* spp. which may gain access to the circulation because of a mucosa damaged by inflammatory bowel disease, and also in AS where gut lesions are often found. Correlation of an elevated humoral response to klebsiella, but not to other gut bacteria, with gut lesions argues in favour of a role for klebsiella in the pathogenesis of AS, and possibly also of arthritis in inflammatory bowel disease (Granfors *et al.* 1995*b*; O'Mahony *et al.* 1992; Sahly *et al.* 1994*b*). However, a convincing T-cell response to klebsiella has not been demonstrated in SpA (Geczy *et al.* 1986; Hermann *et al.* 1995). In any case, these bacteria are extracellular and should therefore preferentially be presented by MHC class II molecules to CD4+ T cells, although a presentation by MHC class I is not excluded (as mentioned above). The same could be true for streptococci or other bacteria which could pass the barrier through psoriatic skin lesions.

Therefore other pathogenetic models should be considered in which CD8 T cells do not play a dominant role.

Hypothesis IV

Another possible form of autoimmunity is suggested by a few recent findings:

1. Naturally processed self-peptides extracted from MHC class II molecules consist predominantly of peptides derived from MHC molecules expressed on the same cell. Furthermore, MHC-derived promiscuous self-peptides, capable of binding to multiple HLA-DR alleles, have been identified. Which self-peptide from which MHC molecule is presented by MHC class II molecules depended on the HLA type (Chicz *et al.* 1993). In another study, self-peptides eluted from HLA-DR4 molecules were derived mainly from HLA class I heavy-chain molecules, preferentially from HLA-B molecules (Hayden and Davey 1994).
2. The B27 transgenic rat SpA model depends on a high-copy number of B27 genes (Taurog *et al.* 1993); and SpA can be transferred to low-copy B27 transgenic rats only by bone-marrow cells expressing a high density of B27 molecules on their surface (Breban *et al.* 1993). T-cell transfer is ineffective, but T cells are needed for the rats to develop the disease (Breban *et al.* 1996). Furthermore, germfree animals do not become ill, indicating that bacteria are needed either to be presented by HLA-B27 or to break tolerance to self-antigens (Taurog *et al.* 1994).

3. B27 transgenic mice have been reported not to develop arthritis unless they also lack the murine β2m gene (Khare *et al.* 1995), although others have described arthritis in B27 transgenic mice with intact β2m (Weinreich *et al.* 1995). The $\beta 2m^{-/-}$ B27 transgenic mice express only low amounts HLA-B27 on their cell surface, making B27-restricted stimulation of CD8 T cells unlikely for the explanation of the immunopathology found in these animals (Khare *et al.* 1995*b*).

Based on these findings, a hypothesis based on the presentation by MHC class II molecules of B27-derived peptides is worth considering. This could depend on the MHC class II allele (an HLA-DR1 association in AS patients has recently been described: P. Wordsworth, personal communication) and/or on the level of HLA-B27 expression, as in the B27-transgenic rat model. The differential expression of MHC class I genes in human tissues has been reported (Daar *et al.* 1984; Garrido *et al.* 1993), and a role in the pathogenesis of diabetes mellitus postulated (Faustman *et al.* 1991). However, the importance of this for the pathogenesis of diseases is less clear. We have reported that HLA-B27 is expressed in inflamed tissue of the sacroiliac joint (Braun *et al.* 1995*a*), but the level of expression in different tissues of B27-positive patients or in B27-positive patients versus healthy B27-positive controls has not been compared. One study performed with peripheral blood mononuclear cells found no significant difference (Creamer *et al.* 1992). Differential B27 expression on cell surfaces could be due to polymorphism in the promotor region, as has been proposed for the W, X, and Y boxes in the promoter-proximal region of MHC class II genes (Benoist *et al.* 1990; Yao *et al.* 1993).

Tolerance to B27 could be broken by cross-reactivity between B27 peptides and bacterial peptides. In this context, two recent reports are of interest which demonstrate that B27 peptides show the highest homology of all MHC class I molecules to Gram-negative enteric bacteria (Scofield *et al.* 1993), and that the 2 Md-plasmid of Shigella, which shows some homology with HLA-B27, was present only in arthritogenic but not in non-arthritogenic shigellae (Stieglitz *et al.* 1993). Support for a crucial role of B27-derived peptides in the pathogenesis of SpA also comes from a study showing the reactivity of peripheral blood mononuclear cells to a B27 peptide in patients with B27-associated uveitis (a disease related to SpA), but not in controls. Furthermore, in an animal model of experimental uveitis oral tolerance could be induced by feeding these animals with the same B27 peptide (Wildner *et al.* 1993). We have recently presented preliminary evidence that a T-cell response can be found in B27-positive individuals against a specific B27-derived self-peptide (Sieper *et al.* 1995).

An alternative possibility, not invoking cross-reactivity, is that cryptic or latent self-epitopes in the B27 molecule or other self-molecules become able to provoke a response as a result of non-specific inflammation (Sercarz *et al.* 1993). This could occur, for example, after bacterial infection or trauma. The hypothesis that B27-derived peptides are presented by MHC class II in the pathogenesis of the spondyloarthropathies has recently been discussed in detail by Parham (1997).

Hypothesis V

Still another possibility could be the interference of invading bacteria with HLA-B27. Although there have been conflicting reports about whether HLA-B27 inhibits bacterial invasion of a cell leading to an assumed inhibition of bacterial elimination (Kapasi and Inman

1992) or not (Granfors *et al.* 1995*a*), preliminary data from an *in vivo* model of HLA-B27 transgenic mice given yersinia intragastrically support the former possibility (Ismail and Inman 1994). These mice showed increased persistence of extracellular yersinia in the early stages of infection and yersinia remained detectable in the gut and the spleen, but not in the joints, at 2 weeks when no bacteria could be found in controls. This inhibitory effect on invasion was mediated by competitive binding of the Yad-A protein of yersinia with either cell-surface integrin or the ME1 epitope of HLA-B27. These observations await confirmation.

Recently, yet another possible relationship between bacteria and HLA-B27 was proposed (Ikawa and Yu 1995). Bacterial infection of B27-transfected cells might lead to an induction of cytokines and to an increase in the expression of total HLA-B27. Furthermore, an increase in the transcription of the LMP2 gene of the proteasome complex, as a consequence of the infection, resulted in a change of the peptide repertoire of the HLA-B27 molecule. Thus bacterial infection of a cell could have a non-specific effect on HLA molecules which might be relevant for Hypothesis IV discussed above.

Summary and conclusions

Based on the data presented above, the following ideas about the pathogenesis of SpA are postulated. (Fig. 13.1).

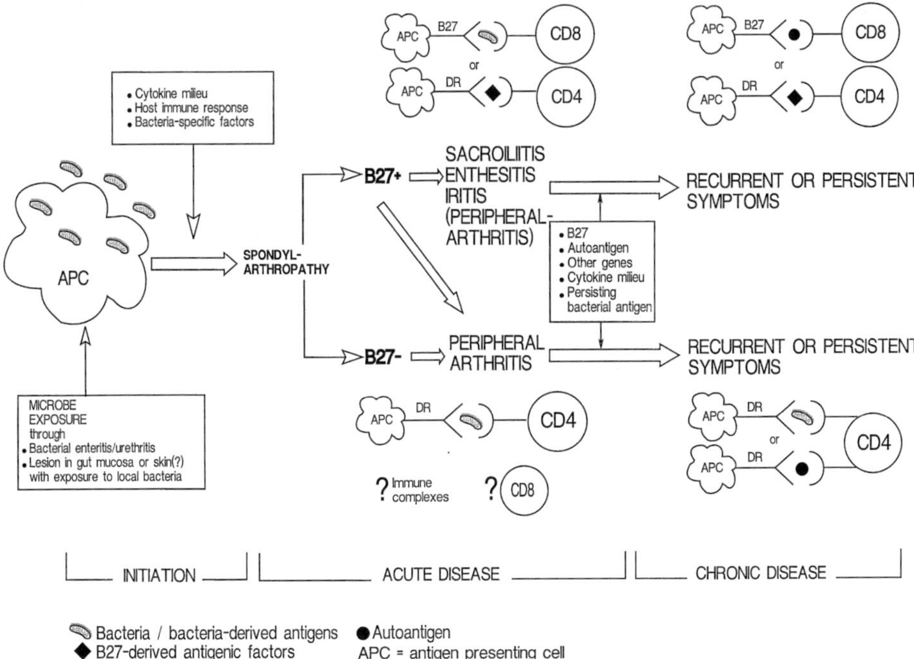

Fig. 13.1 Exposure to microorganisms leads to synovitis of peripheral joints in both HLA-B27 positive and HLA-B27-negative patients, while features such as sacroiliitis, enthesitis, and iritis occur in spondylarthropathies predominantly among B27-positive patients. In synovitis, a CD4+ T-cell response to a local bacterial antigen (either persistent in the joint or constantly transported from elsewhere) seems to be important, whereas for the other features (including chronic synovitis in B27-positive patients) other mechanisms, especially autoimmunity, may be more relevant. Modified, with permission, from Sieper and Kingsley (1996).

Peripheral arthritis is special among the manifestations of SpA. In ReA, peripheral arthritis frequently occurs independently from HLA-B27, perhaps more so if live bacteria persist in the joint (chlamydia) or elsewhere (yersinia). If the infection is only short-lived and bacterial peptides gain access to the joint only temporarily, as can be assumed for shigella infections, HLA-B27 seems to play a more critical role in the development of arthritis, as it does with all triggering bacteria in the case of severe chronic arthritis and for other SpA-specific features such as sacroiliitis, enthesitis, iritis. Chronic arthritis also occurs in B27-negative patients if the triggering bacterium persists inside the joint, as has been shown repeatedly for chlamydia. In this respect, ReA resembles the peripheral arthritis in inflammatory bowel disease and psoriatic arthritis, which has a low HLA-B27 association, and in which a constant supply of bacterial products from the gut or the skin might play a pathogenetic role. The immune response in this type of synovitis may well be explained by a primarily CD4+ T-cell response to bacterial antigen, although a convincing bacteria-specific T-cell response in any of the other SpA besides ReA has not yet been demonstrated. Therefore another pathogenetic mechanism such as immune complexes (containing bacterial antigen from the gut) could be relevant for B27-negative peripheral arthritis. At this stage of the disease, regulatory cytokines, either T_{H1} or T_{H2} or both, might play a role (possibly independently from HLA-B27) in the manifestation and/or the chronicity of peripheral arthritis. Other factors might also be relevant (Fig. 13.1).

Persistence of bacteria in all affected structures seems to be an unlikely explanation for the chronic symptoms of SpA. Rather, it can be assumed that bacteria trigger an autoimmune response. Progress is being made both in the identification of bacteria-derived immunodominant antigens (common for different pathogenetic bacteria) and for as yet unidentified autoantigens for CD4+ and CD8+ T cells. Candidate proteins are those that are highly conserved such as heat-shock proteins, ribosomal proteins, and histone-like proteins. The hypotheses concerning the interaction of bacteria, T cells, and HLA-B27 (mainly for chronic SpA) presently favoured by the authors include: (1) the classical arthritogenic peptide theory involving B27-restricted CD8+ T-cell recognition of self-(rather than bacterial) peptides (Hypothesis III); and (2) the presentation of B27-derived peptides by MHC class II antigens to CD4+ T cells (Hypothesis IV).

14 Mechanisms of arthritis associated with chronic intestinal inflammation

Ulrich Böcker and R. Balfour Sartor

Peripheral arthritis and spondylarthritides are part of a characteristic spectrum of systemic inflammation which accompanies numerous forms of clinical and experimental intestinal inflammatory disorders (Table 14.1) (Sartor and Lichtman 1994). These extraintestinal manifestations, which include arthritis, hepatobiliary inflammation, erythema nodosum, pyoderma gangrenosum, and uveitis, occur in approximately 20–30% of patients with Crohn's disease, ulcerative colitis, and jejunoileal bypass for obesity (Lichtman and Sartor 1994), but are relatively infrequent in the other clinical conditions listed in Table 14.1. Although the aetiologies of the underlying clinical intestinal diseases are different, these disorders share important common features which contribute to the systemic manifestations, namely:

(1) increased mucosal permeability (ulcerative colitis, Crohn's disease, coeliac disease, and collagenous colitis);

(2) relatively persistent bacterial infections (enteric pathogens, Whipple's disease, diverticulitis); or

(3) overgrowth of predominantly anaerobic bacteria (jejunoileal, gastric, or biliary surgical bypass and pouchitis).

Of considerable interest, rodent models of arthritis accompanying experimental intestinal inflammation (Table 14.1) also exhibit enhanced mucosal permeability and/or overgrowth of luminal anaerobic bacteria. In addition, experimental models clearly illustrate the influence of the host genetic background on the incidence, chronicity, and aggressiveness of intestinal and joint inflammation. These observations suggest that resident bacteria play a dominant role in the pathogenesis of arthritis and spondylarthritides that complicate a genetically susceptible host with intestinal inflammation. This chapter discusses clinical and experimental evidence to

Table 14.1 Association of arthritis with intestinal inflammation

Clinical syndromes		Experimental models
Crohn's disease	Jejunoileal bypass	HLA-B27 transgenic rats
Ulcerative colitis	Pouchitis	PG–PS-induced enterocolitis
Coeliac disease	Bacterial overgrowth	Small bowel bacterial-overgrowth (reactivation)
Enteric pathogen[a]	Diverticulitis	Vitamin A-deficient rats
Whipple's disease	Collagenous colitis	Pigs on high-protein diet

[a] Arthritis is frequently associated with *Yersinia* (especially *Y. enterocolitica*), *Shigella*, *Salmonella*, and *Campylobacter spp.*; and infrequently with *Clostridium difficile*, *Giardia*, Amoeba, *Strongyloides*, and *Taenia saginata*.

support the potential mechanisms of arthritis which accompany idiopathic intestinal inflammation and develops a unifying hypothesis to explain this intriguing relationship. Mechanisms of reactive arthritis and spondylarthritides due to enteric pathogens are discussed in previous chapters.

Clinical observations regarding the relationship between intestinal and joint inflammation

Crohn's disease and ulcerative colitis, collectively referred to as idiopathic inflammatory bowel diseases (IBD), are frequently complicated by peripheral and axial arthritis with distinct features (Lichtman and Sartor 1994). Peripheral arthritis occurs without gender preference in 6–20% of patients with IBD (Finch 1989; Gravallese and Kantrowitz 1988; Rankin 1990) and is slightly more frequent in Crohn's disease than in ulcerative colitis. An abrupt onset of non-erosive arthritis is characteristic, predominantly affecting the large joints in an asymmetrical, migratory pattern, with resolution of the majority of cases within 2 months (McEwen *et al.* 1962; Wright and Watkinson 1965*a*). There is no association of peripheral arthritis with possession of the HLA-B27 antigen. Stein *et al.* (1993) reported that 44% of patients with Crohn's disease complained of arthralgia, but only 7% had objective evidence of arthritis. Although the percentage of control patients with arthralgias was similar (46%), the location of pain differed. Control patients complained of back pain in contrast to knee, hip, and wrist involvement in Crohn's patients. Similarly, results of a recent questionnaire demonstrate joint symptoms in 31% of IBD patients (Yahia *et al.* 1996).

Peripheral arthritis correlates with the extent and activity of intestinal inflammation and the presence of colonic rather than small intestinal disease. For example, in the classic study of Greenstein *et al.* (1976), the incidence of arthritis was 26% for ulcerative colitis, 39% for colonic Crohn's disease, 26% for ileocolitis, and 14% for isolated ileitis. Arthritis independently correlates with the extent of colonic inflammation. Wright and Watkinson (1959) documented this correlation by observing arthritis in 22% of patients with extensive ulcerative colitis (transverse colon or greater extent), 12% with left-sided colitis, but only 5% of patients with isolated proctitis. Similarly, Monsen *et al.* (1990) reported that 70% of patients with arthritis had extensive colitis but only 3% had isolated proctitis. Like erythema nodosum and iritis/uveitis, peripheral arthritis is an activity-related extraintestinal manifestation (Table 14.2). It mirrors the activity of the underlying bowel disease, rarely precedes the onset of gut inflammation or follows colectomy, and resolves with total proctocolectomy. The improvement of arthritis after intestinal resection is less apparent in Crohn's disease than in ulcerative colitis, possibly due to persistent or recurring intestinal lesions (Neumann and Wright 1983; van Patter *et al.* 1954). In addition, activity-related extraintestinal manifestations tend to occur

Table 14.2 Correlation of activity of extraintestinal manifestations and idiopathic inflammatory bowel diseases

Activity related:	Peripheral arthritis, erythema nodosum, iritis/uveitis, anaemia
Intermediate:	Pyoderma gangrenosum
Activity unrelated:	Ankylosing spondylitis, sacroiliitis, sclerosing cholangitis

simultaneously in patients with IBD. Monsen *et al.* (1990) reported that 39% of patients with activity-related disorders had multiple complications. For example, 70% of patients with iritis had an associated condition, most frequently arthritis. In Rice-Oxley and Truelove's (1950) description of 129 patients with ulcerative colitis, 42% with skin manifestations had arthritis and 83% of the patients with arthritis presented with skin involvement. Similar observations have been made for the coexistence of erythema nodosum and arthritis (Bywaters and Ansell 1958; Wright and Watkinson 1965*a*).

Axial joint involvement in IBD includes sacroiliitis and ankylosing spondylitis, which are more frequent in Crohn's disease (5–22%) than in ulcerative colitis (2–6%) (Gravallese and Kantrowitz 1988; Schorr and Brandt 1988; Yahia *et al.* 1996). In contrast to idiopathic ankylosing spondylitis, females with IBD are as likely to develop ankylosing spondylitis as males. Furthermore, an increased prevalence of ankylosing spondylitis has been shown for relatives of patients with IBD. Symmetrical sacroiliitis, which is usually asymptomatic, is found radiologically in 5–16% of patients with IBD, but in 18–50% by the more sensitive technetium pyrophosphate scan (Davis *et al.* 1978) and in 32% by CT scan (McEniff *et al.* 1995). It is independent of the HLA status (Hyla *et al.* 1976). Ankylosing spondylitis, however, strongly correlates with the expression of the HLA-B27 antigen, although the 50–70% B27-positivity in IBD-related ankylosing spondylitis is far less than the 90–95% association of HLA-B27 with idiopathic ankylosing spondylitis (Brewerton *et al.* 1974; Russell 1977). Axial joint inflammation is related to the extent of intestinal disease but to a lesser degree than peripheral arthritis (Wright and Watkinson 1965*b*). Neither sacroiliitis or spondylitis parallel the activity of bowel inflammation nor respond to colectomy, in contrast to peripheral arthritis.

The high frequency of clinically silent gut lesions in spondylarthritides (Table 14.3) have led Mielants and colleagues (1988, 1996) to postulate that a significant proportion of patients with 'idiopathic' spondylarthropathies have subclinical Crohn's disease. These results have been confirmed by Leirisalo-Repo *et al.* (1994*b*), who detected endoscopic gut lesions in 44% of 118 patients with various inflammatory and non-inflammatory joint diseases. Mielants *et al.* (1995*b*) identified predominantly chronic histological gut lesions in 68% of spondylarthropathy patients who underwent ileocolonoscopy, with no apparent influence of non-steroidal anti-inflammatory drugs. Furthermore, in prospective studies, these authors identified risk factors for patients with sacroiliitis or ankylosing spondylitis to develop Crohn's disease, which occurred in approximately 6% of patients overall, but in 20% of patients with chronic histological inflammation (Mielants *et al.* 1995*b*). These risk factors included persistently elevated inflammatory serum markers, chronic inflammatory gut lesions by histology, and absence of HLA-B27.

Table 14.3 Occult ileocolitis associated with the spondylarthritides

Clinical syndrome	% prevalence
Ankylosing spondylitis	65
Undifferentiated spondylarthritides	70
Juvenile chronic arthritis	75
Psoriatic arthritis	16
Anterior uveitis	66

Experimental models of arthritis associated with chronic intestinal inflammation

Several rodent models of intestinal inflammation have associated peripheral arthritis (Table 14.1). In each model, intestinal disease generally precedes articular involvement, suggesting that the arthritis is dependent on gut inflammation or increased permeability. Detailed reviews of these models have been recently published (Sartor *et al.* 1996*b*) and some are covered in Chapter 15 of this text, but this present chapter provides an overview upon which to illustrate mechanisms of joint inflammation. These models firmly incriminate normal enteric bacteria, bacterial products, and host genetic susceptibility in the pathogenesis of arthritis associated with intestinal inflammation.

B27 transgenic rats

Rats transgenic for HLA-B27 and human β_2 microglobulin spontaneously develop enterocolitis which is associated with multiorgan systemic inflammation in joints, skin, nails, testes, heart, and stomach (Hammer *et al.* 1990*b*). Disease susceptibility correlates with the level of expression of HLA-B27 and is dependent, to some degree, on genetic background (Hammer *et al.* 1995; Taurog *et al.* 1993, 1996). Non-bloody diarrhoea is first detected around 2 months of age and is associated with a thickened colon with histological features of mucosal hyperplasia, decreased numbers of goblet cells, mononuclear cell infiltration of the lamina propria, and rare crypt abscesses. Arthritis is detectable by 3 months of age in the ankle joints with an incidence of 70% and persists for several days to months (Hammer *et al.* 1990*b*; Taurog *et al.* 1993). Histological features include chronic synovial inflammation with hyperplasia, bony erosions, and neutrophils in the joint space (Fig. 14.1(a)). Disease can be transferred by bone marrow, fetal liver, and either CD4+ or CD8+ lymphocytes (Breban *et al.* 1993, 1996). Importantly, neither arthritis nor colitis occurs when B27 transgenic rats are raised in a sterile environment (Taurog *et al.* 1994) and disease can be attenuated with metronidazole therapy (Rath *et al.* 1996*b*).

PG–PS/blind loop syndrome

Inflammation in ankle joints previously injured with the bacterial cell-wall polymer, peptidoglycan–polysaccharide (PG–PS), is reactivated by experimental bacterial overgrowth in response to a surgically created jejunal self-filling blind loop (SFBL) in Lewis rats (Lichtman *et al.* 1995). Arthritis peaks 4–7 days after surgery and gradually subsides over the next 8 weeks; no arthritis occurs in sham-operated rats or those with self-emptying blind loops which have only moderate increases in luminal bacteria (10^{4-5} bacterial/ml vs. 10^{8-9} predominantly anaerobic bacteria/ml in the self-filling blind loop). Histological features include synovitis, mild pannus formation, and tendonitis, but only mild joint destruction (Fig. 14.1(b)). Joints previously injected with saline rather than PG–PS showed no evidence of inflammation despite the presence of enteric bacterial overgrowth. Luminal anaerobic bacteria are implicated, since metronidazole, but not gentamicin or polymyxin-B, prevents arthritis.

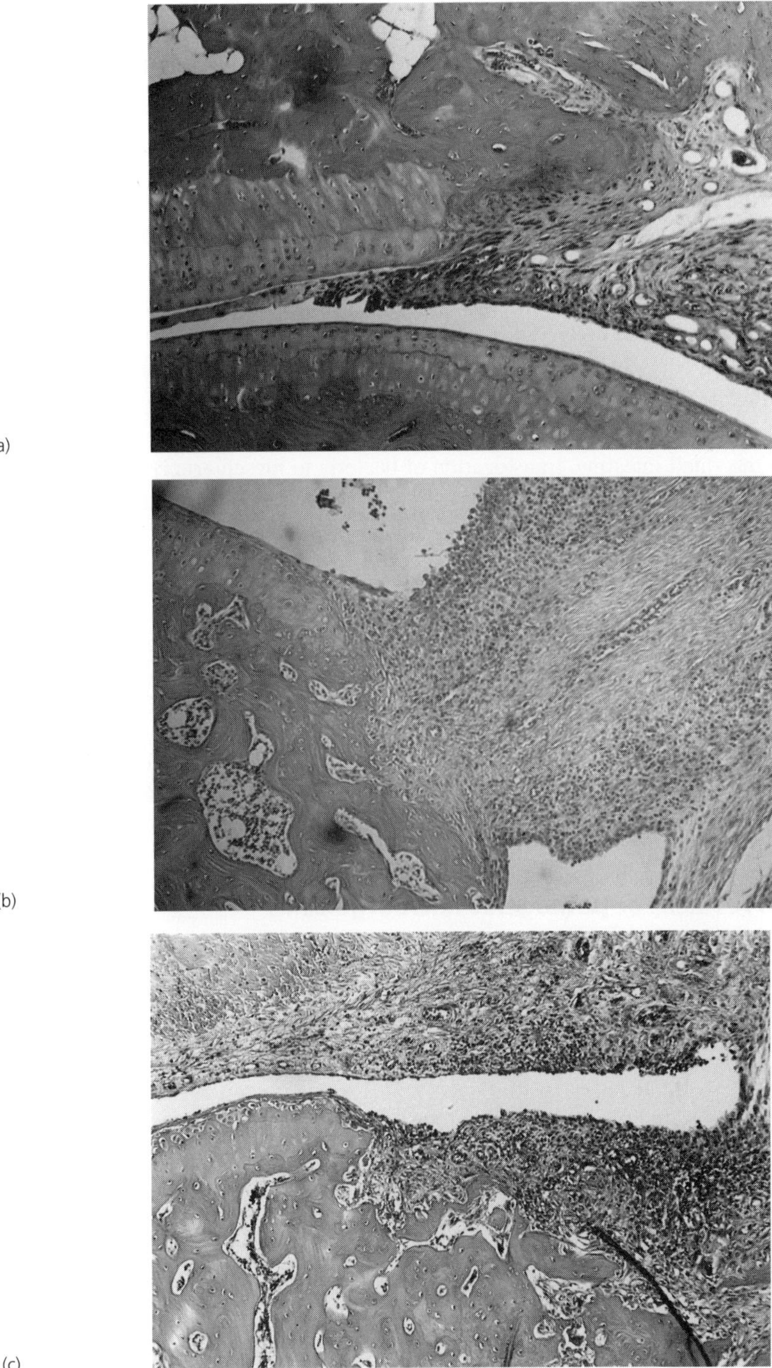

Fig. 14.1 Histological features of arthritis in ankle joints of rats with various forms of intestinal inflammation. (a) Ankle joint of an HLA-B27/β_2 microglobulin transgenic rat raised under conventional conditions. Synovitis, exudate, and articular erosions are present. (b) Marked synovitis in the tibiotalar joint of a Lewis rat injected with PG–PS 11 days prior to surgical creation of a self-filling blind loop, then killed 7 days after the loop was formed. (c) Marked erosive synovitis 6 weeks after ileocaecal injection of PG–PS in a Lewis rat. Reproduced from Sartor *et al.* (1996) with permission of Ballière Tindall.

Intramural PG–PS

Subserosal intramural injection of PG–PS into the distal ileum and caecum of Lewis rats leads to a biphasic granulomatous enterocolitis with associated arthritis, granulomatous hepatitis, anaemia, and leukocytosis that persists for at least 4 months (Sartor *et al.* 1996*b*). Approximately 10–20% of the rats develop acute, self-limited arthritis that peaks 5 days after gut PG–PS injection, but 80% develop chronic, progressively destructive arthritis that leads to ankylosis. Histological features include synovial hyperplasia, cartilage erosions with pannus formation, exudation of neutrophils into the synovial space, and periarticular granulomatous inflammation (Fig. 14–1(c)). The chronic granulomatous phase of enterocolitis and arthritis is T-lymphocyte mediated (Sartor *et al.* 1993).

Several additional models have been described which use dietary manipulations to alter intestinal flora. Pigs fed a high-protein diet develop an overgrowth of klebsiella spp. which leads to arthritis. Vitamin A deficient rats have decreased luminal IgA secretion, overgrowth of bacteria from the small intestine, translocation of bacteria to mesenteric lymph nodes, and associated arthritis (Wiedermann *et al.* 1995). Furthermore, Lewis rats infected with the enteric pathogen *Yersinia enterocolitica* 0:8 also develop combined gut and joint inflammation (Hill and Yu 1988).

Mechanisms of arthritis

A number of theories have been advanced to explain the association of arthritis with chronic intestinal inflammation (Table 14.4). Relevant clinical and experimental evidence supporting or refuting each mechanism is addressed in the context of current knowledge of IBD pathophysiology.

Infection with resident or pathogenic microorganisms

Simultaneous, bacteria-dependent intestinal inflammation and arthritis could be the result of:

(1) concurrent intestinal and joint infection;

(2) increased susceptibility of IBD patients to pathogens with a tropism for the articular surface; or

(3) increased mucosal permeability leading to translocation of resident luminal microflora or pathogens to the joint.

Table 14.4 Mechanisms of arthritis associated with intestinal inflammation

Mechanisms
Primary or secondary infection
Systemic distribution of luminal antigens and toxic bacterial products
Systemic distribution of inflammatory mediators and cytokines produced by the inflamed intestine
Immune complex deposition
Cell-mediated immune response
Autoimmune response
Genetically determined immunoregulatory defects

Although *Mycobacterium paratuberculosis, Listeria monocytogenes*, or measles have been postulated as aetiological agents in Crohn's disease (reviewed by Sartor *et al.* 1996*c*), there is no compelling evidence that a persistent infection with any pathogen causes the majority of cases of Crohn's disease. Moreover, none of these organisms is associated with reactive arthritis. Transient intestinal infections with a number of enteric pathogens, including *Yersinia, Salmonella, Shigella, and Campylobacter* spp., can exacerbate IBD (Sartor 1995*a*). However, there has been no association of these organisms with flares of arthritis or the presence of spondylarthropathy in IBD patients, although enteric infections are capable of reactivating quiescent idiopathic spondylarthritis (Rynes *et al.* 1984). An inability to identify viable bacteria or bacterial antigens from the synovial fluid of IBD patients with arthritis does not exclude transient early infection, particularly since persistently inflamed joints are sterile 1 month after experimental infection with *Y. enterocolitica* (Hill and Yu 1987) or *Salmonella enteritidis* (Volkman and Collins 1975). Arthritogenic potential has been closely related to the ability of *Y. enterocolitica* to persist in lymphatic tissues (Gaede and Heesemann 1995). To date, no such studies have been conducted in arthritis complicating IBD, although bacteria-specific T lymphocytes have been identified in reactive arthritis (Hermann *et al.* 1994), supporting the possibility of persistent antigenic challenge by arthritogenic pathogens.

In intestinal inflammation, there is convincing evidence of mucosal invasion by resident luminal bacteria and translocation of these organisms to mesenteric lymph nodes. However, viable bacteria are not routinely recovered from inflamed joints. Enteric bacteria were cultured from the serosa or mesenteric lymph nodes of 56% of resected Crohn's disease intestines compared with 17% of control tissues (Ambrose *et al.* 1984) and from portal venous blood of 27% of patients undergoing colectomy for ulcerative colitis (Brooke *et al.* 1961). Immunohistochemical evidence of *Escherichia coli* or streptococci in 62% of resected Crohn's disease specimens clearly documents secondary invasion of ulcerated tissues by resident luminal bacteria (Liu *et al.* 1995). Similarly, translocation of viable enteric bacteria to mesenteric lymph nodes develops in 66% of rats with experimental small-intestinal bacterial overgrowth vs. 25% of sham-operated controls (Lichtman *et al.* 1990). The most compelling evidence for a role of resident bacteria in the pathogenesis of enteric-associated arthritis, however, is that arthritis does not occur in the absence of luminal bacterial stimulation. Taurog and colleagues (1994) demonstrated that colitis and arthritis are absent in germfree (sterile) HLA-B27 transgenic rats. Rath *et al.* (1996*b*) incriminated anaerobic bacteria in this model by demonstrating that metronidazole attenuated colitis and arthritis and showed that, in selective colonization studies, *Bacteroides* species were preferentially involved. The latter investigation is particularly important because it documents that all resident flora do not have equal capacities to induce inflammation in this model. Lichtman *et al.* (1995) substantiated the role of anaerobic bacteria, especially *Bacteroides* spp., in the pathogenesis of arthritis associated with intestinal inflammation, by demonstrating that metronidazole completely prevented recurrence of arthritis in the SFBL model, coincidental with the elimination of luminal bacteroides. In these studies, there was no evidence of viable bacteria in the joints, although translocation of luminal *E. coli* in one-third of inflamed joints was evident in a dietary IgA deficiency model (Wiedermann *et al.* 1995).

Collectively, these studies convincingly document the ability of luminal bacteria to secondarily invade ulcerated intestinal tissues and incriminate resident flora in the pathogenesis of experimental enteric-associated arthritis, but viable bacteria are not routinely found within the inflamed joints. It is more likely that toxic or immunologically active constituents of resident luminal bacteria provide the arthropathic stimulus.

Systemic distribution of bacterial constituents

The lumen of the distal ileum and intact colon contains high concentrations of bacterial constituents and antigens capable of inducing local and systemic inflammation (reviewed by Sartor 1995*b*; Sartor *et al.* 1996*c*). PG–PS polymers, endotoxin (lipopolysaccharide, LPS) and chemotactic oligopeptides (formyl–met–leu–phe, FMLP) activate phagocytic cells (monocytes/macrophages and neutrophils) to secrete a wide variety of soluble inflammatory mediators, such as cytokines, reactive oxygen metabolites, nitric oxide, eicosanoids, and proteases, and can activate the complement and kallikrein/kinin cascades. Furthermore, systemic uptake of these phlogistic bacterial products is enhanced by intestinal inflammation due to increased mucosal permeability. Systemic endotoxaemia has been documented in 88% of patients with active ulcerative colitis and in 94% of relapsed Crohn's disease patients; moreover, plasma endotoxin levels correlate with the extent and activity of disease and with anti-LPS core-antigen IgG concentrations (Gardiner *et al.* 1995*a*). IBD patients with extraintestinal inflammation have increased plasma concentrations of FMLP (Anderson *et al.* 1991) and serum anti-peptidoglycan antibodies (Sartor *et al.* 1984) (Table 14.5), which are also found in ankylosing spondylitis (Park *et al.* 1984) and seronegative arthritis (Rahman *et al.* 1990). Similarly, systemic distribution of PG–PS, LPS, and FMLP is dramatically increased following experimental intestinal injury (Gardiner *et al.* 1995*b*; Hobson *et al.* 1988; Lichtman *et al.* 1991; Sartor *et al.* 1988). Indirect evidence that these bacterial products induce joint inflammation accompanying jejunoileal bypass for morbid obesity is provided by the provocative demonstration of radiolabelled bacterial cell walls in circulating immune complexes (Wands *et al.* 1976), *E. coli* antigen in dermal biopsies (Utsinger 1980), and exacerbation of arthritis with peptidoglycan skin tests (Ely 1980).

Rodent models clearly demonstrate that enteric bacterial cell-wall polymers can induce peripheral arthritis in genetically susceptible hosts (Schwab 1993). A single intraperitoneal injection of an aqueous suspension of sterile PG–PS polymers from group A streptococci produces acute synovitis in the ankle joints of rats. Susceptible strains, such as Lewis and Sprague–Dawley rats develop chronic, spontaneously relapsing erosive polyarthritis, which persists for up to 4 months. Chronicity of the response depends on the host genetic background and source of PG–PS. Poorly biodegradable PG–PS polymers from group A streptococci, *S. faecium* (enterococcus), certain *Eubacterium*, *Bifidobacterium*, and *Lactobacilli* species induce chronic arthritis, whereas PG–PS sensitive to lysozyme degradation, such as from *Peptostreptococci* and *Clostridium* species, produce transient or negligible joint inflammation (Severijren *et al.* 1989*a,b*; Stimpson *et al.* 1986). Of considerable interest, PG–PS from *Eubacterium contortum* isolated from a patient with Crohn's disease (Severijnen *et al.* 1989*a*) and PG–PS from an ileostomy effluent (Kool *et al.* 1991) had arthropathic properties.

Table 14.5 Evidence of systemic distribution of luminal bacterial components with intestinal inflammation

Crohn's disease:	↑ Mucosal permeability; bacterial translocation; endotoxaemia; T-cell and Ig responses to enteric bacteria, PG–PS, and LPS
Ulcerative colitis:	↑ Endotoxaemia, IgG response to LPS, T-cell response to enteric bacteria
Experimental enterocolitis:	↑ Bacterial translocation; plasma levels, LPS, PG–PS, FMLP; Ig responses to enteric bacteria, PG–PS; T-cell response to enteric flora

The acute phase of PG–PS-induced arthritis is mediated by complement, IL-1, and the kallikrein/kinin system (Sartor *et al.* 1996*a*; Schwab *et al.* 1991), whereas the chronic phase is T-cell mediated (Wahl *et al.* 1986), with input from the IL-1 and kallikrein/kinin systems (DeLa Cadena *et al.* 1995; Schwab *et al.* 1991). We have demonstrated that subserosal injection of PG–PS induced chronic granulomatous enterocolitis with erosive arthritis identical to the intraperitioneal PG–PS model (Sartor *et al.* 1996*b*). Once arthritis has been initiated by intraperitoneal or intra-articular injection of PG–PS, it can then be reactivated by homologous or heterologous PG–PS, LPS from enteric commensal or pathogenic organisms (*E. coli* or *S. typhimurium*), or bacterial superantigens in concentrations which fail to cause arthritis in naive joints (Schwab *et al.* 1993; Stimpson *et al.* 1987, 1988).

Lichtman *et al.* (1995) have manipulated the intra-articular reactivation model to demonstrate the ability of normal luminal bacterial PG–PS to reactivate arthritis in previously injured joints. Overgrowth of predominantly anaerobic bacteria in jejunal blind loops reactivates peripheral arthritis, apparently due to the systemic distribution of luminal PG–PS. Evidence for endogenous PG–PS involvement is provided by documentation of enhanced absorption of immunoreactive PG–PS polymers from the blind loop, detection of increased serum anti-PG–PS antibody, and the ability of mutanolysin, whose sole known function is to degrade the peptidoglycan polymer, to attenuate arthritis (Lichtman *et al.* 1992, 1995). The role of LPS in this model is less convincing due to the lack of beneficial effects of polymyxin B and anti-lipid A monoclonal-antibody treatments.

Although LPS was not linked to the jejunal bacterial-overgrowth arthritis model, other experimental systems demonstrate the ability of LPS to induce acute and chronic peripheral arthritis. Injection of LPS into rabbit knee joints provoked acute local inflammation indicated by leucocyte infiltration and loss of cartilage proteoglycan (Matsukawa *et al.* 1993). Furthermore, a biweekly subcutaneous injection of LPS or heat-killed *E. coli* in incomplete Freund's adjuvant induced chronic, hyperplastic synovitis in the ankles of rats, but little evidence of inflammation in the paw, elbow, and knees joints (Noyori *et al.* 1994).

Together, these studies indicate the ability of luminal bacterial constituents to cross the inflamed mucosa, to be systemically distributed, and to induce acute and chronic arthritis in genetically susceptible hosts. It is important to note the synergistic activities of PG–PS, LPS, and superantigens in the PG–PS reactivation model, as well as the ability of low doses of FMLP or LPS to trigger cytokine secretion or oxygen bursts by macrophages primed with LPS (Baldassano 1993), given the complex microenvironment of the distal intestine. The important question of organ specificity following systemic uptake of phlogistic bacterial cell-wall polymers is addressed by tropism of PG–PS to the joints (Chetty *et al.* 1982) and selective deposition of high molecular weight particles at the borderline between highly vascularized and avascular tissues such as joints, cardiac valves, and renal mesangium (Schulz *et al.* 1985). The distribution and phagocytosis of high molecular weight substances was altered following joint inflammation, which may explain the ability of circulating PG–PS and LPS to selectively reactivate previously injured joints and the observation that recurrent bouts of arthritis in patients with IBD tend to localize to those joints initially involved.

Systemic distribution of proinflammatory mediators from the intestine

A vast array of proinflammatory soluble mediators, such as cytokines, eicosanoids, reactive oxygen metabolites, nitric oxide (NO), proteolytic enzymes, and complement products, are generated in the intestine during the active stages of Crohn's disease, ulcerative colitis, and

Table 14.6 Reactivation of PG–PS-induced arthritis by soluble inflammatory mediators

Ability to reactivate:	
Interleukin-1	Platelet-derived growth factor
Interleukin-8	Substance P
Tumour necrosis factor-α	
Inability to reactivate:	
Interleukin-6	C_{5a}

experimental colitis (Sartor 1994). Increased circulating levels of tumour necrosis factor-α (TNF-α) and IL-6 have been documented during active IBD (Sartor 1995*d*), due either to the uptake of locally produced mediators from the inflamed intestine or to enhanced production of cytokines by activated circulating monocytes. Similarly, increased plasma levels of TNFα and NO metabolites have been reported in the jejunal self-filling blind loop and PG–PS enterocolitis models, respectively (Lichtman *et al.* 1993, Yamada *et al.* 1993). Paralleling the incidence of accompanying arthritis, IL-1 and TNF-α levels are higher in Crohn's colitis than ileitis (Isaacs *et al.* 1992; Murch *et al.* 1991).

A number of cytokines and neuropeptides (Table 14.6) can reactivate arthritis in joints previously injured by PG–PS at concentrations below those necessary to induce inflammation in naive joints (Stimpson *et al.* 1988*a,b*). Intra-articular injection of IL-1 or transforming growth factor-β TGF-β induces transient non-erosive arthritis, although systemic TGF-β attenuates acute and chronic phases of PG–PS-induced arthritis (Brandes *et al.* 1991). IL-1 and TNF-α can injure the joint by a variety of mechanisms, including activation of macrophages, fibroblasts, and synovial lining cells to secrete collagenase, elastase, proteoglycanase, plasminogen, and eicosanoids (Wahl 1991). The central role of cytokines in gut-associated arthritis is illustrated by the ability of recombinant IL-1 receptor antagonist or anti-TNF-α antibodies to completely inhibit the reactivation of arthritis by experimental, jejunal bacterial overgrowth (Lichtman *et al.* 1995). However, this protection by TNF-α and IL-1 blockade does not identify the source of cytokine production, which could be the gut, circulating monocytes, the joint, or any combination of the three.

Immune complexes

Detection of circulating immune complexes in IBD has yielded conflicting results, attributable both to the indirect methods used and to the prevalence of false-positive results in active IBD arising from the presence of low albumin, elevated globulins, and increased C-reactive protein (Soltis *et al.* 1979). Nevertheless, concentrations of circulating immune complexes have been reported to correlate with the activity of ulcerative colitis and Crohn's disease, to be associated with colonic involvement (47% Crohn's colitis, 28% ileocolitis, and 9% isolated small intestinal disease), and to be increased with concurrent arthritis (Hodgson *et al.* 1977; Lawley *et al.* 1980). Hodgson and colleagues (1977) found that 100% of IBD patients with acute arthritis and two-thirds of those with ankylosing spondylitis had detectable small immune complexes in their plasma, in contrast to none of those with 'chronic arthritis'. In a separate study, Peeters *et al.* (1988) detected serum IgA immune complexes in 75% of ankylosing spondylitis patients followed serially for 9 months. With IBD complicated by ankylosing spondylitis, nephropathy, and leukocytoclastic vasculitis, two patients had circulating IgA immune complexes and perivascular IgA deposits in the skin and renal mesangium (Peeters *et al.* 1990). The well-established association of IgA nephropathy and ankylosing spondylitis argues for the pathogenic potential of circulating IgA complexes in this condition. In a widely quoted study, Wands *et al.* (1976) detected circulating antibody and cryoprotein complexes, some of which contained antibodies against *E. coli* and *Bacteroides* spp., in the majority of patients with arthritis following jejunoileal bypass for morbid obesity. A pathogenic role was suggested in this disorder by the finding of complement activation in the serum, complement deposits in the synovial biopsies, and immune complexes in synovial fluid (Utsinger 1980; Zapanta *et al.* 1979). Although complement deposition is present in the inflamed bowel in both ulcerative colitis and Crohn's disease (Halstensen *et al.* 1993), there is no evidence of chronic activation of the classical complement cascade in the plasma, nor detection of immune complexes in the synovial fluid of IBD patients. Therefore, the causal role of immune complexes in the arthropathies of IBD remains speculative.

Cell-mediated immune response

Although T-lymphocyte activities have not been studied in arthritis complicating IBD, their involvement is likely based on the cell-mediated natures of Crohn's disease, reactive arthritis, and experimental models of chronic intestinal and joint inflammation (reviewed by Sartor 1995*c*, 1996*b*; Sieper and Kingsley 1996). Crohn's disease appears to be a T_{H1}-mediated disorder based on its granulomatous nature and its profile of increased IL-12 and interferon-γ (IFN-γ) expression in the face of low IL-4 production (Mullin *et al.* 1996). The nature of the antigenic drive remains unclear, but a provocative observation by Duchmann *et al.* (1995) suggests that tolerance to resident enteric bacteria is broken in IBD, based on T-cell proliferative responses to autologous flora in patients with ulcerative colitis or Crohn's disease. However, the preservation of tolerance in inactive ulcerative colitis and the presence of the same abnormality in experimental colitis (Duchmann *et al.* 1996) make it likely that this is a secondary rather than a primary process. Klasen and co-workers (1993, 1994) demonstrated proliferative responses of peripheral blood and mesenteric lymph node cells from Crohn's disease patients to bacterial PG–PS polymers. In a preliminary communication, Lügering *et al.* (1996) reported extensive oligoclonality of peripheral-blood T lymphocytes from patients with Crohn's disease and peripheral arthritis or ankylosing spondylitis, but did not investigate synovial T-cell receptor expression.

$CD4^+$ T_{H1} lymphocytes appear to mediate all types of chronic enterocolitis models investigated to date (reviewed by Sartor 1995*c*). Recently, Cong *et al.* (1996) demonstrated a resident caecal flora-specific $CD4^+$ T_{H1} response in mesenteric lymph nodes derived from C_3H/HeJ Bir mice, which spontaneously develop colitis. Of potential pathophysiological importance, neither C_3H/HeJ Bir mice nor any of the genetically engineered mice which develop colitis exhibit peripheral or axial arthritis, despite the reproducible evidence of arthropathy in a wide variety of human intestinal disorders and several rat models of intestinal inflammation (Table 14.1) HLA-B27 transgenic rat colitis and arthritis can be transferred by both $CD4^+$ and $CD8^+$ lymphocytes, although $CD4^+$ cells have been found to be more efficient (Breban *et al.* 1996). Recent data from Taurog's group suggest that dendritic cell function is deficient in this model (Stagg *et al.* 1995*a*). Similarly, cell-mediated responses have been incriminated in the PG–PS model based on the absence of chronic enterocolitis and arthritis in athymic nude rats or following cyclosporin A treatment (Sartor *et al.* 1993). Arthritis can be transferred with PG–PS-specific T lymphocytes and inhibited by antibody to CD4+ T cells (van den Broek *et al.* 1992). Similarly, reactivation of arthritis following experimental, jejunal bacterial overgrowth can be inhibited by cyclosporin A and anti-CD4 antibody (Lichtman *et al.* 1996).

Autoimmune responses

Despite long-term speculation, there is no convincing evidence of pathogenic autoimmune responses in ulcerative colitis or Crohn's disease (Brandtzaeg 1995; Sartor 1995*d*). Circulating and tissue-bound antibodies and lymphocytes which recognize epithelial cell antigens probably are secondary rather than aetiological events. Furthermore, there is no correlation between disease activity and the titre of anti-neutrophil cytoplasmic autoantibody (ANCA) in ulcerative colitis (Saxon *et al.* 1990). The possibility that arthropathies associated with IBD are autoimmune in nature is also speculative, but is plausible due to molecular mimicry between joint-specific epitopes and enteric bacterial antigens. As shown in Table 11.4, a sequence homology exists between several regions of the HLA-B27 protein and a number of enteric bacteria, but the incidence of serum antibodies or cytotoxic lymphocytes recognizing B27 in reactive arthritis or ankylosing spondylitis is quite low. Moreover, although a 40 kDa putative autoantigen in epithelial cells from patients with ulcerative colitis is also found in bile duct and dermal epithelial cells, there is no evidence that this antigen is present in the synovium (Halstensen *et al.* 1993).

A more convincing case can be made for a humoral or cell-mediated response to homologous bacterial and mammalian heat-shock proteins (hsp) or cartilage components. The expression of hsp in human cells is increased by cytokines, including IFN-γ, infections, and reactive oxygen metabolites (Kaufmann 1990). Expression of hsp in inflamed IBD tissues and T-cell responses to hsp in IBD patients are the subjects of conflicting data (Baca-Estrada *et al.* 1994; Winrow *et al.* 1993). However, T-lymphocyte clones recognizing hsp-65 mediate Freund's adjuvant-induced arthritis in rats, and immunization with hsp-65 prevents adjuvant and PG–PS-induced arthritis (van den Broek 1989). Similarly, immunization with hsp-70 blocks the reactivation of arthritis in the jejunal bacterial-overgrowth model (Lichtman *et al.* 1996). Moreover, at least one peptide derived from hsp appears to bind to HLA-B27 (Jardetzky *et al.* 1991). An immune response to cartilage components can also be pathogenic. Balb/c mice immunized with fetal proteoglycan depleted of chondroitin sulphate develop progressive polyarthritis and ankylosing spondylitis (Glant and Mikecz 1991). Furthermore, synovial mononuclear cells from a patient with Crohn's disease and arthritis exhibited proliferative responses to the cartilage components chondroitin sulphate and proteoglycan, as well as to bacterial cell-wall polymers, and PG–PS-primed murine T cells can induce anticartilage responses (van den Broek *et al.* 1988). The actual role of immune responses to hsp and cartilage components in chronic spondylarthritides remains to be determined, but a secondary autoimmune response to structural or inducible proteins could be a mechanism for perpetuating chronic inflammation.

Genetic factors

Between 50 and 70% of IBD patients with ankylosing spondylitis are HLA-B27-positive, but this antigen is not increased in those IBD patients with only peripheral polyarthritis (8–10%). Nevertheless, approximately 25% of B27-positive patients with IBD will develop ankylosing spondylitis compared with only 1% of B27-negative IBD patients, indicating the considerable influence of this HLA molecule in ankylosing spondylitis. Conversely, IBD is also a risk

Table 14.7 Mechanisms of differential susceptibility of inbred rats to chronic inflammation

1. Hypothalamic corticotrophin-releasing hormone production (↓ Lewis) (Sternberg *et al.* 1989; Wilder 1995)
2. Interleukin-1/IL-1 receptor antagonist ratio (↑ Lewis) (McCall *et al.* 1995)
3. Bone-reabsorbing activity of macrophages (↑ Lewis) (Bristol-Rothstein and Schwab 1992)
4. IL-1/PGE_2 ratio (↑ Lewis) (Kandil *et al.* 1994)
5. Kallikrein-kinin system activation (↑ Lewis) (Sartor *et al.* 1996*a*)

factor for ankylosing spondylitis, as illustrated by the observations that only 2% of the general HLA-B27 positive population develop ankylosing spondylitis vs. 25% of those with IBD, and that 6% of the patients with 'idiopathic' ankylosing spondylitis eventually develop clinically apparent Crohn's disease. Clearly, other genetic factors are also involved, since 30–50% of IBD patients with ankylosing spondylitis do not have the B27 marker, and Monsen *et al.* (1990) have identified families comprising multiply-affected individuals with IBD and arthritis.

Animal models of arthritis and intestinal injury also clearly demonstrate the critical importance of host genetic factors in the incidence, chronicity, and aggressiveness of both joint and intestinal inflammation. Inbred Lewis rats develop chronic aggressive granulomatous enterocolitis with fibrosis and extraintestinal inflammation, including erosive peripheral arthritis, after a single injection of PG–PS polymers derived from group A streptococci (McCall *et al.* 1995; Sartor *et al.* 1996*a*). In contrast, Buffalo and Fischer 344 rats, with essentially the same MHC as the Lewis strain, exhibit self-limited acute enterocolitis, but no chronic gut or extraintestinal disease after identical exposure to PG–PS. Similarly, Lewis rats develop extraintestinal lesions such as hepatobiliary inflammation (Lichtman *et al.* 1990) and reactivation of arthritis (Lichtman *et al.* 1995) following experimental, jejunal bacterial overgrowth, but no extraintestinal disease develops in Buffalo or Fischer rats with identical concentrations of jejunal bacteria (Lichtman *et al.* 1990). Variation of a somewhat different nature is seen in HLA-B27 transgenic rats, in which both Lewis and Fischer rats develop arthritis and enterocolitis, but the Fischer rats selectively develop colonic neoplasia (Hammer *et al.* 1995), whereas Lewis rats develop more frequent arthritis. Lewis rats consistently develop arthritis in other models as well, such as following exposure to Freund's adjuvant, *Y. enterocolitica* 0:8, and Salmonella (Brown–Norway × Lewis F_1 crosses) (Hill and Yu 1988). A number of mechanisms have been advanced to explain the heightened susceptibility of Lewis rats to experimental inflammation (Table 14.7). Consistent features are an overly aggressive inflammatory response mediated by defective immunosuppression (lack of appropriate hypothalamic/ pituitary/adrenal, IL-1 receptor antagonist, or PGE_2 responses) or dysregulated proinflammatory pathways (kininogen activation and bone-reabsorbing activity of macrophages). Similar regulatory balances need to be evaluated in human IBD, particularly in light of the parallel abnormalities in the balance of IL-1 and IL-1-receptor antagonist in Lewis rats and in patients with IBD (Casini-Raggi *et al.* 1995; McCall *et al.* 1995).

Conclusions and unifying hypothesis

These clinical and experimental observations stress several recurrent themes which provide important insights into the pathogenesis of arthropathies associated with intestinal inflammation. The following factors are critical components of this pathogenesis.

1. *Colonic anaerobic bacteria*—Peripheral arthritis is associated with colonic disease, active intestinal inflammation, luminal bacterial overgrowth, and enhanced mucosal permeability. Moreover, antibiotics with anaerobic spectra can prevent disease, and *Bacteroides* species are preferentially involved in experimental colitis. Sterile proinflammatory components are probably more important than viable organisms.
2. *Host genetic background*—The presence of arthropathies in a relatively small percentage of IBD patients and rodent models of colitis, the striking role of HLA-B27 in ankylosing spondylitis, and the dramatic differential susceptibility of chronic disease in inbred rat strains demonstrate the requirement for permissive host susceptibility factors.
3. *Defective immunoregulation*—Intestinal and joint inflammation are immunologically mediated, with key contributions from CD4^{+} T_{H1} lymphocytes and macrophages secreting IL-1 and TNF-α. Aggressive inflammation is probably abetted by defective down-regulation of the inflammatory response, possibly genetically determined.

We propose the following hypothesis for the association of intestinal and joint inflammation, yet independent progression of ankylosing spondylitis and underlying IBD. Enhanced mucosal permeability leads to the increased absorption of proinflammatory bacterial com-

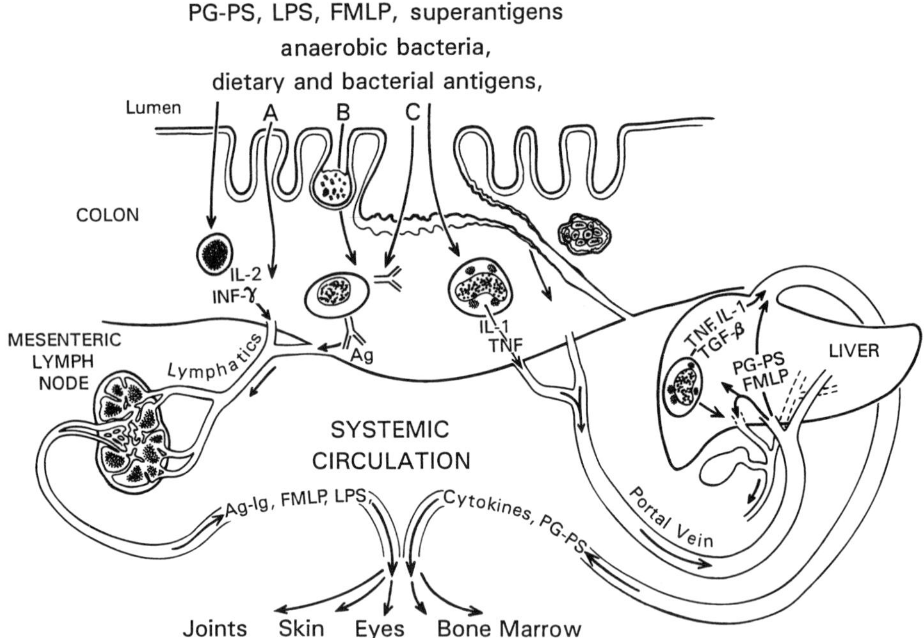

Fig. 14.2 Systemic distribution of phlogistic luminal products. Luminal bacterial products cross the colonic mucosa in areas of enhanced permeability across (A) leaky epithelia, (B) crypt abscesses, or (C) ulcers and fistulae. During transit through the lamina propria and submucosa, antigens complex with immunoglobulin (Ig), and cell-wall polymers stimulate macrophages and lymphocytes, which secrete cytokines. Bacterial products, cytokines, and immune complexes are transported through the mesenteric lymphatics or portal vein to regional lymph nodes or the liver, where further stimulation of immune cells occurs. In the liver, PG–PS and FMLP can be excreted into the bile duct, activate Kupffer cells, or enter the hepatic vein. After entering the systemic circulation bacterial products, immune complexes, and inflammatory mediators are distributed to the joints, skin, eyes, and bone marrow, where local inflammation is incited in genetically susceptible hosts. Reprinted from Sartor and Lichtman (1994) with permission of Williams & Wilkins, Baltimore.

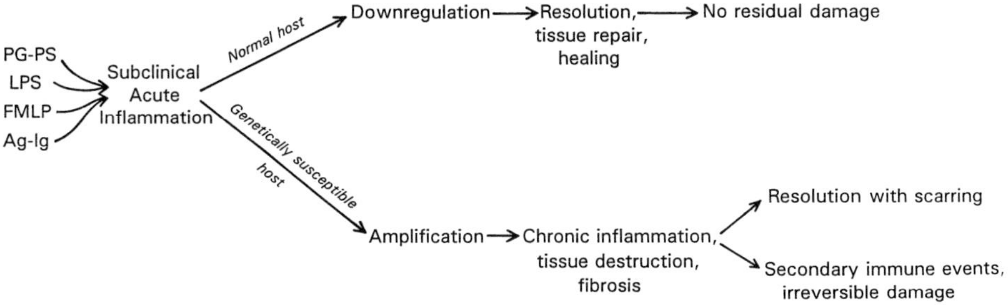

Fig. 14.3 Genetically determined inflammatory response to luminal antigens and bacterial products. Systemically distributed bacterial polymers and immune complexes induced subclinical inflammation in all hosts. The normal response is appropriate down-regulation of inflammation with no residual damage (*upper arm*). However, genetically susceptible hosts (*lower arm*) amplify the inflammatory response leading to joint injury, which either resolves when intestinal uptake of luminal antigen ceases (peripheral arthritis) or pursues an independent, progressive course when secondary immune events become involved (ankylosing spondylitis, sacroiliitis). Reprinted from Sartor and Lichtman (1994) with permission of Williams & Wilkins, Baltimore.

ponents from the distal ileum and colon, with secondary invasion of ulcers and fistulae by viable bacteria (Fig. 14.2). Absorption of these bacterial constituents and locally produced soluble inflammatory mediators through the mesenteric lymphatics and portal circulation leads to the systemic distribution of these phlogistic molecules to articular surfaces. These circulating bacterial polymers, antigens, cytokines, and immune complexes localize in joints under the influence of regional vascular permeability caused by pre-existing injury, trauma, or a particular tropism for the synovial surface. Most patients fail to develop overt inflammation with these stimuli, but a genetically susceptible subset of patients with intrinsically dysregulated immune responses develops clinically apparent aggressive inflammation (Fig. 14.3). These proinflammatory bacterial products and soluble inflammatory mediators probably act synergistically to potentiate the inflammatory response.

Peripheral arthritis resolves when stimuli emanating from the intestine cease to reach the joint because of decreased mucosal permeability due to medical or surgical therapy or because of spontaneous remission. However, additional factors must be invoked to explain the independent course of ankylosing spondylitis. HLA-B27 or other immunoregulatory genes must regulate inflammatory pathways that are independent of those mechanisms that initiate intestinal injury. For example, an autoimmune response may develop to cartilage components or heat-shock proteins which then pursue a separate course from the independently regulated gut disease, leading to progressive, irreversible destruction and ankylosis of the joint–ligament–cartilage junctions of the axial skeleton (entheseopathy).

This hypothesis suggests an interaction between genetic and environmental influences, with each factor being permissive but insufficient for full clinical expression of disease. For example, B27-positive individuals may fail to develop ankylosing spondylitis unless gut inflammation or infection occurs, just as HLA-B27 transgenic rats fail to develop colitis or arthritis unless the appropriate luminal bacteria are present. In addition, factors initiating and perpetuating inflammation may be entirely distinct. Finally, this theory conforms to the clinical observation that genetic susceptibility for chronic intestinal inflammation and arthritis, particularly ankylosing spondylitis, are independent variables. Our understanding of genetic associations in Crohn's disease and ulcerative colitis is expanding rapidly (Hugot *et al.* 1996;

Satsangi *et al.* 1996), and this may soon lead to a more thorough understanding of the immunogenetic regulation of IBD-associated arthropathies. Although mechanistic studies of arthritis associated with IBD have been superficially performed to date, rapid advances from investigations of rodent models, reactive arthritis, and idiopathic spondylarthritides should help direct fruitful research in this under-investigated area.

15 Animal models of the spondyloarthropathies

Joel D. Taurog

Introduction

The study of the pathogenesis, treatment, and prevention of human disease is invaluably aided by animal models. Animal models of human disease have traditionally been divided operationally into two groups, those occurring spontaneously and those requiring experimental induction. However, diseases occurring in genetically manipulated animals, for example transgenic or 'gene knockout' animals, can logically be considered in either of these categories. Ultimately, classification is less important that the utility a particular type of animal or experimental system provides in understanding important aspects of human disease.

The spondyloarthropathies are multisystem diseases, generally considered unique to humans, that are epidemiologically interrelated and share certain characteristic forms of arthropathy and extra-articular lesions. The epidemiological interrelationships are based on:

(1) familial association;

(2) a striking association with HLA-B27;

(3) probable associations with other genes as well; and

(4) certain environmental factors.

With minor exceptions, this review will consider animal diseases that either manifest an arthropathy similar, in an essential way, to the characteristic arthropathies of the spondyloarthropathies, and/or are associated with HLA-B27 (Table 15.1). These are the models deemed most likely to help elucidate the pathogenesis, treatment, or prevention of the spondyloarthropathies. The present level of knowledge derived from these models pertains primarily to pathogenesis; little has been done with regard to prevention or treatment. A wide variety of other animal disease models exist in which there is inflammation in relevant tissues (such as the joints, gut, skin, or eye), or in which there is infection caused by bacteria known to trigger reactive arthritis, but consideration of these is beyond the scope of this review. Aspects of some of these disorders are discussed elsewhere in this book.

Transgenic animals

Basics of transgenic technology in rodents

Two approaches to the introduction of specific genetic alterations into the germline of mice have become widely established: (1) pronuclear microinjection of fertilized ova; and (2) gene deletion or replacement by homologous recombination in embryonic stem cells.

Table 15.1 Animal models of the human spondyloarthropathies

	Resemblance to human spondyloarthropathies			Relationship to		
	Axial arthropathy/ enthesopathy	**Peripheral arthritis/ enthesopathy**	**Extra-articular lesions**	**HLA-B27**	**Arthritogenic bacteria**	**Normal bacterial flora**
B27 transgenic rats	+	+++	++++	++++	?	+++
Ankylosing enthesopathy	–	++	–	+	?	– (?)
B27 mβ2m$^{-/-}$ mice	?	++	?	+++	?	++
Infection of B27 rodents with arthritogenic bacteria	– (?)	– (?)	– (?)	++	++++	?
ank/ank mouse (MPA)	++++	++++	+/–	?	–	– (?)
Proteoglycan-induced arthritis	++	+++	–	?	–	– (?)
Spondyloarthropathies in gorillas	+++	?	?	+	?	?
Reactive arthritis in rhesus monkeys	?	++	(?)	(?)	++	?

Features rated on an arbitrary scale: – absent to ++++ maximal.

? Not examined.

(?) Results suggestive, but not conclusive.

Pronuclear microinjection, which has also been applied to a variety of species in addition to mice, was developed in the early 1980's (reviewed in Palmiter and Brinster 1986). It consists of the microinjection of cloned genes into one of the two pronuclei of fertilized ova, which are then gestated in pseudopregnant foster mothers. For any given injection, varying numbers of copies of the cloned DNA integrate into an apparently random site within the host chromosomes to form a single locus, which may then be transmitted in Mendelian fashion. Whether and how the transgenes are expressed depends upon the *cis*-regulatory elements contained within the injected gene and upon the site of integration within the host genome. This form of genetic manipulation is most useful for studying the effect of dominant-acting genes.

Gene deletion in embryonic stem cells, also called gene knockout technology, came to fruition about a decade after pronuclear microinjection; at the time of writing it has only been applied to mice. In this method, genes can be inactivated through replacement with altered cloned genes by homologous recombination in embryonic stem cells. These cells maintain pluripotency *in vitro*, but when introduced into blastocyst embryos, they give rise to cell lineages within the subsequently developing embryo and can be transmitted through the germline to subsequent generations (reviewed in Ramirez-Solis and Bradley 1994). This technology has proven most useful for examining the recessive effect of gene deletions in animals homozygous for the targeted gene disruption.

HLA-B27 transgenic rats

General description

Rats transgenic for HLA-B27 were produced under the rationale that, since rats are either uniquely susceptible, or more susceptible than mice, to a variety of immune-mediated inflammatory disorders, it would be more likely that rats would develop B27-specific pathology. When lines of rats were produced that were transgenic for genomic clones for HLA-B27 and its associated light chain human β2-microglobulin (hβ2m), two of the lines, 21-4H on the inbred LEW background and 33-3 on the inbred F344 background, were found to develop a spontaneous multisystem inflammatory disease that bears a strong clinical and histological resemblance to the human (Hammer *et al.* 1990; Taurog *et al.* 1993). The clinical features include:

(1) inflammatory gastrointestinal disease, affecting the colon, stomach, and small intestine;

(2) peripheral arthritis;

(3) spinal lesions;

(4) a variety of skin lesions (psoriasiform dermatitis, folliculitis, alopecia, nail dystrophy);

(5) orchitis and epididymitis;

(6) carditis.

Susceptibility to disease is clearly related to the gene copy number and level of expression of B27, with disease developing only in those lines having supraphysiological levels of transgene expression (Taurog *et al.* 1993). The strongest evidence for this was the finding that rats of the 21-3 line, which carry an intermediate number of gene copies, develop disease only if homozygous for the transgene locus, whereas rats of the two high copy lines, 21-4H and 33-3, develop disease when hemizygous.

Clinical and histological features

Of the affected lines, nearly 100% of the rats develop diarrhoea as the earliest clinical manifestation, which correlates histologically with a diffuse mononuclear cell infiltrate in the lamina propria of the colon, stomach, and, more variably, the small intestine. The colitis is associated with the increased production of biochemical markers of an inflammatory response, including cytokines, nitric oxide, and myeloperoxidase (Aiko and Grisham 1995; McLean *et al.* 1995; Rath *et al.* 1996). In the 33-3 line, but not the 21-4H line, the chronic colitis is associated with a high prevalence of adenoma formation, with progression in some cases to locally invasive adenocarcinoma (Hammer *et al.* 1995). This most likely is related to differences between the two inbred backgrounds of these two lines, LEW and F344.

Within several weeks of the onset of intestinal inflammation, most affected rats develop arthritis, and all of the males develop genital inflammation (Taurog *et al.* 1993). Skin and nail changes appear late and more variably (Taurog *et al.* 1993; Yanagisawa *et al.* 1995). Histological examination of the 21-4H line has revealed enthesopathy (Hammer *et al.* 1990). Although fusion of sacroiliac and spinal apophyseal joints was reported in a preliminary communication (Kriegsmann *et al.* 1995), the specificity of these lesions has not yet been established. Occasional myocarditis (Hammer *et al.* 1990), and very rare (and questionably specific) anterior uveitis (Baggla *et al.* 1997) have also been observed. Elevation of acute-phase reactants in serum correlates with disease onset (Taurog *et al.* 1994 and unpublished findings). Although there are some obvious differences between the disease in rats and the spectrum of human spondyloarthropathies (for example, orchitis and dermal folliculitis occur in rats but not typically in humans), there are many clinical and histological similarities.

Specificity for HLA-B27

To examine whether this phenomenon is specific for HLA-B27 as opposed to another HLA class I gene, lines of rats transgenic for HLA-B7 and HLA-Cw6 have been produced with gene copy number and expression similar to the disease-prone B27 lines. These lines show mild testicular abnormalities, occasional late alopecia, and a very low incidence of transient peripheral arthritis, but most of the rats in these lines have remained healthy. These data provide fairly convincing evidence for the relatively strong specificity of B27 in the rat disease.

Role of bacteria

As described elsewhere in this volume, the role of bacteria in the pathogenesis of the spondyloarthropathies is of great interest. Two fundamental questions remain to be answered: (1) what specific molecular events underlie the role of bacteria in reactive arthritis; and (2) do bacteria play any role at all in ankylosing spondylitis or any of the other spondyloarthropathies? Since the microbial environment of laboratory animals can be experimentally manipulated, the disease-prone B27 transgenic rats have provided a model system in which these questions can be approached experimentally.

To this end, rats of the disease-prone B27 lines were rederived in a germfree environment to test the hypothesis that normal gut flora are involved in the pathogenesis of the disease of the B27 transgenic rats (Taurog *et al.* 1994). The germfree rats showed no evidence of gut or joint inflammation, even after a year, and it was thus concluded that normal environmental flora, most likely within the gastrointestinal tract, contribute a critical factor to the pathogenesis of these aspects of disease. Typical skin lesions and male genital lesions appeared in the germfree B27 rats, suggesting that the pathogenesis of these aspects of the disease is distinct from that of the arthritis and bowel disease. This result suggests that reactive arthritis, which is triggered by mucosally invasive pathogens, may represent one end of a spectrum of disease pathogenesis, with rheumatic disease induced by normal bacteria lying elsewhere on the spectrum.

The entire disease complex returns once the germfree rats are reconsituted with gut flora from specific pathogen-free or conventionally housed rats (Rath *et al.* 1996; Taurog *et al.* 1994). Moreover, initial reconstitution experiments indicate that not all bacteria are equal in contributing to disease pathogenesis, with anaerobes appearing to favour the development of colitis (Rath *et al.* 1996). It remains to be determined whether spondylitis in the rats is also dependent upon the presence of a gut flora.

Rats with low copy numbers and physiological expression of the B27/hβ2m transgenes have also been used to examine the response to bacteria associated with reactive arthritis in humans. Rats of the 21-4L line on the LEW background were compared with their non-transgenic littermates for the arthritic response to the intravenous administration of a *Yersinia enterocolitica* O:8 isolate that is known to induce arthritis in LEW rats by a mechanism thought to require persistence of viable bacteria within the host (Gaede and Heesemann 1995; Hill and Yu 1987). Arthritis developed equally in transgenic and non-transgenic rats, with no difference in incidence, severity, or course (Taurog *et al.*, unpublished results). Interestingly, when rats of this transgenic line were infected intragastrically or intraperitoneally with a virulent *Y. pseudotuberculosis* isolate, yersinia-specific CD8+ cytolytic T cells (CTL) were induced, but these were shown to be restricted only by rat class I, and not by B27 (Falgarone *et al.* 1996).

Very recently, a quantitative correlation between the severity of colitis and the level of *E. coli* and *Enterococcus* spp. in the cecum has been observed in B27 transgenic rats (J. Taurog and A. Onderdonk, unpublished observations). The cause-and-effect relationship of these observations remains to be investigated.

The cellular basis of the disease

The major disease manifestations can be reproducibly transferred from either 21-4H or 33-3 donors to irradiated, normally healthy rats, either transgenic or non-transgenic, by bone-marrow stem cells (Breban *et al.* 1993). Transfer of spleen cells alone is effective only if there is accompanying bone-marrow stem cell engraftment, whereas lymph node cells alone are ineffective. These results suggest that one or more cell(s) arising from transgenic precursors plays a critical role in the transferred disease, whereas mature lymphocytes found in spleen or lymph node are not sufficient. This has suggested that the critical cell arising from the bone marrow of the disease-prone lines may be an antigen-presenting cell.

A critical role for T cells is indicated by the finding that athymic *rnu/rnu* (nude) rats bearing the 33-3 transgene locus fail to develop disease, whereas their transgenic euthymic *rnu/+* littermates develop disease (Breban *et al.* 1996). Transfer of T cells from euthymic 33-3 donors to 33-3 *rnu/rnu* rats induces disease, as does engraftment of a thymus (Breban *et al.* 1996 and unpublished data). The phenotype of the transferring T cells is still somewhat uncertain. The most efficient transfer occurs with purified CD4+ T cells. Disease also occurs in most recipients of CD8+ T cells, but the phenotype is somewhat milder and there is considerable *in vivo* expansion of contaminating CD4+ T cells. It is curious, but unexplained, that arthritis is much less common in T cell-reconstituted 33-3 nude rats than in euthymic 33-3 rats (Breban *et al.* 1996 and unpublished data).

Characterization of the evolving lesions has indicated that the T-cell infiltrate is polyclonal from the earliest time points on, as assessed by T-cell receptor Vβ gene usage (McLean *et al.* 1994). Moreover, the cytokine pattern varies considerably between different sites of inflammation. The most prominent cytokines in inflamed intestine are interleukin-2 (IL-2) and interferum-gamma (IFN-γ), whereas the inflamed synovium shows little of these cytokines but abundant IL-6 and transforming growth factor-β 1 (TGF-β1) (McLean *et al.* 1995). IL-1 is also prominent in the inflamed gut (Rath *et al.* 1996), although in vivo administration of an IL-1 receptor antagonist preparation had no effect on disease in line 33-3 rats (unpublished results).

The transfer of disease to non-transgenic rats by B27 bone-marrow cells establishes that B27 need not be expressed in non marrow-derived elements in the intestinal mucosa, synovium, or skin in order for B27-mediated disease to be induced in these sites. Fetal liver cells and bone-marrow cells from nude animals also transfer disease into normal or thymectomized non-transgenic rats. This suggests that B27 also does not need to be expressed on thymic epithelium, since these cell sources presumably lack post-thymic T cells. The thymus itself may not be necessary, although the role of radioresistant host T cells has not yet been identified. This has been supported by experiments in which disease has been reproducibly transferred to lethally irradiated, adult-thymectomized rats with T-cell depleted bone marrow or fetal liver cells from disease-prone donors (Breban *et al.* 1996). Thus, despite the characteristic organ-specificity of B27-associated disease, the pathological process appears to be carried out within the immune system itself, driven by bone marrow-derived cells with high B27 expression.

These data implicate antigen-presenting cells in disease pathogenesis. However, preliminary experiments to examine the function of dendritic cells have shown an unexpected lack of competence in dendritic cells from disease-prone, but not disease-resistant, B27 transgenic lines (Stagg *et al.* 1995). Similarly, lymph node cells from ageing males of the 21-4H line lose the ability to present the HY minor histocompatibility antigen *in vivo* and *in vitro* (unpublished results). The significance of these findings is unclear, but may reflect a loss of central or peripheral tolerance that permits disease expression.

Peptide presentation by B27

A fundamental unanswered question regarding the role of B27 and disease concerns whether this role requires that B27 binds a specific peptide or group of peptides, or conversely whether the participation of the B27 molecule is independent of its binding specificity. One experimental approach to this has taken advantage of a naturally occurring polymorphism in the cellular machinery that loads rat class I MHC molecules with peptides. Two genes encoded within the class II region of the MHC, termed *Tap-1* and *Tap-2*, have been characterized in rats, mice, and humans, which encode the two chains of a heterodimer that transports peptides from the cytosol into the endoplasmic reticulum, where the transported peptides, or peptides derived from them, are bound to nascent class I MHC molecules.

The rat version of *Tap-2* has two alleles, *Tap-2A* and *Tap-2B*, that differ substantially in coding sequence. These correlate with two previously described functional alleles, *cim*^{a} and *cim*[b] (Joly *et al.* 1994). The *Tap-2B* allele recessively encodes for altered peptide loading and slow intracellular processing of the rat class I allele RT1.A[a]. The *Tap-2* alleles, or linked MHC-encoded alleles, were found to have a profound effect on peptide binding and presentation by B27 (Simmons *et al.* 1996). None the less, rats bearing the 33-3 transgene locus developed typical disease, regardless of the *Tap-2* genotype. Thus, if peptide binding to B27 plays a role in disease pathogenesis in B27 transgenic rats, the critical peptide(s), unlike HY and many other peptides, seem(s) little influenced by the *cim* phenomenon that largely correlates with *Tap-2* polymorphism. Such peptides could conceivably be acquired by recently described alternative pathways to class I peptide binding (Rock 1996). Alternatively, the role of B27 in disease may have little to do with peptide binding. However, recent preliminary evidence from B27 transgenic rats also expressing a transgene encoding a B27-binding influenza protein suggests that the specificity of peptide bound to B27 may be important in the pathogenesis of arthritis in these rats (Zhou *et al.* 1997).

Background genetic influence

Interestingly, although backcrossing the 33-3 transgene locus on to the PVG strain showed little effect on the disease, backcrossing on to the DA strain completely attenuated the disease within two to three generations (Taurog *et al.* 1996). This result indicates that alleles within the DA background are protective. Intriguingly, collagen-induced arthritis shows the opposite strain specificity: DA rats are highly susceptible, whereas F344 rats are resistant (Remmers *et al.* 1996).

Summary of HLA-B27 transgenic rats

The spontaneous disease in rats with high expression of HLA-B27 bears a strong resemblance to the spectrum of disease in the spondyloarthropathies. Assuming that the pathogenic molecular recognition events in which the B27 molecule participates are similar in humans and rats, the lessons learned from the rats so far include:

1. B27 itself, not a linked gene, is the disease marker.
2. B27 need not be expressed on non-haematopoietic cells in order for disease expression.
3. The disease is T-cell dependent.
4. Gut inflammation precedes peripheral arthritis.
5. Background genes can completely suppress disease expression.
6. The specific role of B27 in disease, particularly whether a specific B27-bound peptide is required, remains to be determined, with evidence from different experiments pointing in both directions.

HLA-B27 transgenic mice

Introduction

Mice transgenic for HLA-B27, with or without hβ2m, have been described by a number of groups during the past decade (Ismail *et al.* 1994; Kalinke *et al.* 1990; Krimpenfort *et al.*

1987; Nickerson *et al.* 1990; Taurog *et al.* 1988*b*; Weiss *et al.* 1990). Although no phenotype has been observed that is as dramatic as that of B27 transgenic rats, interesting pathology has been observed in B27 mice that has at least some specificity for B27.

Ankylosing enthesopathy

The first report of mice transgenic for HLA-B27 described mice carrying 5–10 copies of a genomic clone for the B*2702 gene, and an independent line was made bearing human β2m (Krimpenfort *et al.* 1987). These transgene loci have been backcrossed on to numerous backgrounds, and immune responses in the B27 and B27/hβ2m transgenic mice have been extensively investigated (Frangoulis *et al.* 1993). When the mice were rigorously examined for evidence of spontaneous disease (Weinreich *et al.* 1995), a curious arthropathy was discovered in both the transgenic mice and in non-transgenic controls. This consisted of a rigidity of one or both ankles noted upon flexion or extension, which correlated histologically with an inflammatory process culminating in cartilagenous proliferation and ankylosis of one or more of the tarsal joints. The investigators termed this process ankylosing enthesopathy (ANKENT), because the cartilage proliferation was observed primarily at the insertions of the ligamentous parts of the joint capsules (namely at entheses), with subsequent ossification proceeding from the same site. No pathological abnormalities were found in the spine or in any extra-articular tissues.

The condition was found to occur almost exclusively in male mice 3 months of age or older. An initial, apparently acute, inflammatory process affecting one ankle would be observed, with clinical stiffness and histological ankylosis supervening over several weeks. In 25–50% of mice, depending on the cohort, the process would subsequently develop in the contralateral ankle, but often months after the initial unilateral involvement.

Three interacting genetic risk factors were found for ANKENT. Mice transgenic for HLA-B*2702 were found to have a higher prevalence of the process (irrespective of the presence or absence of the hβ2m transgene), than were mice bearing the MHC haplotypes H-2^k or H-2^b, and mice with various C57BL backgrounds. The highest prevalence was seen in male C57BL/10.BR (H-2^k) mice, with an overall prevalence of about 30%, ranging from 2 to 50% in different cohorts. In this population, the presence of the B27 transgene carried a relative risk for ANKENT of approximately 1.5, whereas in C57BL/10 and (C57BL/10 × C57BL/10.BR)F_2 mice, in which the overall prevalence of ANKENT was somewhat lower, the aggregate relative risk associated with B27 was approximately 2.5–3. B27 was not a severity factor, but tended to increase the likelihood of bilateral disease. No association was found between the prevalence of ANKENT and either the nature of the housing environment or specific bacteria. Immunosuppressive treatment had no effect on the process, although elevated serum IL-6 levels could be shown to precede its clinical onset by several weeks.

Perhaps the most surprising thing about this process is that it had not been previously described, since it was found in common inbred strains of laboratory mice. It seems unlikely that geographic factors can explain this, since the process was seen in mice of the same stock in Paris, Amsterdam, and Prague. It is intriguing that the process in mice resembles the progression of events in ankylosing spondylitis, namely, the relatively sudden and apparently spontaneous onset of inflammation primarily at entheses, progressing to chondrocyte hyperplasia and ankylosis in conjunction with an apparent waning of inflammation. The process also resembles the ankylosing tarsitis that tends to accompany juvenile-onset B27-related joint disease in the Mexican Mestizo population (Burgos-Vargos and Granados-Arriola 1990). As usual with spontaneous animal models, more needs to be learnt about the pathogenesis of the process before its relative merit as a model of human disease can be reliably judged.

Spontaneous arthritis in HLA-B27 mice lacking mouse β2m

A novel report (Khare *et al.* 1995) describes spontaneous peripheral arthritis in mice in which a transgene locus bearing a low copy number of HLA-B*2705 was backcrossed on to a background homozygous for deletion of the endogenous (mouse) β2m gene. The arthritis was seen predominantly in males and only when the mice were housed in a conventional, as opposed to a specific pathogen-free, environment. Nail lesions were also noted. No abnormalities in the gut or spine have been described. As would be expected in the absence of β2m, there was no normally folded B27 detectable on lymphoid cell surfaces, but there was surface staining with an antibody that recognizes the denatured free HLA-B heavy chain. Since the $\beta 2m^{-/-}$ mice lack CD8 T cells, these results add to the evidence obtained in B27 transgenic rats which suggests that the role of B27 in arthritis involves something other than the conventional presentation of a peptide to CD8 T cells.

Subsequently, these authors reported a similar phenotype in B27 transgenic $m\beta 2m^{-/-}$ mice that also expressed a human β2m transgene (Khare *et al.* 1996).

Preliminary results suggest that CD4 but not MHC class II is essential for arthritis in B27 transgenic, $m\beta 2m^{-/-}$ mice (Khalil *et al.* 1997). Rather elaborate hypotheses to explain these results have been put forward by these authors (Khare *et al.* 1995, 1996). It should be noted that other groups who have produced B27 transgenic $m\beta 2m^{-/-}$ mice, with or without hβ2m, have not been able to confirm the frequency or B27-specificity of these findings (Taurog *et al.*, Colbert *et al.*, unpublished results), although varying environmental or genetic factors may account for the different results.

Infection of HLA-B27 transgenic mice with *Yersinia enterocolitica*

Nickerson *et al.* (1990) infected B*2705 transgenic mice and their non-transgenic littermates intravenously with a *Y. enterocolitica* O:8 isolate, described above in the section on B27 transgenic rats. They observed enhanced mortality and a tendency to paraspinous abscesses in the transgenic mice, in comparison with the non-transgenic controls. Ismail *et al.* (1994) infected a different line of B*2705 transgenic mice intragastrically with another *Y. enterocolitica* O:8 isolate. They observed delayed clearance of the infection in the transgenic rats, evidenced by persistence of culturable bacteria in the spleen and liver several weeks after the bacteria could no longer be cultured from these organs in the non-transgenic mice. These studies lend support to the hypothesis that B27 may interfere with some form of host defence, permitting the persistance of certain types of bacterial pathogens. The absence of arthritis in the chronically infected B27 mice may reflect the low susceptibility of mice to arthritis of any type, rather than a lack of relevance to the spondyloarthropathies.

Infection of HLA-B27 transgenic mice with *Chlamydia trachomatis*

Transgenic mice expressing B27 have recently been used to study the immune response to infection with *C. trachomatis*. These mice mounted a strong HLA-B27-restricted cytolytic

T-cell response that lysed chlamydia-infected targets (Kuon *et al.* 1997). This contrasts with the situation alluded to above in which B27 transgenic rats infected with *Y. enterocolitica* mounted a CTL response to the organism that was RT1-restricted but not B27-restricted.

Murine progressive ankylosis

General description and clinical features

Murine progressive ankylosis (MPA) is a spontaneous disorder of mice resulting from a homozygous recessive single gene defect at a locus, *ank* (Sweet and Green 1981), which produces an arthritis of peripheral and axial joints that eventually results in joint ankylosis. The gene, which has yet to be isolated, maps near the centromere of Chromosome 15, closely linked to the coat colour locus *uw* (Sweet and Green 1981). The predominant pathological process in MPA appears to be the intra-articular deposition of calcium hydroxyapatite (Hakim *et al.* 1984, 1986; Mahowald *et al.* 1989; Sampson *et al.* 1991), but whether this is the primary process resulting from the genetic defect is not known. The disorder in *ank/ank* mice shows 100% penetrance and fairly uniform expressivity.

MPA shows several similarities to the human spondyloarthropathies, clinically, radiographically, and histologically (Hakim *et al.* 1984, 1986; Krug *et al.* 1989; Mahowald *et al.* 1988, 1989; Sampson 1988*a,b*; Sampson and Davis 1988; Sampson and Trzeciakowski 1990). Peripheral joints are inflamed initially, but the subsequent progressive ankylosis appears largely non-inflammatory. Ankylosis in the extremities begins distally and proceeds proximally. In contrast to most rodent arthropathies, forefeet are involved before hindfeet. The process also involves essentially all of the axial joints and produces severe spinal ankylosis. Extra-articular manifestations include balanitis and crusting skin lesions, which perhaps are a consequence of an inability of the affected mice to groom themselves (Mahowald *et al.* 1988).

Pathology

Radiographically evident bony erosions and calcification of articular and periarticular tissues are extensive and vertebral syndesmophytes produce a 'bamboo spine'. Under light microscopy, the earliest synovial lesion observed is inflammatory, followed by synovial proliferation and cartilage erosions. Later changes include progressive joint ankylosis by fibrosis and ossification of articular and periarticular tissues and new bone proliferation. Electron microscopy reveals synovial cell proliferation and hypertrophy with collagen deposition during the early inflammatory phase before the appearance of intracellular and extracellular hydroxyapatite (HA) crystals. After this proliferative phase, chondrophytes form (bridging the joint), mineralize, and are replaced by bone.

Pathogenesis

Although inflammatory lesions can be found early in the course of the disease, the evidence does not favour an immune pathogenesis (Krug *et al.* 1997). Disease is not transferable to normal mice with bone-marrow cells, spleen cells, or serum from *ank/ank* mice, or to SCID mice with *ank/ank* spleen cells. Moreover, *ank/ank* mice that are congenitally athymic and

T-cell deficient as a result of homozygosity for the *nu* (nude) gene (Nehls *et al.* 1994) are phenotypically identical to non-nude *ank/ank* mice.

Disease progression exhibits brief, transient delays when homozygote animals are treated with total body irradiation, parenteral IL-1, or indomethacin. When mice were treated with high-dose hydrocortisone, synovitis receded, chondrophytes and osteophytes stopped forming, but calcium hydroxyapatite continued to accumulate in synovial spaces. Disease progression is markedly delayed by parenteral treatment with phosphocitrate, a potent inhibitor of calcium phosphate crystallization and an inhibitor of the *in vitro* mitogenic response of fibroblasts to basic calcium phosphate crystals.

It is unclear whether this disorder shares any fundamental molecular pathways with the human spondyloarthropathies, but the phenotypic similarity to AS is striking and clearly merits continued investigation.

Proteoglycan-induced arthritis in mice

General description and clinical features

Proteoglycan-induced arthritis is a chronic, immune-mediated, inflammatory, erosive peripheral arthritis and spondylitis that has been studied predominantly in BALB/c mice. In the original experiments, mice were immunized with high-bouyant density proteoglycan monomers (aggrecan) from human fetal cartilage, emulsified in complete Freund's adjuvant, followed by several subsequent immunizations in incomplete Freund's adjuvant (Glant *et al.* 1987; Mikecz *et al.* 1987). The same syndrome was also seen if incomplete Freund's adjuvant was used for all the immunizations. Arthritis occurred in 100% of females with onset 5–6 weeks after the initial injection, whereas in males only 70% developed arthritis, with onset at about 7 weeks. Extra-articular disease has not been found to be a part of this disorder.

Pathology

The peripheral arthritis in this disorder is characterized histologically by an inflammatory infiltrate of mononuclear cells and neutrophils, followed sequentially by pannus formation with erosion of cartilage and bone, destruction of the growth plate, chondrocyte proliferation with ankylosis, and osteophyte formation (Glant *et al.* 1987). Spondylitis has been described in the lumbar spine and tail, consisting of perivertebral inflammation and pannus eroding the intervertebral disc, followed by a remarkable degeneration of the cartilaginous growth plate, resorption of the endplate and destruction of the intervertebral disc (Glant *et al.* 1987).

Pathogenesis

Much of the work on this model has focused on immunopathogenesis. The primary pathogenic response appears to be mediated by CD4 T cells specific for an antigen contained within the G1 (hyaluronate binding) domain of the murine aggrecan molecule (Leroux *et al.* 1992, 1996; Mikecz *et al.* 1987, 1988, 1990). This concept is supported by the finding that a proteoglycan-specific, MHC class II (I-A^{d})-restricted CD4 T-cell hybridoma of the Th1 type (secreting IFN-γ and IL-2, but not IL-4) can mediate arthritis upon adoptive transfer to irradiated

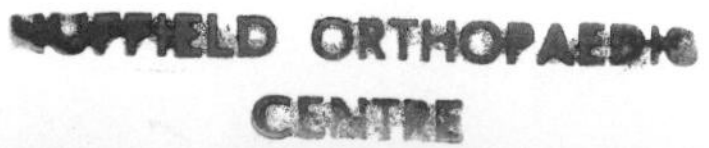

BALB/c recipients (Buzas *et al.* 1995). A strong antibody response to mouse aggrecan accompanies the disorder, and there is some evidence that antigen-specific B cells may play a role in amplifying the T-cell response (Brennan *et al.* 1995; Mikecz *et al.* 1990). Consistent with this is the finding that arthritis develops only in those mice that develop autoantibodies to self-cartilage proteoglycans following immunization (Glant *et al.* 1995).

The immunizing proteoglycan is arthritogenic typically only upon treatment with chondroitinase or hyaluronidase, and the presence of keratan sulphate or chondroitin sulphate on the aggrecan moiety inhibits both arthritis development and *in vitro* T-cell responses (Leroux *et al.* 1996). Only a select group of proteoglycans have been found to be arthritogenic in this model, namely, those from fetal and newborn human, fetal pig or canine articular cartilages, human osteophytes, or human chondrosarcomas (Glant *et al.* 1987, 1995; Mikecz *et al.* 1987). The disease has generally not been inducible in mouse strains other than BALB/c, including other strains such as DBA/2 that share the H-2^d MHC haplotype with BALB/c (Mikecz *et al.* 1987).

Relationship to the spondyloarthorpathies

The principal resemblance of proteoglycan-induced arthritis to the human spondyloarthropathies resides in the fact that both show dramatic vertebral pathology together with peripheral arthritis. Only limited information is available regarding the axial pathology of the murine disorder, however, (Glant *et al.* 1987), and the extent to which this reproduces that of ankylosing spondylitis remains to be clarified. Although both conditions show early perivertebral inflammation and enthesitis, with subsequent ankylosis, the destruction of the vertebral endplates and intravertebral discs seen in the murine disorder is not characteristic of ankylosing spondylitis, so the question remains whether any histological similarity in the initial process reflects a common molecular or cellular pathogenesis.

Regarding immunopathogenesis, the investigators who developed the murine proteoglycan-induced arthritis model have reported evidence of proteoglycan-specific T cells in patients with ankylosing spondylitis (Mikecz *et al.* 1988). However, this intriguing finding has largely been neglected, and the precise role that immunity to this (auto)antigen may play in the pathogenesis of ankylosing spondylitis remains to be investigated.

Adjuvant arthritis

Adjuvant arthritis in the rat is an extensively studied, experimentally induced inflammatory arthritis that is widely studied by investigators in many disciplines, including drug discovery, cellular immunology, inflammation, and neurobiology. The disease is typically induced by an intradermal injection of complete Freund's adjuvant (Taurog *et al.* 1988*a*). In the past, it has been suggested that adjuvant arthritis might serve as model of reactive arthritis; in part because it is an arthritis of acute onset that follows exposure to bacterial products, and partly because of a somewhat superficial resemblance of extra-articular features to those of reactive arthritis (Calin 1984; Rosenbaum 1981). However, in recent years it has become evident that the primary immunological events in adjuvant arthritis most likely involve a CD4 T cell-mediated response to mycobacterial heat-shock protein (Hogervorst *et al.* 1992; Pelegri *et al.* 1996), and the suggestion has been made that this response is somehow cross-reactive with cartilage components (Feige *et al.* 1994). It remains conceivable that critical and unique pathogenetic mechanisms are shared by adjuvant arthritis and the human spondyloarthropathies. However, in practice, the rat disease, while widely studied as a model of rheumatoid arthritis, has largely been abandoned by investigators interested primarily in the spondyloarthropathies.

Spondyloarthropathies in non-human primates

Evidence has been found to support the concept that non-human primates may be susceptible to the spondyloarthropathies. A captive, adult female gorilla has been described with clinical and radiographic findings fairly classic for ankylosing spondylitis, including hip disease requiring total hip replacement (Adams *et al.* 1987). Moreover, this gorilla had an offspring who developed peripheral arthritis at 2 years of age. Although this case report stated that the animal was typed as B27 by alloantisera, this has little significance in a xenogenetic context. Subsequent DNA sequencing of the B-locus alleles of this gorilla is discussed below.

In an examination of skeletal material from 99 lowland gorillas that had been free-living, evidence suggestive of spondyloarthropathy was found in 20, including erosive peripheral arthritis, spondylitis, sacroiliitis, and enthesitis (Rothschild and Woods 1989). In relation to human disease, the lesions were most reminiscent of psoriatic arthritis, although no precise correlation could be drawn to a distinct human condition.

The sharing of enteric pathogens between humans and non-human primates provides another approach to the study of the spondyloarthropathies. In a colony of rhesus macaques in which *Shigella flexneri* was enzootic, a self-limited asymmetrical arthritis of acute onset was noted in 14 out of 35 infected animals, including one animal with a probable sausage digit (T. J. Rowell and J. D. Taurog, unpublished results). All of the infected animals carried the same *S. flexneri* isolate, which was found to contain a plasmid which correlates with arthritogenicity in shigella (Stieglitz and Lipsky 1993).

It is an obvious, but still unanswered, question whether HLA-B27-like genes that predispose to disease might exist in primates. A number of studies have examined the homologies of class I MHC molecules between humans and other primates. MHC class I genes evolve primarily by recombination within loci, creating allelic lineages, and it is thought that certain allelic lineages antedate the separation of the modern primate species (Parham and Ohta 1996; Watkins 1995). The closest relationship between human and non-human primate class I sequences is a sharing of certain A locus allelic lineages between humans and chimpanzees (Watkins 1995). Moreover, considerable homology in the $\alpha 1$ domain of the B locus was been found when chimpanzee and pygmy chimpanzee sequences were compared with HLA, and HLA-B homologues from the pygmy chimpanzee that resemble B27 in the $\alpha 1$ domain were described in this study (McAdam *et al.* 1994). To date, no evidence for disease resembling the spondyloarthropathies in these species has come to our attention.

Gorilla alleles have generally been found to have less similarity than chimps to HLA, with the exception of sequences resembling HLA-B27 and -A2 (Lawlor *et al.* 1991). The homology between the gorilla (Gogo)-B*0101,-0102, and -0103 alleles and HLA-B*2702 is rather striking (Fig. 15.1). The amino-acid sequence homology in the $\alpha 1$ and $\alpha 2$ domains between B*2702 and Gogo-B*0101 is 91.8%, compared with 88.5% between B*2702 and the serologically cross-reactive allele B*0702, and compared with 86.3% between Gogo-B*0101 and

```
        α1 domain
        1
B*2702  GSHSMRYFHT SVSRPGRGEP RFITVGYVDD TLFVRFDSDA ASPREEPRAP WIEQEGPEYW DRETQICKAK AQTDRENLRI ALRYYNQSEA
GB*0101 --------D- A--------- ---------- -Q-------- ----M----- ---------- -----TS--Q ---------- ----------
B*0702  --------Y- ---------- ---S------ -Q-------- ---------- ---------- --N---Y--Q ------S--N LRG-------

        α2 domain
        91
B*2702  GSHTLQNMYG CDVGPDGRLL RGYHQDAYDG KDYIALNEDL SSWTAADTAA QITQRKWEAA RVAEQLRAYL EGECVEWLRR YLENGKETLQ RA
GB*0101 ----I-R-F- ---------- ---S-S---- ---------- ---------- ---------- -E-------- --T------- -----R---- --
B*0702  ------S--- ---------- --HD-Y---- ---------- R--------- ---------- -E---R---- ---------- ------DK-E --

        α3 domain
        183      191
B*2702  DPPKTHVT HHPISDHEAT LRCWALGFYP AEITLTWQRD GEDQTQDTEL VETRPAGDRT FQKWAAVVVP SGEEQRYTCH VQHEGLPKPL TLRW
GB*0101 -T------ ---------- ---------- ---------- ---------- --------G- ---------- ----E----- ---------- ----
B*0702  -------- ---------- ---------- ---------- ---------- ---------- ---------- ---------- ---------- ----

        TM domain                                    IC domain
        275    281                                   314
B*2702  EPSSQS TVPIVGIVAG LAVLAVVVIG AVVAAVMCRR KSS   GGKGGSY SQAACSDSAQ GSDVSLTA
GB*0101 ------ -I-------- ---------- ---T--I--- ---   ------- ----S----- --------
B*0702  ------ ---------- ---------- ---------- ---   ------- ---------- --------
```

Fig. 15.1 Comparison of amino-acid sequences for HLA-B*2702, HLA-B*0702, and the gorilla MHC B locus allele Gogo-B*0101. In the α1 and α2 domains, B*2702 is more closely related to Gogo-B*0101 than to B*0702 (see text for details). TM, transmembrane domain; IC, intracytoplasmic domain.

B*0702. Moreover, Gogo-B*0101 shares amino-acid identity with B*2702 at residues 71–94, including the most variable part of the α1 domain, although the B pockets of the two molecules differ at three of four residues (9, 45, 67), with identity at residue 24. The gorilla described by Adams *et al.* (1987), mentioned above, was found to carry Gogo-B*0101 and -B*0301 (J. Urvater and D.I. Watkins, unpublished observations) but B*0101 appears to be quite common in gorillas, so whether it confers risk for spondyloarthropathy is unclear.

The class I molecules of rhesus and other Old World monkeys bear less overall similarity to HLA alleles than those of apes (Watkins 1995, Boyson *et al.* 1996). None the less, characterization of class I alleles and continued investigation of anecdotal spondyloarthropathic disease in these and other primates may ultimately provide information that complements the disease-related epidemiology of the B27 subtypes and other HLA-B alleles.

Conclusions

A variety of animal models of the spondyloarthropathies is under investigation. Additional information may be achieved by combining experimental systems. For example, proteoglycan-induced arthritis or the *ank* gene can be studied in B27 transgenic mice, and disease-related primate alleles can be introduced as transgenes into rodents. There is good reason to hope that these animal systems will provide answers to many questions regarding the pathogenesis of the spondyloarthropathies. However, as in any experimental science, it will only be possible in retrospect to know which systems will turn out to have been the most fruitful.

16 Disease and outcome indices/instruments for the spondylarthropathies

L. Gail Kennedy

Introduction

Every disease requires some method of assessment. This may be to evaluate aspects such as disease status, progression, or response to treatment. Irrespective of the reason for performing the analysis, the method used has to comply with certain standards.

Bombardier and Tugwell (1982) defined a methodological framework for the development of indices. They listed five criteria which should be fulfilled:

1. Content validity—are the components of the index and their weighting appropriate for the analysis they are to be used for?;
2. Face validity—is the combination of the components sensible?;
3. Criterion validity—are the results reliable and able to reflect the true state of the disease?;
4. Discriminant validity—does the method detect even the smallest change in status?;
5. Construct validity—do the results of the index agree with the expectations of the study's hypothesis?

Although these guidelines were set out to aid the formation of indices, they can be used in assessing the suitability of any instrument involved in evaluating different aspects of disease.

Many methods of assessing patients, either in research or clinical situations, are performed out of tradition rather than having been properly evaluated and proven to be reliable, valid, and practical. This chapter looks at various forms of assessment, and reviews their suitability for collecting information on the diseases for which they are used.

As there is very little information on standard methods of assessment in many of the spondylarthropathies, this chapter concentrates on ankylosing spondylitis and psoriatic arthritis. Some, but not all, of the comments and conclusions may apply to the other spondylarthritides.

Ankylosing spondylitis

For many years assessing disease activity and outcome in ankylosing spondylitis (AS) has been notoriously difficult. As pointed out in the *Lancet* (1987) this is not made any easier by the fact that AS is a heterogeneous disorder.

When assessing disease activity in any disease, either to study progression or to chart treatment responses, objective measures are judged to be the most suitable and reliable. For a

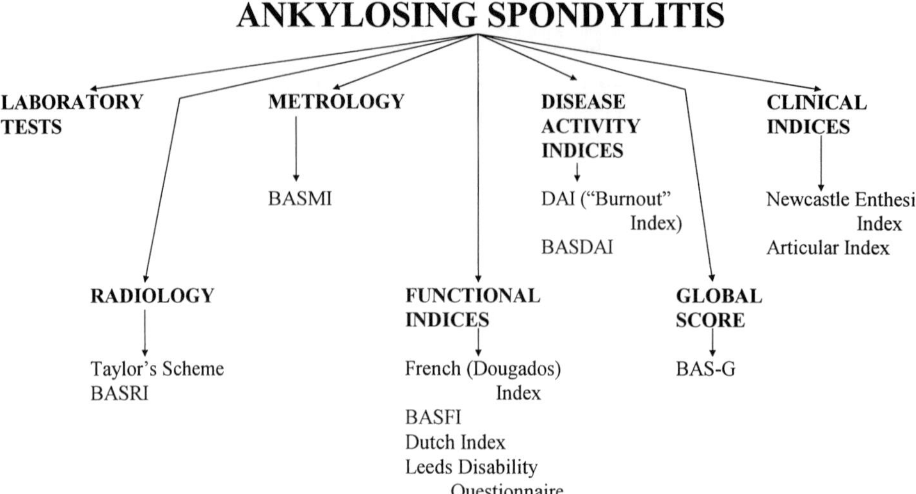

Fig. 16.1 Methods of assessing disease and outcome in AS that are discussed in this Chapter.

disease such as rheumatoid arthritis both laboratory variables and radiology play a major part in evaluating progression, but for ankylosing spondylitis the story may be different.

Laboratory tests

There are many different analyses that can be performed in the laboratory to assess disease processes, but for ankylosing spondylitis, erythrocyte sedimentation rate (ESR) and C-reactive protein levels (CRP) are the two best documented.

ESR is thought to be the conventional laboratory index of inflammation even though it can be altered in response to other variables, such as changes in the red blood cell morphology and the presence of abnormal serum proteins, which make the results unreliable (Carr 1983). Also, the ESR reading may be lowered if the test is not performed immediately after the blood is collected.

CRP does not suffer from these problems. The exact biological function of CRP is unknown, but the levels of the protein can increase rapidly (within hours) and may rise to high levels in response to infections, tissue injuries, and inflammatory processes.

Both ESR and CRP estimations are widely used in rheumatoid arthritis, where they are sensitive markers of disease activity (Amos *et al.* 1977; McConkey *et al.* 1972; Mallya *et al.* 1982). In AS, however, there are reports both for and against the value of these two variables in determining disease activity.

Cowling *et al.* (1980) reported that their patients with AS had raised CRP and ESR values which were comparable to the values found in patients with rheumatoid arthritis (Amos *et al.* 1978). They also reported a correlation between the CRP and ESR values and clinically assessed disease activity. Nashel *et al.* (1986) found CRP to be valuable in differentiating between active and inactive disease, although their results were not as great as has been reported for active rheumatoid arthritis. They did not find a relationship between ESR and active or inactive AS.

Other studies have reported no such correlation between ESR or CRP and disease activity. Sheehan *et al.* (1986), using a scheme of clinical assessment similar to Cowling *et al.* (1980) and Nashel *et al.* (1986), reported no statistically significant results between the laboratory variables and activity of the disease. Laurent and Panayi (1983) and Taylor *et al.* (1991) also found a lack of correlation similar to that found between clinical disease activity and ESR by Kendall *et al.* (1973).

Unfortunately, clinical assessment of disease activity has frequently been gauged on the presence or absence of uveitis or peripheral joint involvement (Cowling *et al.* 1980; Laurent and Panayi 1983). If these are then used to evaluate laboratory measures (Cowling *et al.* 1980; Nashel *et al.* 1986), the results are open to question.

It may be the peripheral synovitis which causes the raised CRP and ESR rather than the spondylitis *per se.* Laurent and Panayi (1983) found CRP to be raised only marginally in a group with spondylitis alone, whereas it was significantly elevated in those who also had peripheral arthritis or uveitis. ESR was only raised in the subset of patients with spondylitis and uveitis. Sheehan *et al.* (1986) also found ESR and CRP results to be higher in patients with peripheral arthritis or secondary forms of AS.

A possible reason for the lack of correlation between laboratory variables and axial disease may be due to the difficulty in accurately assessing the activity of the clinical process in these patients. It is also possible that the inflammation involved in the spondylitic disease may not stimulate a response in these particular variables. In disorders in which several acute-phase proteins (APP) have been measured, there was not always a simultaneous increase in all. This has been reported in systemic lupus erythematosus (Becker *et al.* 1980) and subgroups of Behcet's syndrome (Adinolfi and Lehner 1976). It is possible that each APP requires a different type of inflammatory stimulus and each could have a specific physiological function. However, Laurent and Panayi (1983) failed to show a correlation between other APP (such as α1-antitrypsin, fibrinogen and the ninth component of complement (C9)) and disease activity as did Sheehan *et al.* (1986) with orosomucoid, α1-antitrypsin and α2-macroglobulin.

Radiology

The scoring of plain radiographs is thought to be unreliable and non-reproducible (Hollingsworth *et al.* 1983; Taylor *et al.* 1991), but due mainly to their inclusion in both the Rome (Kellgren *et al.* 1963) and New York (Bennett and Burch 1968*c*) criteria for the diagnosis of AS (although their inclusion for this purpose has also been criticized (Calin *et al.* 1977; Rigby and Wood 1993)) they are widely used as a 'gold-standard' in evaluating the disease process.

The scoring of the sacroiliac joints alone has proven unreliable for inter- and intraobservations. For example Kappa statistic results[1] range from 0.38 to 0.84 in the report of Taylor *et al.* (1991). Hollingsworth *et al.* (1983) had similar problems, and even attempts to reach agreement by consensus did not offer a greatly improved solution. Assessing the hips and lumbar and cervical regions in the same way increases the problems four-fold. Pande *et al.* (1995)

[1]Kappa statistic—an index which defines the proportion of agreement above or below that expected by chance alone: 1 indicating total concordance of the results, 0 indicating that concordance is equal to that expected by chance alone, and –1 being absolute discordance.

have compared the old scoring methods with a new BASRI system (Bath Ankylosing Spondylitis Radiology Index). They report less inter-and intraobserver variation, and greater speed and simplicity than the system described by Taylor *et al.* (1991). However, no further details have yet been published.

Another problem is that, as pointed out by Laurent *et al.* (1991), a measure of disease needs to be potentially reversible as well as reliable and valid. Radiographs can only record progressive worsening of the skeleton, irrespective of treatment or results of other measures indicating improvement. In addition, any alteration in the radiographic results are likely to occur only over long periods. Certainly, no change is likely to be noticeable over weeks or months. Taylor *et al.* (1991), comparing radiographs taken 12 months apart, reported significant progression in their scores, but said that the magnitude of change was too small to be clinically useful. Also, viewing the 12-month films in conjunction with the initial ones may have produced observer bias toward progression. Unfortunately, therefore, new methods of assessment have to be compared to a 'gold-standard' which is flawed in itself.

The use of magnetic resonance imaging (MRI) has been explored for assessing spinal changes in AS. Although the radiation exposure is reduced compared with plain X-rays, and has the benefit of revealing soft-tissue involvement, the inter-and intraobserver reliability is no better than for the normal radiographs (Doherty *et al.* 1992). In contrast, there was good intraobserver reproducibility reported for computed tomographic (CT) scans of the sacroiliac joints (Taylor *et al.* 1991). This was not the case for the interobserver analysis, but this may have been due to a systematic error which could be overcome by prior training, according to the authors. However, there is concern over the higher radiation exposure, cost, and availability of the equipment. Therefore, standard radiographs still remain the 'gold-standard'.

Metrology

There have been numerous methods proposed for measuring spinal movements, many of which use special instruments or even radiology. These methods have rarely been assessed for reliability or validity at the time of publication.

Two large studies have been performed in recent years to address this subject. The first, by Pile *et al.* (1991), investigated inter- and intraobserver variation and reliability in 17 different spinal measurements. For analysis of the cervical spine they concluded that lateral flexion (measured by goniometer as opposed to the tragus-to-acromioclavicular-joint distraction) and rotation were reliable and had no significant interobserver variability. However, extension and flexion measures were not reliable and had little clinical use.

The authors rejected the measurement of spinal flexion by finger-to-floor distance (Kraus and Eisenmenger-Weber 1945). Although it is a reliable and easy method to perform, it is invalid as a measure of vertebral flexion (Kippers and Parker 1987). This is because it is influenced by structures other than the spine, so making changes in the measurements difficult to interpret. Thoracic and upper lumbar movement was better assessed by C_7-to-iliac crest line distraction (flexion) as reported previously (AAOS 1965), while lateral flexion of the same area was reliably measured by the finger-to-floor distance taken laterally (this did not have the same problems as finger-to-floor distance on sagittal flexion). The modified Schober index (Macrae and Wright 1969; Schober 1937) was judged to be a reasonably reliable measure of lumbar flexion.

Pile and colleagues (1991) felt that although the tragus-to-wall distance (Tomlinson *et al.* 1986) had the highest ranked coefficient of reliability, it was not considered to be a clinically useful measurement since it was only relevant in patients with severe disease (Calin 1985).

Chest expansion is not reliable, as has been shown by Moll and Wright (1972) and Mackay *et al.* (personal communication).

None of the hip-mobility measurements involving a goniometer (AAOS 1965) were shown to be reliable (as Boone *et al.* (1978) have previously reported), and the authors suggested that intermalleolar distance should be investigated as an alternative. They concluded that, as a minimum number of measurements, the following assessments should be performed to assess spinal function in patients with ankylosing spondylitis: cervical rotation; lateral cervical flexion using a goniometer; C_7-to-iliac crest line distraction; modified Schober index, and lateral flexion by finger-to-floor distance.

Jenkinson *et al.* (1994*b*) have also analysed the reliability of various measurements. Having evaluated the metrology results from 20 movements, they intuitively chose those five which were considered to reflect axial status most accurately: tragus-to-wall distance (Tomlinson *et al.* 1986); modified Schober index (Macrae and Wright 1969; Schober 1937); intermalleolar distance (Calin 1985); cervical rotation (AAOS 1965); and lumbar side-flexion (measured by finger-to-floor distance: Pile *et al.* 1991). These five measurements have been collectively named BASMI—the Bath Ankylosing Spondylitis Metrology Index. Each measurement was given a scoring system. Originally this was on a 0, 1, 2 scale with each score being added together to give a 0–10 range. This has since been improved to give a 0 through 10 scale for each measurement, and a mean of the five results gives the overall BASMI score (Jones *et al.* 1995). The BASMI was tested both for reliability and inter- and intraobserver variation, for which it performed well (the range of inter-and intraobserver correlation values = 0.94–0.99). In addition, the BASMI was shown to be sensitive to changes in patients' mobility over a 3-week intensive in-patient treatment course.

The two papers agree on three of the measurements: cervical rotation; lateral side-flexion (by the finger-to-floor method) and the modified Schober's index. Jenkinson and colleagues (1994)*b* did not have the measurements of lateral cervical flexion and C_7-to-iliac crest line distraction in their original list, so it is unknown if the two groups would have come to the same conclusions. The Bath group assessed intermalleolar distance, which proved to be highly reliable and valid, as Pile *et al.* (1991) had suggested. Tragus-to-wall distance was included, without comment, as a good measure by Jenkinson *et al.* (1994*b*) but was rejected by Pile *et al.* (1991) with doubts about its clinical utility.

An attempt has been made to validate the metrology index (BASMI) by comparing it to radiology (Kennedy *et al.* 1995). The correlation between the two instruments was poor. This was attributed to the sensitivity of metrology to factors other than pure radiological changes, such as normal individual physical limitations, soft-tissue changes, and enthesopathic involvement, all of which would be expected to reduce correlation. Another obstacle in attempting to correlate the two methods was the well-documented unreliability of the radiographic scoring itself, discussed above (Hollingsworth *et al.* 1983; Taylor *et al.* 1991).

Although metrology lacks good correlation with the radiographs, its obvious advantages over X-rays may make it more useful in assessing disease progression. For example, metrology is quickly performed and does not require expensive equipment. The measurements can be repeated as often as required without any risk of irradiation. However, probably the most important point is that metrology examines parameters that are potentially reversible, unlike radiographic changes, which largely either stabilize or deteriorate.

Questionnaires and indices

In the early 1980s, the concept of self-administered questionnaires became more acceptable for the assessment of rheumatic diseases, with the publication of the Health Assessment Questionnaire (HAQ: Fries *et al.* 1980) and the Arthritis Impact Measurement Scales (AIMS: Meenan *et al.* 1980). These were primarily designed to evaluate health status in patients with rheumatoid arthritis. Subsequently, numerous studies have shown both instruments to be reliable, valid, and sensitive to change for both research and clinical purposes. They have also been translated into other languages and assessed in diseases other than rheumatoid arthritis. The HAQ has been modified for use with spondylarthropathies (HAQ-S: Daltroy *et al.* 1990) by adding items of daily living which were reported to be troublesome by patients with AS. However, there is still a general feeling that the instruments which have been designed for use with rheumatoid arthritis are not appropriate, even with modifications, to assess fully and accurately spondylarthropathy in general, and ankylosing spondylitis in particular. Therefore, a variety of disease-specific instruments have now been produced for use in patients with ankylosing spondylitis.

Functional questionnaires

Dougados *et al.* (1988) were the first group to produce a functional index specifically designed for patients with ankylosing spondylitis. The questionnaire consists of 20 actions taken from an original list of 29 suggested by a team of rheumatologists. A score of 0 was given if the action could be accomplished without difficulty, 1 if it was possible but with difficulty, and 2 if it was impossible. The index was scored by an interviewer after a verbal response from the patient. The index, with a scale of 0–40, is reported to take approximately 2 minutes to complete and to have inter-and intraobserver reliability. A high correlation was found between the change in the index after 2 weeks of treatment and the overall judgement of the patient and clinician. A second analysis, during an evaluation of non-steroidal anti-inflammatory drugs, found the index to be appropriate for use in such studies (Dougados *et al.* 1990).

Three further papers were published in 1994 on the subject of functional assessment in AS. The first, the Bath Ankylosing Spondylitis Functional Index (BASFI), is a completely new instrument (Calin *et al.* 1994). It consists of ten questions, eight on activities relating to the functional anatomy of the patients and two assessing the patient's ability to cope with everyday life. The self-administered questionnaire has the results recorded on 10 cm visual analogue scales, the final score being a mean of the ten results (0–10 scale). The questions were designed by a team of rheumatologists, physiotherapists, and research associates, and included input from patients with AS. This index was compared to the previous functional index (Dougados *et al.* 1988). The two indices were comparable in all aspects except for two—the BASFI scores covered more of the available range than the older index, and only the BASFI was able to show a significant change in the scores over a 3-week treatment period. BASFI has since been found to have a high internal consistency when the Cronbach's alpha score[2] was calculated (Jones *et al.* 1996*a*).

[2]Cronbach's alpha score is a measure of internal consistency to give an indication of an index's reliability. An index with a score of >0.7 is regarded as suitable for use in group comparisons as a research tool, whilst a score of >0.9 indicates the index can be also used as a clinical tool with individuals (Cronbach 1951).

The second paper concerned the development and validation of a Dutch version of the original French index (Creemers *et al.* 1994*a*). This also involved various health professional groups and patient opinion. Activities were added to the questionnaire which had a specific duration, for example sitting for 10 and 30 minutes. Other items were included to correspond with the Dutch way of life, such as riding a bicycle. In total, 15 items were added. Questions such as getting in and out of the bath were split into two separate actions, so giving a total of 37 items. This version was self-administered in contrast to the original questionnaire. The scoring system was also altered from 0,1, and 2 to 0,2, and 4. The main three responses remained essentially the same. However, if patients answered with more than one response per question the scores were adapted accordingly. For example, 'possible' plus 'possible but with difficulty' = 1, while 'possible with difficulty' plus 'not possible' = 3. It is not made clear how the patients were asked to indicate their responses. If they were instructed to only tick one answer then the adapted scores (1 and 3) are only used when patients complete the questionnaire incorrectly. The results from this system may be quite different if compared to a defined five-point scale. The authors also suggest that up to three items can be omitted by the patients, and the end score is calculated from only those questions answered. This indicates that patients may have trouble answering some of the questions. The index was reported to be reproducible, have criterion validity, and be sensitive to the changes which occurred during a 12-week drug study. In addition to this, the index had a very high Cronbach's alpha score.

The third paper described yet another new index (the Leeds Disability Questionnaire: Abbott *et al.* 1994). This is based upon a previous paper by Badley *et al.* (1984). Questions were extracted from the mobility, bending-down, and reaching-up sections, with the addition of a posture category based on another paper (Dougados *et al.* 1986). The questions within each section deal with tasks that are scaled in increasing order of difficulty. Alterations were made in accordance with patients' suggestions, giving a final 19 questions in the four functional areas. This was reduced further to 16, since three items which rarely caused any problems were removed. The scoring system is similar to that of the Health Assessment Questionnaire, or HAQ (Fries *et al.* 1980), but with an alternative category of 'only able to do using unusual movements or gadgets' as the authors felt that the third category of the HAQ, namely only able to do 'with some help from another person' (as it was in the original paper) or able to do 'with much difficulty' (as in a modified version of HAQ; Pincus *et al.* 1983) did not provide enough discrimination between 'able to do with difficulty' and 'unable to do'. Each individual item is then scored from 0–3, and the highest score within each section is recorded. The total score is divided by the number of sections answered, giving an overall score between 0 and 3. The self-administered questionnaire was reproducible and had external validity. High internal consistency was also measured using the Cronbach's alpha test. The authors showed changes in the scores after a treatment regimen.

To date, the three functional instruments proposed in 1994 have not been directly compared with each other. There is agreement amongst the authors, however, that there are several problems with the French index (Dougados *et al.* 1988). For example, some patients found difficulty in answering without qualification, due to either a lack of specificity of the questions or the fact that the index did not account for the possible use of help or aids. Patients can often 'circumvent' difficulties by adopting 'unusual' movements or techniques (Calin *et al.* 1994). However, the index was originally designed to be used as part of an interview where the questions can be clarified. Unfortunately, this can lead to interobserver, and even intraobserver, variation if strict procedures and instructions are not adhered to. Additional problems arise from the wording of the middle category, in which the patient can perform the activity, but with difficulty. This covers a broad range of subjects from those who have minimal difficulty to those who are only just able to complete the task. Thus it lacks sensitivity both to small variations in individual patients' status and to differences between patients.

Each group has attempted to overcome problems such as these by altering the original index or by proposing a new instrument. Each one reports good validity and reproducibility, and claims to show a sensitivity to changes relating to treatment. All three involved patient's views in the design and preliminary testing of the instruments as suggested by Bakker *et al.* (1993). Finally, all had very high Cronbach's alpha scores, showing them to be useful as both research tools in group comparisons and for assessing individual patients in a clinical situation (Jones *et al.* 1994*a*).

Disease activity questionnaires

Single measurements may not be valuable in assessing various aspects of disease on their own, but when combined with other variables the overall index has a number of advantages, such as improvement in validity (van der Heijde *et al.* 1993), avoidance of duplicity, and an increased sensitivity to change (Boers and Tugwell 1993; Roberts 1993). Such composite indices may then form a more powerful outcome indicator (Goldsmith *et al.* 1993), provided the final product is reliable and valid, as depicted by Bombardier and Tugwell (1982).

Two instruments have used a combination of measures to evaluate disease activity in ankylosing spondylitis. The first was designed originally to evaluate the phenomenon of 'burn out'[3] in ankylosing spondylitis. The disease activity index consisted of three questions and a global visual analogue scale, and was given to patients in the form of a self-administered questionnaire (Kennedy *et al.* 1993*a*). Of the three questions, two concentrated on the severity and frequency of pain, and one question concerned the activity of the AS. The questions were originally taken, with slight modification, from the Arthritis Impact Measurement Scale questionnaire (Meenan *et al.* 1980). The limitations of this index relate to the absence of morning stiffness and fatigue (Calin *et al.* 1993), and a lack of validation.

A year later the same group developed and published a new disease activity scale (Garrett *et al.* 1994). This consists of six questions relating to five major symptoms of AS: fatigue; spinal pain; joint pain/swelling; areas of localized tenderness; and morning stiffness. The last symptom is measured in terms of both quality (degree of stiffness) and quantity (length of time for which the stiffness persists). In all, 10 cm visual analogue scales are used to measure a patient's response to each question. The mean of the two scores relating to morning stiffness is used in calculating the final 0–10 score, giving equal weighting to each symptom.

This Bath Ankylosing Spondylitis Disease Activity Index (BASDAI) is reported to take an average of 1 minute to complete, and has been tested for its reliability in terms of consistency and sensitivity to change.

The original disease activity index (Kennedy *et al.* 1993*a*) was validated at the same time as the BASDAI, on the same patients. Both indices performed equally well in all the criteria assessed, but the BASDAI was deemed to be the superior index in terms of face and content validity due to its comprehensive assessment of symptoms and their equal weighting.

---

[3]This refers to an indefinite period without disease activity as opposed to remission, a self-limiting state that may be followed by a relapse (Kennedy *et al.* 1993*a*).

BASDAI is deemed appropriate for use as a research tool in group comparisons (Jones *et al.* 1996*a*) since it has a Cronbach's alpha score of 0.8.

Global assessments

A single item (global) assessment of patients with AS tends to occur frequently in the literature. Bakker *et al.* (1993) reported that physicians used such a method in 7 out of 34 studies. A recent study (Jones *et al.* 1996*b*) has focused on formalizing and validating this approach. A self-administered question (in two versions) asks patients to indicate the effect of ankylosing spondylitis on their well-being over the previous week and 6 months, using 10 cm visual analogue scales to record the answers.

The main purpose of the study was to 'provide health professionals with a quick, quantifiable and valid way to obtain the patient's perspective and monitor it over time'. The greatest use of BAS-G, as it has been named (Bath Ankylosing Spondylitis Global Score), may be in a clinical setting where a numerical score indicating the patient's well-being can be compared to previous scores. This would be particularly useful where patients do not necessarily consult the same rheumatologist at each visit.

The BAS-G is not designed to stand alone. The authors recommend that it should be taken as only one element in a complete assessment of patient status. The BAS-G is reported to correlate well with the BASDAI (Garrett *et al.* 1994) and the BASFI (Calin *et al.* 1994). The BAS-G is not disease-specific in content and so may be applicable to other chronic and rheumatic diseases, but it would obviously require revalidation in each case.

Clinical indices

Two similar indices, published within a year of each other, have been designed to evaluate tenderness of the entheses (Mander *et al.* 1987) and tenderness of the joints (Dougados *et al.* 1988).

The Newcastle-based group (Mander *et al.* 1987) constructed a list of entheses that are known to be involved in ankylosing spondylitis and those that are possibly involved. Some sites were scored individually and some as a group (the highest scoring site being recorded for the group as a whole). The scoring system (0, no pain; 1, mild tenderness; 2, moderate tenderness; and 3, wince or withdraw) allows a total possible score of 90.

Although there was an indication that the index was sensitive to changes in clinical state, there was a high degree of interobserver variability, despite attempts to reduce it. The authors maintained that this was to be expected with a subjective method of assessment. However, no such variation was produced with the visual analogue scales which the patients completed in the same study to record their level of pain and stiffness, even though these are also subjective in nature. It was suggested that sequential measurements of the same patient would need to be made by the same observer. However, the level of intraobserver variability was not addressed in the original study. The authors report that the index is non-invasive, acceptable to patients, and is designed to take 3 minutes to perform.

The Newcastle enthesis index has been compared to a new disease activity index (Garrett *et al.* 1994), with poor results in the enthesis index's ability to monitor changes in activity during a physiotherapy in-patient treatment course, in contrast to the self-administered questionnaire (Calin 1995).

The second instrument assessed tenderness in a slightly different way by concentrating on the joints as opposed to the entheses (Dougados *et al.* 1988). In all, three rheumatologists formed a list of 18 sites to be assessed, 10 of which remained in the final index. Firm digital pressure or movement was used at each site and scored as follows: 0, no tenderness; 1, painful; 2, painful and the patient winced, and 3, the patient said it was painful, winced, and withdrew the limb. This index, which takes 2–5 minutes to perform, was reported to be reproducible with little inter-and intraobserver variation, and reflected a clinical change over 2 weeks of treatment.

Neither of these indices appear to be in widespread use for research purposes, although this may not be true in clinical practice.

Psoriatic arthritis

At least as much as ankylosing spondylitis, psoriatic arthritis is highly variable. Some patients have a few episodes and then recover completely, but others have severe, persistent skin and joint problems. Since there have been relatively few studies into the most appropriate methods for assessing disease progression and outcome of psoriatic arthritis/spondylitis, this has hampered efforts to define the natural history of the disease, and it is only recently that this issue has begun to be addressed.

Clinical and radiological assessments

Gladman *et al.* (1990*a*) have proposed and validated a method of assessing inflammatory activity and damage in the joints of patients with psoriatic arthritis. The inflammation was documented by the number of joints with stress pain and/or effusions (ARA 1965), while clinical damage was recorded by the number of deformed joints and the number with ankylosis, loosening, or limitation of movement of more than 20% of the range. This was compared with radiographs, both of the hands and feet (Steinbrocker *et al.* 1949) and the sacroiliac joints (Bennett and Burch 1968). The clinical measurements of inflammatory activity and damage were reliable, with little observer variability. This was in contrast to radiological analysis, which again proved to be unsatisfactory.

In contrast, Hanly *et al.* (1988) reported reliable results with radiographic scoring. Reliable intraobserver readings were shown, but no statistical values were given. There was said to be complete agreement between the two evaluators on all radiographs except three. However, it is not clear if the readings were performed separately and later compared, or whether the researchers scored the films together, so increasing the likelihood of agreement.

It should be noted here that 'clinical' evidence of sacroiliitis is mentioned frequently in some published work (Gladman *et al.* 1987; Hanly *et al.* 1988) as opposed to, or in addition to, 'radiological' evidence. The 'clinical' evidence is obtained by the use of specific tests—the Gaenzlen's manoeuvre, the Patrick-Fabere test, or by direct pressure over the sacroiliac joints (Hoppenfeld 1976). These techniques are of dubious value in assessing ankylosing spondylitis and are not widely used.

Laboratory variables

There are no specific laboratory tests for psoriatic arthritis, either for diagnosis or for monitoring disease progression. Raised levels of white blood cell counts and other acute-phase reactants may occur (Gladman *et al.* 1987), indicating an inflammatory reaction, but this is not necessarily specific for joint disease in the setting of psoriasis. An elevated ESR has been found in 40% of patients with psoriatic arthritis, but this may also reflect both skin and joint inflammation (Gladman *et al.* 1986, 1987). ESR is thought to be a poor indicator of both disease activity (Duffy *et al.* 1992) and functional outcome (Coulton *et al.* 1989) in patients with psoriatic arthritis.

Metrology

Some patients with psoriatic arthritis are reported to have a restricted range of back movements (Gladman *et al.* 1987, Hanly *et al.* 1988), showing a reduction in flexion–extension, lateral flexion, and rotation. However, these patients generally do not have as many symptoms from their back disease or the same degree of limitation of back movements as patients with ankylosing spondylitis (Hanly *et al.* 1988, Scarpa *et al.* 1988). Therefore, using metrology to assess spinal function may not be applicable in patients with psoriatic arthritis.

Questionnaires

The Arthritis Impact Measurement Scales (AIMS: Meenan *et al.* 1980), originally designed to assess health status in rheumatoid arthritis, has been assessed for use in psoriatic arthritis (Duffy *et al.* 1992).

The authors reported that AIMS is a valid instrument for psoriatic arthritis. They concluded that the physical-function scales reflected not only physical-function impairment but also the degree of disease activity and severity. The pain scale was said to 'highly' reflect disease activity. However the r values for the correlations concerned (Pearson's product–moment correlation) were never higher than 0.6 (the lowest being 0.09) so, although the p values look highly significant, there is concern regarding the usefulness of the scales in real terms.

Stern (1985), while studying the epidemiology of joint complaints in patients with psoriasis, designed a short questionnaire to be used during an interview between the patient and a nurse. Although this has not been formally validated, the author showed that the proportion of patients with psoriatic arthritis who reported a limiting effect on daily activities increased in direct relation to the number of anatomical sites involved.

Concluding remarks

The last 5 years have seen a large increase in the number of methods for assessing disease activity, impact, and outcome in the field of spondylarthropathy. Previously, it was assumed that instruments designed for other rheumatic diseases could be used satisfactorily, either with or without additions to increase the sensitivity. However, disease-specific instruments are now being developed and are becoming more acceptable. It is likely that even within the group of spondylarthropathies, different diseases will require slightly different approaches. Many of the methods summarized in this chapter are still in their infancy and will need further investigation and testing. The various means of assessing disease and outcome in AS are summarized in Fig. 16.1

The measurement of 'health-related quality of life' or 'health status,' as well as of outcomes, is becoming a major component in all aspects of health care. Bowling (1995) summarized various definitions of health and health-related quality of life (including that of the World Health Organization (WHO 1947, 1948) by defining health status as the:

> Optimum levels of mental, physical, role (e.g. work, parent, career, etc.) and social functioning, including relationships and perceptions of health, fitness, life satisfaction and well-being. It should also include some assessment of the patient's level of satisfaction with treatment, outcome and health status and with future prospects. It is distinct from quality of life as a whole, which would also include adequacy of housing, income and perceptions of immediate environment.

There is still much to be done before we are able to assess fully the health status of patients with spondylarthropathies, but the indices and instruments which are already available provide a good basis on which to work and expand.

17 Ankylosing spondylitis—the patient's point of view

Fergus J. Rogers

Ankylosing spondylitis (AS) is such a variable condition that every patient's experience is different. The first major problem encountered by patients worldwide is misdiagnosis. For the young spondylitic patient with a recent disease onset this can become a lonely, painful, and humiliating experience: an ideal sequence of events would be the following:

1. The family doctor suspects ankylosing spondylitis.
2. Referral to a rheumatologist confirms the diagnosis, and appropriate medication is prescribed, with referral to the physiotherapist.
3. The physiotherapist is aware of the latest stretching techniques, and any recent loss of posture and mobility is regained.
4. Either the rheumatologist or the physiotherapist acquaints the patient with the AS patient association in his country (such as the National Ankylosing Spondylitis Society (NASS) in the UK), membership of which brings the patient into contact with the society's literature, etc., and the local weekly evening supervised group physiotherapy. A national network of physiotherapy support groups is the aim of most European societies.

Unfortunately the reality is often quite different and any or all of the following may occur.

1. The disease goes unsuspected, despite years of symptoms, either by the primary physician or by the specialists. Improvements have now been made in this area (Calin *et al.* 1988).
2. Repeated visits to physicians lead to the suspicion of neurosis. The undiagnosed patient feels frustrated, isolated, and angry at being considered neurotic or a malingerer. After several years, some patients also experience additional loneliness due to the withdrawal of sympathy from friends and members of their family who begin to sympathize with the physician's misdiagnosis.
3. The patient develops uveitis, which may be misdiagnosed and mistreated as conjunctivitis. Eventually the patient visits an ophthalmologist, who diagnoses uveitis.
4. Loss of spinal posture leads to referral to a physiotherapy department for mechanical back damage, and inappropriate interventions are performed.
5. Surgery is performed for presumed disc disease.
6. Upon diagnosis the patient is given only a brief description of the disorder, most of which is rapidly forgotten. The primary physician knows little about the condition and either cannot give advice or gives inappropriate advice. This leads some patients to suspect that the doctor is withholding information to protect them against knowledge of an appalling prognosis. The patient is not referred to a patient organization.

7. Even after diagnosis there is no referral to physiotherapy and loss of posture continues. Unaware of his own role in disease management, the patient feels helpless and this feeling is reinforced by the family doctor informing him that, apart from anti-inflammatory medication, nothing can be done.

Historical aspects of AS prior to the foundation of AS self-help societies

The recorded history of ankylosing spondylitis is a long and fascinating story dealt with by Bywaters and others in previous publications. However, the disease has slowly and logically emerged over three centuries to the present day. First, there were the published observations of skeletal remains by Bernard Connor in 1691.

> ....the Body of this Perfon muft have been immoveable, that he could neither bend or fretch himfelf out, rife up nor lye down, nor turn upon his Side, having only the Head, Feet, and Hands moveable... and it is likely this Perfon breathed very fhort...
>
> An Extract of a Letter from Bernard Connor, M.D. to Sir Charles Walgrave, Publifhed in French at Paris: Giving an Account of an Extraordinary Humane Sceleton, whofe Vertebrae of the Back, the Ribs, and feveral Bones down to the Os Sacrum, were all firmly united into one folid Bone, without Joynting or Cartilage.
>
> Philosophical Transactions. Royal Society (1695) London Vol 19, p 21.

The first clinical descriptions were made by Benjamin Travers in 1824, and the first clinical and pathological correlations drawn by Charles Fagge 1877, also from Guy's Hospital, London. At about the same time, observations were being made on the continent of Europe by people whose names, until halfway through this century, were synonymous with the condition in their own countries: Adolf Strümpell in Germany, Pierre Marie in France, and Wladimir M. Bechterew in Russia (Benoist 1995). The disease is still known as *Morbus Bechterew* in Scandinavia, Germany, Austria, Russia, and Russia's former satellite countries.

During the first half of this century patients were erroneously treated by immobilizing they in plaster jackets, to prevent the 'hoop-like deformity' associated with the condition (a term used by Benjamin Brodie in the fifth edition of his book *Pathological and Surgical Observations on the Diseases of Joints* published in 1850). In 1906 radiography was used by Schlayer to look at the living spine, which by 1930 was used as an aid to diagnosis by recognizing the important role of sacroiliitis in the onset of the condition. Deep X-ray therapy was introduced by Kohler in 1926 which, for many patients, produced a noticeable decrease in pain.

Drafting so many young men into the British (and other) armed forces during the Second World War, combined with the 23-year-old average age of disease onset, increased the disease profile. Some military patients, when being referred to civilian doctors (especially in the Westminster Hospital) expressed their feelings that they would be happier out of their plaster 'prisons' and mobilized through exercise. Fortunately, the rheumatology specialists listened to them, their plaster casts were removed, and they were referred to the military remedial gymnasts. The improvement in mobility was immediately apparent, and the patients' instincts were well founded. During those years the military did much to spearhead a change of attitudes and treatment.

At the United Services Section meeting in 1966, Group Captain C. B. Wynn Parry reviewed 176 military cases (Wynn Parry 1974). It was demonstrated that with a regime of exercises, drug therapy, and periodic admission to a rehabilitation centre for intense mobility treatment the majority of patients were able to follow a full service career.

He reported on a further 66 cases treated between 1966 and 1973: 62 were still on full-time duty. The remainder had been invalidated from the services but had physically highly demanding jobs and did not wish to change to a less exacting trade (Wynn Parry 1974).

Aspirin had for decades been the only common form of pain control. However, the 1950s saw the introduction of phenylbutazone—the first anti-inflammatory agent—and this was quickly followed by a host of others, and new ones are still being developed. Deep X-ray therapy was the next accepted treatment to be discarded following early observations and an adverse report by Sir Richard Doll (Court-Brown and Doll 1965).

Population surveys during the 1950s and 1960s (Emery and Lawrence 1967) began to establish familial associations. Observations leading to the naming by Wright *et al.* in 1974 of the seronegative spondylarthritides finally put an end to the insistence in some parts of the world that the disease was as a variation of rheumatoid arthritis.

A fresh explosion of interest occurred in 1973 when ethnic and familial interest came sharply into focus with the discovery of the association between AS and HLA-B27—first, at the Westminster Hospital (Caffrey and James 1973), and in the same year by a team in California (Schlosstein *et al.* 1973). The findings were first published in the journal *Nature*, but were largely ignored until a few months later details appeared in *the Lancet* (Brewerton *et al.* 1973*a*), which is usually erroneously quoted as the first publication to announce this discovery.

Developments leading to the foundation of AS self-help societies

This 300-year accumulation of information since Bernard Connor's paper made it abundantly clear that here was a separate disease, needing specific treatment.

For instance, in the United Kingdom during the early 1970s Dr A. St.J. Dixon, the consultant rheumatologist at the Royal National Hospital for Rheumatic Diseases (RNHRD) in Bath, instigated a 3-week inpatient, intensive physiotherapy programme. There the importance of patient education as a key aspect of better disease management became obvious to both doctors and patients.

The discovery of the association of AS with HLA-B27 became a recurrent theme in patient/rheumatologist discussions, especially since the average age of disease onset (23 years of age) coincides with the age group of marriage and potential parenthood. Uveitis was another important and frequent topic of discussion. Patients must be told how to recognize the symptoms, and how to react, to save what can be crucial time, and to avoid the common experience of misdiagnosis.

The exchange of views between patients and hospital medical staff focused an awareness that as patients they were collectively victims of, and experts on, certain social problems. Due to an ignorance of the condition in the general population there were prejudices by some of the statutory bodies, employers, and life-insurance companies (outlined later in this chapter).

There is no doubt that this increased awareness of patients, viewing themselves as a group, together with newly acquired knowledge, acted as a catalyst towards mutual patient self-help.

In addition, the condition seems to be tailor-made for a patient-led organization. These patients, who became the founder members, viewed themselves as a privileged and fortunate group. They knew that they could all return to the remedial course on an annual basis, and the more politically realistic ones were aware that this could not be provided across the country. It might be unfashionable, but given these realities I believe that their intentions were altruistic, and not symbiotic. They saw the foundation of the society as an addition to the statutory health service, and not a replacement. When viewed at a distance of 20 years, this is undoubtedly the case.

The NASS was founded in 1975 and officially recognized in 1976, having patient education and support at its core. By 1978, societies had been formed in Sweden and Switzerland; France and The Netherlands in 1979; and Germany in 1980. In 1980, a Danish society which had been in existence since 1973 made contact with the NASS. The foundation of these organizations heralded a dramatic worldwide explosion of like-minded societies.

The foundation of the Ankylosing Spondylitis International Federation (ASIF)

Within a few years of the founding of the NASS in the UK, many similar patient-led organizations were set up across Europe, the USA, and Canada.

The majority of these societies are run by people in full-time work, who devote most of their free time to these societies. Today, there are 32 societies in 26 countries, only 5 of which are run by full-time office staff. A current list of their addresses is to be found at the end of this chapter.

In 1988, representatives from 12 of these organizations met in Bath, England, and formed the Ankylosing Spondylitis International Federation (ASIF). Since its foundation it has held four meetings in Switzerland, Austria, Portugal, and Norway attended by 60–80 delegates representing the different societies. These meetings act as a forum where views are exchanged relating to disease treatment, overcoming problems associated with the condition, the attitude of statutory bodies to health care, insurance, etc. Helpful exchanges of information also take place into the mechanics of running such organizations, including funding.

Two cooperative research projects are in progress: the first looking into pregnancy and the disease. A questionnaire has been finalized and carefully translated into several languages representing most of the member societies' membership. The results from several thousand responses are being analysed by a team under the direction of Prof. Monika Østensen at the University Hospital in Trondheim, Norway.

The second research project by a team in Denmark is taking a more detailed look at the problems of head restraints in cars (see below).

Research and ankylosing spondylitis societies

People who have AS, especially due to genetic susceptibility, are comforted by the knowledge that there is active and vigorous medical research taking place into their condition. As the memberships increased some societies started to make a contribution by using their members as a rapidly growing compliant group suitable for epidemiological research, this has been especially true of the British society whose membership has contributed to many published research papers. A comprehensive survey of 1600 members of the German AS society has recently been completed (Feldtkeller 1997*a,b*).

Psychosocial aspects of AS

Until recently very little attention had been paid to this aspect of the condition. There have been studies in this area relating to rheumatoid arthritis, but patients with spondylitis do not view the conclusions as being relevant to themselves.

Recent work has been carried out at Conventry University with the willing cooperation of NASS members (Barlow *et al.* 1992). Some studies looked at AS patients' attitudes and beliefs in the efficacy of their treatment. Another focused on the differences between patients who either do or do not attend NASS evening physiotherapy groups. This latter study found that group members gained more satisfaction from their available support than did AS non-members. Not only did they appreciate the joint therapeutic activity, but meeting others with the same condition who more readily understood their AS-related problems and limitations reduced their sense of isolation.

The study found that group members have a greater belief in the importance of exercise, and therefore exercise more regularly than those who do not participate.

Patient education through publications

The guidebook

A total of 70 000 copies of this publication produced by the NASS has provided the readers with essential patient education on all important aspects of the disease, including their own role in its management. The book has been translated into many languages, the most recent being Arabic.

Most sister societies also produce patient-information booklets and some also produce a physiotherapy cassette tape. Physiotherapy video films, such as *Fight back* which is produced by the NASS, have worldwide sales and they are also produced by the American sister society. *Fight back* has proved to be a useful tool in patient home-disease-management and the training of physiotherapists. During 1996 a similar video was produced by the German society, especially welcome for patients in Austria, Germany, and Switzerland.

AS news

All the AS societies produce their own journals. These are essential tools in the continuous management of the disease and its associated conditions and consequences. They deal with all social, psychological, and medical aspects of the disease (including research), and the individual society's affairs. The NASS journal, *AS News*, has an extensive correspondence section which is popular with its readers. For some reason most other societies have not ventured down this avenue, and those who have underestimate its appeal. These publications are considered by their organizations to be their flagship, signalling their ethos and corporate self-image.

The patient societies' branch network

One key objective of many patient societies is to instigate a network of branches to provide regular, supervised evening physiotherapy treatment. This is a popular time of the day for the working person. Few AS patients could attend regular daily therapy sessions and expect their employers to remain sympathetic. Others would prefer not to reveal that they have a problem as they feel that such knowledge might adversely influence promotion opportunities in the workplace. Evidence of the popularity of these branch activities is illustrated by the fact that over 2500 patients each week attend these therapy sessions in the UK. However, there is a surprisingly high drop-out rate, possibly for some of the reasons listed below.

1. Some patients are active sportsmen and sportswomen and therefore prefer to continue participating in their sporting activities, maintaining their mobility and posture thereby.
2. Exercise sessions often overlap with working hours, club or evening-class commitments.
3. Exercises involve a degree of effort and possible discomfort. Many people find that when they first join an exercise class there is an increase in pain, although the pain will eventually decrease once the muscles and ligaments have been stretched. For some, this represents an austere and unattractive approach to disease management, and their attitude is at variance with the active, positive, and motivated image of the AS patient, who has a high pain threshold.
4. Persuading people to adopt a regular exercise programme is like persuading people to give up smoking or alter their eating habits. The rewards are not always immediately apparent.
5. Some non-participants often do not wish to take responsibility for their own disease. They desire more powerful others (for instance, their doctor) to have control. They feel they cannot influence disease outcome since it is influenced by chance, fate, or luck. However, many previously reluctant people have been converted by a society and its branch leaders.

What, therefore, is the attitude of those people who regularly attend remedial groups?

1. They integrate these sessions into part of their normal week, because they feel that they are immediately benefiting by maintaining their posture and mobility.
2. The group influences and encourages others. They enjoy and benefit from the mutual supportive sharing of problems and anxieties as well as the companionship during the group's remedial activities and social occasions with members of their families. The importance of this socializing should not be overlooked by the medical profession as 'the dwindling of old friendships is a common consequence of any chronic illness' (Williams 1989). Through their tenacity, group members realize that they can, and do, derive pleasure in helping to foster a positive attitude, especially in the newly diagnosed. It demonstrates that they as patients have a positive role to play and that they have a large degree of control which boosts their self-confidence.
3. Membership leads to a reduction in a sense of isolation, frequently expressed by people on first contacting patient groups. People who are able to talk about their condition will do better than those who are unable to express their feelings.

A unpublished NASS survey of 1500 members revealed that 69.5% of those questioned felt that exercise is beneficial, and that it is a vital part of disease management.

Benefits to the health-care providers of organized patient groups

1. Patient groups providing regular group exercise programmes out of health-service hours provide a cost-effective way of treating people with AS. Since there is increasing pressure on budgets, including health-professionals' time, these branches directly address that problem. This is true in many countries as the last few years have witnessed an undeniable financial crises in western health-care systems.
2. Regular exercise leads to an improvement in posture and mobility. Many people who exercise on a regular basis are able to reduce or eliminate their drug intake, leading to a lessening of the side-effects of NSAIDs.
3. Groups can act as a compliant research bank for local rheumatologists, physiotherapists, and other health professionals. There are many examples of research papers using NASS groups as a patient bank.
4. Groups allow physiotherapists and physiotherapy students to gain experience in treating people with AS. They and other health professionals often express the opinion that they see their AS patients as rewarding, feel that they are physically active (Wynn Parry 1966), conscientious people (Wynn Parry and Deary 1980), cheerful, uncomplaining, and motivated, with a high pain threshold (Huskisson and Hart 1972). This seems to be the stereotypical model AS patient derived from those influential early studies, but these are opinions often expressed today by experienced rheumatology physiotherapists.
5. Groups are often seen as hospital or department supporters. Many branches of the society have made significant contributions towards equipment for their physiotherapy departments.

Patient educational symposia

Many of the patients' organizations organize day-long series of lectures for their members, and these have proved to be popular events. They provide the opportunity for their members to hear guest specialists and consultants lecture on the many different aspects of the disease and its associated conditions.

Some important medical and social problems of AS

Acute interior uveitis

Surveys of 1500 NASS members in the UK, indicate that 53.3% of patients experience this complication, making it the most common feature of AS. Edmunds and co-workers (1991*b*) found patients had one attack, 12% had two, and 47% had five or more. Misdiagnosis by family doctors is frequently a major problem associated with uveitis, therefore it is vital that patients learn to suspect this condition. Because of the swift onset of uveitis, patients should be advised to visit the emergency department of a hospital which has an ophthalmology department without delay.

Pregnancy, nursing, and children

Until the 1980s this was a relatively under-researched area and reports tended to be scanty and anecdotal, resulting in confusing and conflicting counselling. Norwegian studies in the early 1980s produced reassuring information for patients (Ostensen *et al.* 1982).

Fortunately, severe involvement of the sacroiliac joints and limited hip abduction are generally complications of long-disease duration, therefore most mothers with AS will not experience complications. The Norwegian studies confirmed that fertility is not affected by the condition. Ostensen *et al.* (1982) found that the disease runs a mild course during the first pregnancy, but that in subsequent pregnancies there is a risk of flare-ups and an increase in peripheral joint involvement in some cases.

However, when associated with other spondylarthropathies with widespread peripheral joint involvement, amelioration occurs during pregnancy as with rheumatoid arthritis.

Pregnancy and NSAIDs

Patients receive much conflicting advice and would appreciate less confusion within the medical profession on this topic. Norwegian studies of 28 pregnancies found that the use of NSAIDs was intermittent in 15 cases, and that no harmful effects to the fetus or mother were observed. They recommended that the lowest possible dose of NSAIDs should be given, in the evening to minimize night-time pain.

As NSAIDs have the potential to prolong gestation and labour, medical opinion suggests that patients should discontinue medication during the last 4 weeks of pregnancy. The use of analgesics is preferred in those pregnancies where pain control is needed.

NSAIDs and breast-feeding is another area where information is scant. Reports do exist showing the minimal excretion of naproxen, ibuprofen, and piroxicam in human breastmilk. However, the Østensen and Husby (1990) reported that: 'Salicylates and indomethacin are found in substantial amounts in breast milk and should certainly be avoided during lactation'.

Physiotherapy and pregnancy

As the dependence on NSAIDs is reduced, or eliminated, during pregnancy, so the importance of regular physiotherapy in the home should be emphasized. A programme of exercises designed to stretch ligaments, strengthen muscles, and maintain lung capacity should be suggested. It is important that patients realize that this will not only contribute to the maintenance of posture and mobility but will also assist in pain reduction.

Motherhood and nursing

Most AS mothers found the year following childbirth to be particularly demanding. They felt dependent on the assistance of others for the first 3 months, and during AS flare-ups. Because of this demand many mothers feel that successive pregnancies should not follow too closely. Since one of the major problems frequently experienced by mothers with AS is lifting, nursing, and playing with their children, they should look at ways of overcoming their physical restrictions, by for example purchasing baby-baths set on a plinth which can be adjusted to the appropriate height. Reconstructing a baby's cot so that the sliding sides are converted into double outward-swinging gates is not a difficult carpentry task, and greatly assists the mother who has a stiff spine.

Relationships and sexual activity

Love-making can be affected in AS, especially during flare-ups in the spine, sternum, and hips. The Norwegian study, and a study by Dudley Hart in 1980 found that sexual activity was more adversely affected by AS in women than in men. However, it has been found that the disease, although recognized by patients as problematical, seldom affects love-making in the average person with AS. Both men and women with AS tend to have similar scores to healthy controls on the sexual motivation scale (Elst *et al.* 1984).

Generally, uncomplicated total hip replacement does not adversely affect sexual activity, with the exception of the first 3 months after surgery. People with widespread axial and peripheral joint involvement may need individual counselling.

Misunderstandings can be caused between couples as symptoms, such as pain, fatigue, irritability, anxiety, and depression, can be misinterpreted. Not recognizing or acknowledging these causes leads to the breakdown of normal relationships. It is therefore necessary that couples should be aware of these problems and maintain an open and honest dialogue.

The most recent information has arisen from a report given to the NASS for publication by research workers at the RNHRD (Garrett 1994). The hospital issued a self-administered questionnaire which was returned by 100 spondylitic patients. The information below is a précis of their conclusions. However, it does produce a less optimistic picture than any previous and smaller studies.

Over two-thirds of the respondents stated that the frequency of sexual contact had diminished as a result of their condition. Intercourse was limited by stiffness in 81% of patients (usually in the neck, back, and hips), and by pain, particularly in the neck and pelvis in 72% of cases. Diminished libido caused by fatigue affected the sexual relationships of nearly 50% of the respondents. For over one-third of respondents, physical difficulties had led to a change in sexual positions used. Patients reported using a variety of sexual positions, and certain positions were highlighted as being more painful than others (for example the 'missionary' position and the 'standing' position). Approximately 25% of patients maintained that sexual relationships had become less enjoyable due to their disease, but none stated that any of their relationships had failed because of it. The majority agreed that (1) their partner understood the difficulties caused by AS during intercourse, and (2) they were able to discuss any difficulties with their partner. However, 50% of the respondents have reduced social contact and lower self-esteem as a result of AS.

Fatigue and early morning stiffness

Until recently the potential severity of fatigue had been overlooked by the medical profession. A study at the RNHRD of 1950 patients indicated that 6% felt that fatigue was their worst symptom, 34% pain, and 25% stiffness whereas, 32% could not distinguish among the three (Calin *et al.* 1993). The society has found that patients are relieved to have fatigue acknowledged as being a feature of the condition, and that it is not caused by some other medical condition.

At some stage fatigue is a feature in almost all spondylitic patients, especially when the disease is flaring and there is additional pain in the joints. Under these circumstances sleep deprivation caused by additional pain is, for many people, a fact of life. Anaemia can also play role, but can, to some extent, be treated.

Like flare-ups of the disease itself, there seems to be no logical pattern and no way of determining the severity or duration of fatigue. But greater acknowledgement by the medical profession can go a long way to help sufferers come to terms with the problem, and allow their family, friends, and employers to make allowances.

A common experience shared by many AS patients is early morning stiffness. For some patients this can last until midday. In others it passes more rapidly and in some it is seldom a problem. Many of those patients who find this problematical habitually take an early morning bath or shower followed by posture-maintaining stretching exercises, which rapidly reduce nocturnal stiffening. There are cases where people with even relatively severe AS are able to hold down some sort of a job. However, some find that the prolonged severity of their morning stiffness precludes them from employment as they simply can not guarantee the regular and prompt time-keeping expected by most employers.

Non-steroidal anti-inflammatory drugs

Because of the long-term nature of the disease, patients need to be able to discuss this important topic fully with their doctors. Patients are concerned about any possible drug side-effects, but especially gastrointestinal problems and the effect of NSAIDs in pregnancy. There is little point in telling patients to take their medication during, or after meals, if the reasons are not explained. Patients are far more likely to comply if they understand the reasoning behind the advice. Often, insufficient warning is given that some of the agents can cause drowsiness and dizziness, and since their occupations reflect those of an average cross-section of the population, including operating dangerous machinery, and public transport, this issue needs to be addressed.

A survey of 2500 NASS members illustrates that 85% of our membership take medication; 57.7% of them throughout the year. The same unpublished survey revealed that a similar percentage of members of the Swedish sister society (DVMB) were taking anti-inflammatory medication, but there the percentage taking medication continuously throughout the year dropped to 40.3%. The survey revealed that British rheumatologists' NSAIDs' preferences are indomethacin, naproxen, piroxicam, and diclofenac sodium (in that order). Follow-up surveys from new members over the years have revealed no changes in the order, and only slight variations in the percentages of each prescribed.

Alternative therapies and medication

Part of the cultural changes within the general population in the western world since the 1960s has been the growing attraction of alternative therapies. It is therefore not surprising that many patients have explored this avenue. NASS surveys have revealed that the most popular is acupuncture, followed by osteopathy, and then homeopathy, However, the great majority will return to conventional treatment.

Again reflecting recent trends, many people question prescribed medication, and 34% of NASS members have tried herbal alternatives. There is a misinformed belief in the general population that because this type of medication is extracted from nature it must be safe and harmless. Sometimes, unknown to their doctors, people take herbal medication and their prescribed anti-inflammatory agents concurrently.

Driving and public transport

Driving may be difficult due to spinal and especially cervical limitations. There has been conflicting advice regarding when a patient with AS should inform the driving licence authorities. In the UK, there are obligations of disclosure when there is severe neck restriction, or peripheral joint involvement. In many countries, however, this is not an issue either with the driving licencing authorities or the vehicle insurance companies.

In cases of significant impairment of cervical movement cars should be equipped with additional external and internal mirrors. Fortunately, most modern cars possess outside mirrors adjustable from the driver's seat. We also advise these patients to visit car-accessory shops to inspect the wide range of mirrors available. Unfortunately, the problem of turning at a T-junction and also entering a main road at a tangent remain unresolved. Here, many car drivers find that they have to move to the left and right in their seats in order to increase their field of vision. This naturally takes more time and they can sometimes find themselves under pressure from drivers queuing behind them. A passenger can act as a useful lookout.

Head restraints are an obvious area for attention, and these should be adjested so that the back of the head is in contact with the restraint. Patients should understand that setting the restraint at a lower level turns it into a neck rest which, on impact, will act as fulcrum and increase the danger of cervical fracture. The Ankylosing Spondylitis International Federation are conducting a survey through one of its Scandinavian member' organizations with the valuable assistance of a motor manufacturer.

For many people with AS, travelling by public transport can present them with additional problems and anxieties. The first problem is often found when boarding a bus or train as the step is often too high and can only be mounted with difficulty. Fears are often expressed by the patient that once on the bus it often moves away before they have reached the safety of a seat, thus increasing the risk of injury due to a fall. Some find that jolting buses and uneven road surfaces cause them discomfort. Some avoid this problem by opting, when practical, for the more expensive taxi.

Life and health assurance

Many people with AS experience problems in obtaining unloaded insurance quotations. In the UK this is a significant topic where loans for purchasing a house are frequently underpinned by life policies.

A study of 3310 NASS members in the UK revealed that 1160 (35%) had taken out life-assurance policies after diagnosis (Jones 1994). Of those 842 (73%) had declared their AS, and 293 (35%) of those had a loaded policy, and only 41 (4.8%) were refused a policy by at least one insurance company.

In the home

Beds and mattresses

Patients should be advised to choose a firm mattress, not a hard or a soft one. and should consider replacing their mattresses more frequently, depending on the quality of the mattress and the total weight. Beds should have a firm base, and if necessary a three-quarter inch (2.0 cm) piece of chipboard can be placed between the base and mattress.

Chairs

A large number of people with AS have their own chair. Low, soft furniture encourages bad posture and increases pain. Many chairs are suitable, although they should have sufficient lumbar support, a high back to provide head support, a firm (not hard) seat, and arms at the correct level. Sufferers should shop around for the most comfortable and appropriate office chair.

Other home modifications

A top-loading washing machine is recommended; dustpans and brushes with extended handles are readily available; and duvets or quilts, rather than sheets and blankets, simplify bed-making. Upright vacuum cleaners are better than the cylinder type. An additional bannister at the correct height can be a great assistance for many people; bannisters and good stair illumination are also essential to prevent falls at home. Some people raise the height of their sinks and worktops by inserting plinths at ground level. Patient-organization literature will also give advice about daily domestic chores and home modifications.

Employment

The majority of patients are able to carry on with their occupation until retirement age, but as the condition is very variable some will be obliged to make early adjustments to their working lives. During recessionary times a change of occupation can be difficult, and the disease will decrease choice, especially for those with a reduced range of movement in their peripheral joints.

NASS surveys in the UK found that during any one year 36% of their members had not taken sickness-related time off work; 16% had taken less than 1 week, 17% between 1 and 4 weeks, 6% 1–3 months, and 9% more than 3 months. The remaining 16% were temporarily unemployed, had been made redundant, or were permanently off work for medical reasons. This survey was carried out among people with an average age of 44 years and included the period between disease onset and diagnosis.

Another report of 100 patients from the Oxford region found no evidence of a higher incidence of unemployment among patients with AS, compared with the average population in the same area. The authors did, however, acknowledge that their area is not normally associated with heavy engineering and many available jobs were more suited to these patients than occupations in more industrialized areas of the country (Wordsworth and Mowat 1986).

Many patients choose not to reveal their condition to their employers. They are fearful that they might be judged in a negative light either when being assessed for promotion, or when the company is looking to make redundancies. The same fears emerge when these people fill in job application forms or when they attend for job interviews.

Obviously the best type of occupation is one in which the working day can be divided between periods of sitting and moving around. As the occupation of each NASS member is known through the membership form, a surprising number of people are shown to be in active occupations including the armed forces, police, and rescue services. On diagnosis, many patients have been badly advised by their doctors to change careers. This is unnecessarily gloomy without sufficient information a disease progression.

Conclusions

NASS, and its sister societies, claim that an early diagnosis, followed by patient education, and branches' physiotherapy programmes will significantly contribute to a better disease outcome for the patient. This is especially true when compared with a patient who is diagnosed late and is passive about the condition. We have found that the family is generally supportive, but to be effective they must also participate in the educational process.

The disease is not well understood except by rheumatologists, and members of the AS societies know that they can best turn to their rheumatologist or to the Society for answers to their questions. Visits to their rheumatologists are infrequent. A glance at the correspondence section of the NASS twice-yearly journal *AS News* illustrates the broad brush of patient experiences, anxieties, and concerns.

At one of the NASS symposia, a rheumatologist guest speaker told the audience that, in his opinion, the foundation of NASS and corresponding societies in other countries was one of the most significant events in the history of ankylosing spondylitis.

Addresses of worldwide ankylosing spondylitis self-help societies

Australia

Ankylosing Spondylitis Group: c/o Arthritis Foundation of Western Australia, PO Box 34, Wembley WA6014

Ankylosing Spondylitis Group of Western Australia: Ben Saraceni, 35 Wesley St., Balcatta, WA6021; tel. 344 5857

Tasmanian Ankylosing Spondylitis Association, C/RAFT (Rheumatoid Arthritis Foundation of Tasmania): Stuart K. Hadrill, Battery Point, Tasmania 7004

Austria

Österreichische Vereinigung Morbus Bechterew (ÖVMB): c/o Herta Taschner, Obere Augartenstr. 26–28, A-1020 Wien; tel. (Mi 15-17h) (1) 33 22 810, fax. (1) 33 22

Belgium

Vlaamse Vereniging voor Bechterew-patiënten (VVB): François Waumann, Potaaredestraat 50, B-9140 Temse; tel. (3) 771 08 22

Canada

Ankylosing Spondylitis Association of British Columbia (ASABC): Andrew Hobbs, 2283–132nd St., Surrey, British Columbia V41 9A9

Manitoba Ankylosing Spondylitis Association: Lorne Ferlay, 19 Carolyn Bay, Winnipeg, Manitoba R2J 2Z3; (204) 256 5320

Ontario Spondylitis Association (OSA): 393 University Ave. Suite 1700. Toronto, Ontario M5G 1E6; tel. (416) 979 7228 fax (416) 979 8366

Ankylosing Spondylitis Support Group of Nova Scotia, c/o Arthritis Society: Kathleen Vallis, 2745 Dutch Village Road, Suite 100, Halifax, Nova Scotia B3L 1GY; tel. (902) 429 7025 fax. (902) 423 6479

Croatia

Hrvatsko drus⁄tvo za ankilozantni spondilitis: Prof. Ivo Jacic, Vinogradska c. 29, HR-41000 Zagreb; tel. (1) 572 440, fax. (1) 172 453

Czech republic

Klub bechtereviku, c/o Revmatologický ústav, Na slupi 4, 128 50 Praha 2

Denmark

Landsforeningen af Morbus Bechterew-Patienter: v/ Advokat Per Lignell Rosenvaenget 58, DK-8362 Horning; tel. 86 92 33 00, fax. 86 92 30 65

France

Association Contre la Spondylarthrite Ankylosants et ses Conséquences: Dominique Baguet, Clinique Rhumatologique, CHRU de Nancy-Brabois, ave du Morvan, F-54500 Vandoeuvre-les-Nancy; tel. (3) 83 22 68 71

Germany

Geschäftsstelle der Deutschen Vereinigung Morbus Bechterew: Ludwig Hammel, Metzgergasse 16, 97421 Schweinfurt, tel. (09721) 22033, fax. (09721) 22955

Hungary

Mozgáskoriátozottak Egyesületeinek Országos Szövetsége, Bechterew section: c/o Dr -Ing, Majtényi Sándor, Rákóczí utca 29, H-1196 Budapest; tel. + fax. (1) 178 16 53

Iceland

Hryggiktarfélagiõ: c/o Emilía Sigurdardóttir, Gigtarfélag Íslands, Ármúli 5, IS-108 Reykjavik

Ireland

Ankylosing Spondylitis Association of Ireland: Edward Witter, 111 Briarfield Grove, Kilbarrack, Dublin 5; tel. (1) 839 35 12

Italy

Associazione Italiana Spondiloartrite Anchilosante: Favio Fornasari, Via Elisabetta Sirani, 3/2, I-40129 Bologna; tel. (51) 37 23 23, fax. (51) 63 30 067

Japan

Japan Ankylosing Club: Dr Hisashi Inoue, 1-11-5, Shinkawa Mitaka-shi, Tokyo 181; tel. (422) 45-7985, fax. (422) 49-6817

The Netherlands

Nederlandse bond van verenigingen van patiënten met reumatisch aandoeningen, Commissie Morbus Bechterew: D. Martens, Postbus 1370, 3800 BJ Amersfoort; tel. (33) 61 63 64, fax. (33) 65 12 00

Norway

Norsk Revmatikerforbund/Bekhterev: Else-Brit Froytlog, Postboks 2653 Solli, N-0202 Oslo; tel. 22 55 72 16, fax. 2243 12 51

Bechterew-Gruppen I Trondheim: Kari Baekker, Postboks 421, N-7001 Trondheim; tel. 73 91 98 41

Portugal

Associação Nacional da Espondilite Anquilosante: Dr Filipe Gonçalves da Rocha, Bairro Social de Alcoitão, Lote 18, P-2765 Estoril; tel. (1) 460 2511, fax. (1) 460 2509

Singapore

Singapore Ankylosing Spondylitis Club, c/o National Arthritis Foundation: Yin Peng Low, 336 Smith St., # 06-302 New Bridge Centre, Singapore 050336; tel. 227 9726, fax. 227 0257

Slovenia

Društvo bolnikov I invalidov ankilozirajoim spondilitisom slovenije: Marjan Hudomalj, Pot na Fuzine I, Ljubljana; tel. 61 455 169

Spain

Associación Codobesa de Enfermos Afectados de Espondondilitis: Jose Roman Lopez, Apartado de Corroes 762, 14080 Córdoba

Sweden

Bechterewreumatikernas Intresseorganisation: Anita Berg, Seglaregatan 29/Box 12031, S-402 41 Göteborg; tel. (Mo-Fr 10-15h) (31) 147 147, fax. (31) 122 305

Switzerland

Schweizerische Vereinigung Morbus Bechterew: Peter Straub, Röntgenstr. 22, CH-8005 Zurich; tel. (1) 272 78 66, fax. (1) 272 78 75

Taiwan

c/o Dr Wha-Tsung Liu, Medical Centre, National Taiwan University, I Jenai Rd., Section 1, Taipei; tel. (2) 321 2258

UK

The National Ankylosing Spondylitis Society: Fergus J. Rogers, 3 Grosvenor Crescent, London SWIX 7ER; tel. (0171) 235 9585, fax. (0171) 235 5827

Ukraine

c/o OSIRSKIJ: Victor Dmiitrijewitsch, Boulevard Gagarina 13/8, Solotonoscha, Ukraine 258100

USA

Spondylitis Association of America: Jane Bruckel, PO box 5872, Sherman Oaks, CA 91413; tel. (818) 981 1616, fax. (818) 981 9826

18 HLA-B27 subtypes, disease susceptibility, and peptide binding specificity

Joel D. Taurog

As documented in Chapters 2 and 12, a great deal of effort has been expended in the investigation of the subtypes of B27. Although the demonstration of disease association with multiple B27 subtypes supported the concept that the B27 molecule itself is a susceptibility factor, until recently it could accurately be stated that B27 subtyping was unhelpful in favoring any particular disease mechanism (MacLean 1992). However, recent application of powerful methodologies, including PCR-based DNA typing of large populations, X-ray crystallography, and sequence analysis of peptides eluted from HLA molecules, has generated epidemiologic and biochemical data regarding the HLA-B27 subtypes that should prove valuable in guiding further research. These recent data are reviewed in this chapter.

The HLA-B27 subtypes

From the standpoint of genetic inheritance, the concept of subtypes as applied to HLA alleles is somewhat artificial. This is so because one subtype of a given specificity bears no closer relationship to another than it does to another specificity of the same locus; they are all merely alternative alleles of that locus. Thus, for example, HLA-B*2702, HLA-B*2705, and, say, HLA-B*4401 are all alleles of the HLA-B locus, although the first two are 'subtypes' of HLA-B27. The concept of subtypes arose originally when HLA alleles were defined serologically, to indicate variants that were serologically identical but could be distinguished from one another in some other manner, for example by T cell reactivity.

It subsequently became clear that all such variants differed from one another by one or more residues in their primary structure (that is, amino acid sequence) (Parham *et al.* 1995). Conversely, as more and more HLA alleles were examined at the protein (or more commonly, cDNA) sequence level, it became clear that the basis for serologic cross-reactivity between HLA subtypes was primarily due to shared segments of primary structure. It also became clear that the primary structure of HLA class I heavy chains can often be viewed as encoded by a patchwork of casettes which are thought to be exchanged within and between loci in the course of time, a process termed *microconversion* (Parham *et al.* 1995). More recently, with the widespread use of DNA-based histocompatibility typing, new HLA specificities and subtypes have tended to be identified solely by cDNA sequencing, almost irrespective of whether the product reacts with antisera that originally defined the parent specificity. The naming of these newly identified subtypes is then based on a guess as to which parent specificity was the recipient in a microconversion event. The B27 subtypes HLA-B*2708 and B*2712 are examples of this process. By the time these alleles were identified, it was recognized that the most significant structural feature shared by all of the serologically cross-reactive B27 subtypes was the B pocket within the peptide binding groove, containing the characteristic residues His9, Thr24, Glu45, and Cys67, with adjacent residues Ala69, Lys70, and Ala71 (Benjamin & Parham 1990; Buxton *et al.* 1992). B*2708 shared these features, and was therefore designated as a B27 subtype, even though it serologically seemed more closely related to HLA-B7, based mainly on the shared Ala69-X70-Ala71 and B7-like Ser77-Asn80-Arg82-Glu83 motifs. This latter motif confers the HLA-Bw6 supertypic determinant, unlike all of the previously identified B27 subtypes, which are Bw4. Even more dramatic in terms of deviation from the 'fundamental' B27 sequence is the most recently described subtype, B*2712 (Marsh 1997), which shares all residues with B*2708 except for the motif Thr69-Asn70-Thr71, which is carried by many HLA-B alleles but not by any of the previously identified B27 subtypes. Not surprisingly, B*2712 does not react with many of the antisera and monoclonal antibodies that react with other B27 subtypes (K. Hurley, personal communication). Table 18.1 shows the amino acid sequence variation among the B27 subtypes. The orientation of these sites within the three dimensional structure of the antigen-binding cleft is shown in Figure 12.1.

Table 18.1 The amino acids that distinguish the twelve known HLA-B27 subtypes

Subtype	Amino acid residue															
	59	69	70	71	74	77	80	81	82	83	97	113	114	116	131	152
B*2705	Y	A	K	A	D	D	T	L	L	R	N	Y	H	D	S	V
B*2701	—	—	—	—	Y	N	—	A	—	—	—	—	—	—	—	—
B*2702	—	—	—	—	—	N	I	A	—	—	—	—	—	—	—	
B*2703	H	—	—	—	—	—	—	—	—	—	—	—	—	—	—	—
B*2704	—	—	—	—	—	S	—	—	—	—	—	—	—	—	—	E
B*2706	—	—	—	—	—	S	—	—	—	—	—	—	D	Y	—	E
B*2707	—	—	—	—	—	—	—	—	—	—	S	H	N	Y	R	—
B*2708	—	—	—	—	—	S	N	—	R	G	—	—	—	—	—	—
B*2709	—	—	—	—	—	—	—	—	—	—	—	—	—	H	—	—
B*2710	—	—	—	—	—	—	—	—	—	—	—	—	—	—	—	E
B*2711	—	—	—	—	—	S	—	—	—	—	S	H	N	Y	R	—
B*2712	—	T	N	T	—	S	N	—	R	G	—	—	—	—	—	—
Pocket	*A*	—	*B*	—	*C*	*F*	*F*	*F*	—	—	*C*	*D*	*E*	*F*	—	*E*

A dash indicates identity at that position with the B*2705 sequence. Residues 59–83 are in the $\alpha 1$ domain, 97–152 are in the $\alpha 2$ domain. B*2708 and B*2712 are homologous with HLA-B7 at positions 77–83, B*2712 is homologous with many other HLA-B alleles at positions 69–71. B*2707 and B*2711 are homologous with HLA-B8 at positions 97–131. B*2704 and B*2706 have a Gly at position 211 in the $\alpha 3$ domain, whereas the other subtypes have Ala (B*2710 and B*2712 have not yet been sequenced in this region). This substitution is not thought to affect peptide binding.

One letter amino acid code: A, alanine; D, aspartic acid; E, glutamic acid; G, glycine; H, histidine; I, isoleucine; L, leucine; N, asparagine; R, arginine; S, serine; T, threonine; V, valine; Y, tyrosine. From Hildebrand *et al.* 1994; Fiorello *et al.* 1995; Marcos *et al.* 1996; Gonzalezs-Roches *et al.* 1997; Hasegawa *et al.* 1997; Marsh 1997; López de Castro 1998.

Disease associations of the B27 subtypes

Firm associations with AS, reactive arthritis, and acute anterior uveitis have been established for B*2702, –04, and –05, based on many large populations surveys over the last 16 years. A few similar studies have also recently implicated B*2707 (Kanga *et al.* 1996; Gonzalez-Roces *et al.* 1997) and probably B*2703 (Gonzalez-Roces *et al.* 1997). There is anecdotal disease association reported with B*2701, –06, and –10 (Feltkamp *et al.* 1996; Marcos *et al.* 1996; Gonzalez-Roces *et al.* 1997; P. Stastny, personnel communication). There are very few data for the rare subtypes B*2708 –11, and –12, and to my knowledge no cases of association with spondyloarthropathy have been reported for these subtypes. As discussed in Chapter 12, B*2708 was found in two of 147 B27+ controls but none of 169 B27+ AS patients in a recent large survey in Britain.

Of significant interest are recent population studies that have convincingly documented a relatively low disease association for B*2706, and a similar but less extensively documented lack of association for B*2709. As shown in Table 18.2, three separate studies carried out in four Asian populations have found a relative lack of association of B*2706 with AS, and apparently with the other SpA as well (Gonzalez-Roces *et al.* 1997; Nasution *et al.* 1997; Ren *et al.* 1997). Regarding B*2709, the data showing a lack of association have been obtained by one group of investigators, and are based primarily on the absence of AS among individuals with this subtype residing on the island of Sardinia, where B*2709 was found in 10 of 40 healthy B27+ subjects, but so far not in any of 50 B27+ Sardinian AS patients (p<0.0002), (D'Amato *et al.* 1995 and R. Sorrentino, personal communication). Proper epidemiologic studies of the association with AS have only been possible in Sardinia, the prevalence of B*2709 being too low elsewhere, even in mainland Italy (Gonzalez-Roces *et al.* 1997 and R. Sorrentino, personal communication).

These data strongly suggest that the peptide binding specificity of the B27 molecule is of critical importance in determining disease susceptibility. This is so because B*2706 differs from disease-prone B*2704 by only two residues in the $\alpha 1$ and $\alpha 2$ domains, residues 114 and

Table 18.2 Low association of HLA-B*2706 with SpA in Asian populations

Location	Patients (*n*)					Controls (*n*)				
B*27 subtype	–02	–04	–05	–06	–07	–02	–04	–05	–06	–07
Indonesia[a]	0	23	8	0	2	0	4	1	21	0
Singapore[b]	0	48	2	0	0	0	40	1	4	0
Thailand[c]	0	41	2	0	2	0	8	1	10	0
China[c]	2	31	16	2	2	0	21	5	0	0
Total (*n*)	2	143	28	2	6	0	73	8	35	0
Total (%)	1.1	79.0	15.5	1.1	3.3	0.0	62.9	6.9	30.2	0.0

[a] Nasution *et al.* 1997. Patients met ESSG criteria for SpA.

[b] Ren *et al.* 1997. All patients had AS.

[c] Gonzalez-Roces *et al.* 1997. All patients had AS.

B*2706 in 2/181 patients vs. 35/116 controls, $\chi^2 = 54.8$, $p < 1.4 \times 10^{-13}$.

Table 18.3 Association of HLA-B27 subtypes with the spondyloarthropathies

Subtype	Association with SpA	Comments
B*2701	+	rare; SpA only reported in a kindred
B*2702	++++	established by epidemiology
B*2703	++	provisionally established by epidemiology
B*2704	++++	established by epidemiology
B*2705	++++	established by epidemiology
B*2706	+/–	low association by epidemiology
B*2707	+++	provisionally established by epidemiology
B*2708	?	rare; epidemiology so far not helpful
B*2709	—	no association by limited epidemiology
B*2710	+	rare; SpA only reported in a kindred
B*2711	?	rare; no epidemiology yet done
B*2712	?	rare; no epidemiology yet done

Adapted from Gonzalez-Roces *et al.* 1997

116, and similarly, B*2709 differs from disease-prone B*2705 only at residue 116. As discussed below and shown in Table 18.1 and Figure 12.1, residues 114 and 116 lie in the floor of the antigen-binding groove, where they have no exposure to the T cell receptor, and where their allelic influence is thought to be solely on peptide binding specificity.

A summary of the disease associations for the B27 subtypes is shown in Table 18.3.

Peptide binding specificities of the B27 subtypes

The concept that antigen presentation by class I molecules involves peptide fragments of intracellular antigens was first proposed by Townsend and coworkers (Townsend *et al.* 1986), based on experiments with influenza virus. Impetus for this concept was provided by the crystal structure of HLA-A2, which suggested the presence of a binding cleft carrying extra protein density (Bjorkman *et al.* 1987a,b). Biochemical confirmation of this concept through extraction of immunologically active peptide was achieved by van Bleek and Nathenson (1990) and by Rammensee and coworkers (Rötzschke *et al.* 1990a,b). The latter group pioneered the methodology of pool sequencing by Edman degradation of whole peptide populations eluted from class I MHC molecules, which led to the observation that each class I allele binds peptides with characteristic 'anchor' residues at one or a few peptide positions (Falk *et al.* 1991; Rammensee *et al.* 1995). Jardetsky *et al.* (1991) extracted peptide from purified B*2705 molecules and used Edman degradation of HPLC-purified peptide peaks to identify endogenously bound peptide and define a characteristic B27 peptide motif with Arg at P2 as as strong anchor residue, confirming earlier work with B27-presented viral peptides by McMichael and coworkers (Huet *et al.* 1990). The peptide specificity of class I alleles was also investigated by a variety of binding assays, which were applied to studying HLA-B27 (Carreno *et al.* 1993; Colbert *et al.* 1994; Parker *et al.* 1994; Galocha *et al.* 1996). Meanwhile, Hunt and co-workers

(1992) pioneered the sensitive methodology of sequencing MHC-bound peptides using tandem mass spectrometry.

Elucidation of the crystal structure of HLA-B*2705 (Madden *et al.* 1991, 1992) and other class I molecules (Fremont *et al.* 1992; Garrett *et al.* 1989; Guo *et al.* 1993; Young *et al.* 1994), with a clear image of the bound peptide, together with the results of numerous biochemical studies of peptide binding, has led to a detailed model of the interaction between bound peptides and the class I binding groove (reviewed in Matsumura *et al.* 1992; Madden 1995). The main features of this include (i) sequence-independent interactions, principally hydrogen bonding, between conserved residues in the peptide binding groove and the N- and C-termini of the peptide, and (ii) formation of 'pockets,' i.e., extensions within the peptide-binding cleft, by the allelically variable MHC residues lining the cleft, the side chains of which form non-covalent bonds with the side chains of the residues of the bound peptide. It is the three dimensional structure of these pockets that confers allelic specificity to the peptide binding cleft and determines the specific motifs and anchor residues of the bound peptides.

As has been previously noted by many authors and discussed in Chapter 12, the B27 subtypes share a unique B pocket but differ amongst themselves in the other five pockets within the peptide binding cleft. The most prominent differences are in the F pocket, the variable residues of which interact with the side chain of the C-terminal residue of the bound peptide. In this regard, the B27 subtypes differ markedly in their tolerance for different C-termini, as indicated in Table 18.4, which shows data from pool sequencing and peptide elution studies. B*2705, B*2703, and B*2710 show the broadest range, binding peptides with C-terminal basic, aliphatic, and aromatic residues, including Tyr. The acceptance of positively charged C-termini has been attributed to the acidic residues at positions 77 and 116 in B*2705. In contrast, B*2702 and B*2704, which carry Asn or Ser, respectively, rather than Asp at position 77, show a more restricted binding, that largely excludes positively charged C-termini.

Recent studies have suggested that the two subtypes with little or no disease association, B*2706 and B*2709, show an even more restricted peptide C-terminal repertoire, permitting only aliphatic residues or Phe at this position, but specifically not Tyr. This has led to the hypothesis that B27-related disease may involve binding to B27 of one or a few specific peptides that carry C-terminal Tyr (Fiorillo *et al.* 1997; García *et al.* 1997b). Although attractive, this hypothesis may be an oversimplification, since the one investigation that has been carried out of endogenous peptides bound to B*2707, which as noted above is rather clearly disease-associated, found only aliphatic C-terminal residues and no aromatic residues (Tieng *et al.* in press). Nonetheless, the combined epidemiologic and structural data suggest that the allelic differences within the binding cleft exert *some* sort of major influence on the peptide preferences of the B27 subtypes that affects disease susceptibility. Further discussion of this topic is reviewed in López de Castro (1998).

Implications

These recent data suggest a strong correlation between peptide binding specificity and disease association for B27 subtypes. Similar data have been obtained for HLA-DR4 subtypes associated with rheumatoid arthritis, pemphigus vulgaris, and insulin-dependent diabetes mellitus (Wucherpfennig & Strominger 1995; Friede *et al.* 1996; Davenport *et al.* 1997; Undlien *et al.* 1997). In all of these cases, the implication is that at some particular point in time and at

Table 18.4 Relationship of B27-subtypes to C-terminal peptide motifs

Subtype	C-terminal amino acid residues of B27-bound peptides		Consensus C-termini		
	Pool sequencing	Isolated peptides	basic	aliphatic	aromatic
B*2701	Y	L, Y, F, W		L	F, Y, W
B*2702	F, Y, I, L, W	F, Y, W		L, I	F, Y, W
B*2703	F, R, M, W, L, Y	L, R, Y, F, W	R	L, M	F, Y, W
B*2704	Y, L, F, M	Y, F, L		L, M	F, Y
B*2705	L, F, Y, M, I, R, H, K	F, R, Y, H, L, K	R, K, H	L, I, M	F, Y
B*2706	L, F	L, F, V		L, V	F
B*2707	L,	L, V		L, V	
B*2709	—	L, I, V, F, M		L, I, V, M	F
B*2710	Y, F	K, R, F, L, Y	R, K	L	F, Y

One letter amino acid code: A, alanine; F, phenylalanine; H, histidine; I, isoleucine; K, lysine; L, leucine; M, methionine; R, arginine; V, valine; Y, tyrosine; W, tryptophan.

References: Jardetzky *et al.* 1991; Rojo *et al.* 1993; Rötzschke *et al.* 1994; Tanigaki *et al.* 1994; Fruci *et al.* 1995; Rammensee *et al.* 1995; Villadangos *et al.* 1995; Boisgerault *et al.* 1996; Galocha *et al.* 1996; Fiorillo *et al.* 1997; García *et al.* 1997a, b, c; Simmons *et al.* 1997; Griffin *et al.* 1997; García *et al.* in press; Tieng *et al.* in press.

some particular anatomic location, the binding of some particular peptide or group of peptides to the HLA allele in question participates in the pathogenesis of the disease in question. For all of these diseases, it remains to be determined whether the peptide specificity of the implicated HLA alleles involves classical peptide presentation to antigen specific T cells or some less straightforward mechanism.

The sources of putative B27-bound arthritogenic peptides have been speculated upon at length (see Chapter 13, for example). If T cell recognition of B27-peptide complexes is indeed a critical factor, it still may not be strictly necessary that all subtypes present exactly the same peptide, and it almost certainly would not be necessary that the arthritogenic T cells restricted by one subtype be able to recognize the same peptide presented by other subtypes. Nonetheless, presentation of the same immunodominant viral peptide by B*2702, –04, and –05 has been reported (Brooks *et al.* 1993), and even crossreactivity among different B27 subtypes by B27 allospecific and B27-restricted CTL clones has been documented (Aparicio *et al.* 1987; Brooks *et al.* 1993; López *et al.* 1994).

It is noteworthy that HLA-B*2706 has been found in a few patients with AS, as reported in the epidemiologic study of Gonzalez-Roces *et al.* 1997 (Table 18.2) and anecdotally by others (Feltkamp *et al.* 1996), although it clearly confers a lower relative risk than the other major subtypes, whereas in contrast, as of this writing not a single case of B*2709-associated spondyloarthropathy has been reported. If this pattern continues to be confirmed, it would suggest that there is a hierarchy of functional affinity for the relevant peptide(s), with B*2702, –04, and –05 together at one end of the spectrum, B*2709 at the other, and B*2706 in between, but closer to B*2709. As a first approximation, the search for disease-related peptides might then be reasonably confined to the set of peptides fitting these criteria. The series of studies showing weak disease associations for TAP and LMP alleles also suggest that allelic effects on peptide binding may influence disease susceptibility (Ploski *et al.* 1995; Maksymowych *et al.* 1994; 1995a,b,c).

Summary

The convergence of recent epidemiologic and biochemical data has confirmed the intuitively attractive hypothesis that the peptide binding specificity of the disease-related B27 subtypes is an important key to understanding the role of B27 in the pathogenesis of the spondyloarthropathies. The search for disease-related peptides, ongoing for several years, should continue to receive high priority in the investigation of these disorders, and should be facilitated by these findings.

References

Aabaikken, L., Larsen, S., and Osnes, M. (1989). Cimetidine tablets or suspension in the prevention of gastrointestinal mucosal lesions caused by non-steroidal anti-inflammatory drugs. *Scandinavian Journal of Rheumatology*, **18**, 647–55.

AAOS (1965). Joint motion. In *Method of measuring and recording*, pp. 44–64. American Academy of Orthopaedic Surgeons, Chicago, Illinois.

Abbott, C. A., Helliwell, P. S., and Chamberlain, M. A. (1994). Functional assessment in ankylosing spondylitis: evaluation of a new self-administered questionnaire and correlation with anthropometric variables. *British Journal of Rheumatology*, **33**, 1060–6.

Abu-Shakra, M., Gladman, D. D., Thorne, J. C., Long, I., Gough, J., Farewell, V. T. (1995). Longterm methotrexate therapy in psoriatic arthritis: clinical and radiologic outcome. *Journal of Rheumatology*, **22**, 241–5.

Ackermann, B., Yu, D. T. Y., Kuipers, J. G., Meyer zum Büschenfelde, K.-H., Märker- Hermann, E. (1995). A Yersinia urease *β* subunit derived peptide is recognized by HLA-B27- restricted cytotoxic T cells in Yersinia-induced reactive arthritis. *Arthritis and Rheumatism*, **38**, S200.

Adams, R. F., Flinn, G. S., Jr., and Douglas, M. (1987). Ankylosing spondylitis in a nonhuman primate: a monkey tale. *Arthritis and Rheumatism*, **30**, 956–7.

Adinolfi, M. and Lehner, T. (1976). Acute phase proteins and C9 in patients with Behçet's syndrome and aphthous ulcers. *Clinical and Experimental Immunology*, **25**, 36–9.

Agner, E., Eriksen, M., Hollnagel, H., Larsen, J. H., Mørck, H. I., and Schroll, M. (1981). Prevalence of raised Yersinia enterocolitica antibody titres in unselected, adult populations in Denmark during 12 years. *Acta Medica Scandinavica*, **209**, 509–12.

Aho, K., Ahvonen, P., Alkio, P., Lassus, A., Sairanen, E., and Sievers, K., (1975). HLA-27 in reactive arthritis following infection. *Annals of the Rheumatic Diseases*, **34** (Suppl.1), 29–30.

Aho, K., Leirisalo-Repo, M., and Repo, H. (1985). Reactive arthritis. *Clinics in Rheumatic Diseases*, **11**, 25–40.

Ahvonen, P., Sievers, K., and Aho, K. (1969). Arthritis associated with *Yersinia enterocolitica* infection. *Acta Rheumatologica Scandinavica*, **15**, 232–53.

Aiko, S. and Grisham, M. B. (1995). Spontaneous intestinal inflammation and nitric oxide metabolism in HLA-B27 transgenic rats. *Gastroenterology*, **109**, 142–50.

Aki, M., Shimbara, N., *et al.* (1994). Interferon-gamma induces different subunit organizations and functional diversity of proteasomes. *Journal of Biochemistry, Tokyo*, **115**, 257–69.

Alarcon, G.S. (1995). Tetracyclines in the treatment of rheumatoid arthritis: they work but we do not know the reason(s). *Journal of Clinical Rheumatology*, **1**, 190–3.

Albertella, M. R. and Campbell, R. D. (1994). Characterization of a novel gene in the human major histocompatibility complex that encodes a potential new member of the I kappa B family of proteins. *Human Molecular Genetics*, **3**, 793–9.

Alexeeva, L., Krylov, M., Trurin, V., *et al.* (1994). Prevalence of spondylarthropathies and HLA-B27 B27 in the native population of Chukotka, Russia. *Journal of Rheumatology*, **22**, 2298–300.

Alibert, J. L. (1818). *Précise Théorique et practique sur les maladies de la peau*. Caille et Ravier, Paris.

Allison, M. C., Howatson, A. G., Torrance, C. J., Lee, F. D., and Russel, R. I. (1992). Gastrointestinal damage associated with the use of non-steroidal anti-inflammatory drugs. *New England Journal of Medicine*, **327**, 749–54.

Alpuche-Aranda, C. M., Racoosin, E. L., Swanson, J. A., and Miller, S. I. (1994). Salmonella stimulate macrophage macropinocytosis and persist within spacious phagosomes. *Journal of Experimental Medicine*, **179**, 601–8.

Altomonte, L., Zoli, A., Veneziani, A., Mirone, L., Santacesaria, G., Chiarelli, C., *et al.* (1994). Clinical silent inflammatory gut lesions in undifferentiated spondyloarthropathies. *Clinical Rheumatology*, **13**, 565–70.

Ambrose, N. S., Honson, M., Burdon, D. W., and Keighley, M. R. B. (1984). Incidence of pathogenic bacteria from mesenteric lymph nodes and ileal serosa during Crohn's disease. *British Journal of Surgery*, **71**, 623–5.

Amor, B. (1983). Arthrites réactionelles. *Revue du Rhumatisme*, **50**, 825–6.

Amor, B., Bouchet, H., and Delrieu, F. (1983). Enquete nationale sur les arthrites ráctionelles de la Société Française de Rhumatologie. *Revue du Rhumatisme*, **50**, 733–43.

Amor, B., Dougados, M., and Mijiyawa, M. (1990) Critères de classification des spondylarthropathies. *Revue du Rhumatisme*, **57**, 85–9.

Amor, B., Dougados, M., Listrat, V., Menkes, C. J., Dubost, J. J., Roux, H., *et al.* (1991). Evaluation des critéres de spondylarthropathies d'Amor et de l'European spondyloarthropathy study group. Une étude transversale de 2228 patients. *Annales de Medicine Interne—Paris*, **142**, 85–9.

Amor, B., Dougados, M., and Khan, M. A. (1995*a*). Management of refractory ankylosing spondylitis and related spondyloarthropathies. *Rheumatic Diseases Clinics of North America*, **21**, 117–28.

Amor, B., Dougados, M., Listrat, V., *et al.* (1995*b*). Are classification criteria for spondyloarthropathy useful as diagnostic criteria? *Revue du Rhumatisme* (English edn), **6**, 10–15.

Amor, B. (1987). La spondyonkrite ankylo-sante. Est-elle mons graves en 1986 – les rôles de facteurs d'environmental. *Revue du Rhumatisme*, **54**, 269–71.

Amor, B., Santos, R. S., Nahal, R., Listrat, V., and Dougados, M. (1994). Predictive factors for the long-term outcome of spondylarthropathies. *Journal of Rheumatology*, **21**, 1883–7.

Amos, R. S., Constable, T. J., Crockson, R. A., Crockson, A. P., and McConkey, B. (1977). Rheumatoid arthritis: relation of serum C-reactive protein and erythrocyte sedimentation rates to radiographic changes. *British Medical Journal*, **1**, 195–7.

Amos, R. S., Crockson, R. A., Crockson, A. P., Walsh, L., and McConkey, B. (1978). Rheumatoid arthritis: C-reactive protein and erythrocyte sedimentation rate during initial treatment. *British Medical Journal*, **1**, 1396.

Anderson, R. P., Friend, G. M., Ferry, D. M., and Chadwick, V. S. (1991). Formyl peptidemia in patients with inflammatory bowel disease and primary sclerosing cholangitis. *Gastroenterology*, **100**, 557A.

Andrews, B. S., McIntosh, J., Petts, V., and Penny, R. (1979). Circulating immune complexes in acute uveitis: A possible association with the histocompatibility complex locus antigen B27. *International Archives of Allergy and Applied Immunology*, **58**, 313–21.

Ansell, B. M. (1978). Diagnostic criteria, nomenclature and classification of juvenile chronic arthritis. In *The case of rheumatic children* (ed. E. Munthe), pp. 42. Eular publishers, Basle, Switzerland.

Ansell, B. M. (1980). Juvenile spondylitis and related disorders. *Ankylosing spondylitis*, (ed. J. M. H. Moll), pp. 120–36. Churchill Livingstone, Edinburgh.

Ansell, B. M. (1992). Hypertrophic osteoarthropathy in the pediatric age group. *Clinical and Experimental Rheumatology*, **10** (Suppl), 15–18.

Aparicio, P., Rojo, S., Jaraquemada, D., López de Castro, J. A. (1987). Fine specificity of HLA-B27 cellular allorecognition. *Journal of Immunology* **139**, 837–41.

Apple, R. and Erlich, H. (1996). HLA class II genes: structure and diversity. In *HLA and MHC: genes, molecules and function*. (ed. M. Browning and A. McMichael), pp. 97–112. BIOS Scientific Publishers Ltd, Oxford.

ARA (Co-operating Clinics Committee of the American Rheumatism Association). (1965). A seven-day variability study of 499 patients with peripheral rheumatoid arthritis. *Arthritis and Rheumatism*, **8**, 302–32.

Archer, J. R., Whelan, M. A., *et al.* (1990). Effect of a free sulphydryl group on expression of HLA-B27 specificity. *Scandinavian Journal of Rheumatology*, **19** (Suppl 87), 44–50.

Armstrong, R. D., Panayi, G. S., *et al.* (1983). Histocompatibility antigens in psoriasis, psoriatic arthropathy, and ankylosing spondylitis. *Annals of Rheumatic Diseases*, **42**, 142–6.

Aranson, J. A., Patel, A. K., Rahko, P. S., and Sundstrom, W. R. (1996). Transthoracic and transesophageal echocardiographic evaluation of the aortic root and subvalvular structures in ankylosing spondylitis. *Journal of Rheumatology*, **23**, 120–3.

Arnett, F. C., Jr., Schacter, B. Z., *et al.* (1977). Homozygosity for HLA-B27. Impact on rheumatic disease expression in two families. *Arthritis and Rheumatism*, **20**, 797–804.

Arnett, F. C. (1993). Pathogenesis of the spondyloarthropathies. *EULAR Bulletin*, **22**, 4–6.

Asakawa, Y., Akahane, S., Kagata, N., Noguchi, M., Sakazaki, R., and Momose, T. (1973). Two community outbreaks of human infection with *Yersinia enterocolitica*. *Journal of Hygiene*, **71**, 715–23.

Atkins, C., Reuffel, L., Roddy, *et al.* (1988). Rheumatic disease in the Nuu-Chah-Nulth native Indians of the Pacific Northwest. *Journal of Rheumatology*, **15**, 684–90.

Autenrieth, I. B., Tingle, A., Reske-Kunz, A., and Heesemann, J. (1992). T lymphocytes mediated protection against *Yersinia enterocolitica* in mice: characterization of murine T cell clones specific for *Y. enterocolitica*. *Infection and Immunity*, **60**, 1140–9.

Autenrieth, I. B., Beer, M., Bohn, E., Kaufmann, S. H. E., and Heesemann, J. (1994). Immune responses to *Yersinia enterocolitica* in susceptible BALB/c and resistant C57BL/6 mice: an essential role for gamma interferon. *Infection and Immunity*, **62**, 2590–9.

Avakian, H., Welsh, J., Ebringer, A., and Entwistle, C. C. (1980). Ankylosing spondylitis HLA-B27 and klebsiella. II. Cross-reactivity studies with human tissue typing sera. *British Journal of Experimental Pathology*, **61**, 92–6.

Averns, H. L., Oxtoby, J., Taylor, H. G., Jones, P. W., Dziedzic, K., and Dawes, P. T. (1996). Smoking and outcome in ankylosing spondylitis. *Scandinavian Journal of Rheumatology* **25**, 138–42.

Axon, J. M. C., Hawley, P. R., and Huskisson, E. C. (1993). Ileal pouch arthritis. *British Journal of Rheumatology*, **32**, 586–8.

Azad Khan, A. R., Pizis, J., and Truelove, S. C. (1977). An experiment to determine the active therapeutic moiety of Sulphasalazine. *Lancet*, **ii**, 892–3.

Azouz, E. M. and Duffy, C. M. (1995). Juvenile spondyloarthropathies: clinical manifestations and medical imaging. *Skeletal Radiology*, **24**, 399–408.

Azzini, M., Girelli, D., Olivieri, O., Guarini, P., Stanzial, A. M., and Frigo, A. (1995). Fatty acids and antioxidant micronutrients in psoriatic arthritis. *Journal of Rheumatology*, **22**, 103–8.

Baca-Estrada, M. E., Gupta, R. S., Stead, R. H., and Croitoru, K. (1994). Intestinal expression and cellular immune responses to human heat-shock protein 60 in Crohn's disease. *Digestive Diseases and Sciences*, **39**, 398–506.

Badley, E. M., Wagstaff, S., and Wood, P. H. N. (1984). Measures of functional ability (disability) in arthritis in relation to impairment of range of joint movement. *Annals of Rheumatic Diseases*, **43**, 563–9.

Baggia, S., Lyons, J. L., Han, Y. B., Angell, E., Barkhuzian, A., Planck, S. R., *et al.* (1996*a*). HLA-B27 transgenic Lewis rats and iritis after gram-negative infection. *Investigative Ophthalmology and Visual Science* (in press), (Abstract)

Baggia, S., Lyons, J. L., Angell, E., Barkhuizen, A., Han, Y. B., Planck, S. R., Taurog, J. D., and Rosenbaum, J. T. (1996*b*). A novel model of bacterially-induced acute anterior uveitis in rats: lack of effect of HLA-B27 expression. Submitted.

Baird-Parker, A. C. (1990). Foodborne salmonellosis. *Lancet*, **336**, 1231–5.

Baker, H. (1966). Epidemiological aspects of psoriasis and arthritis. *British Journal of Dermatology*, **78**, 249–61.

Baker, H., Golding, D. N., and Thompson, M. (1963). Psoriasis and arthritis. *Annals of Internal Medicine*, **58**, 909–25.

Bakker, C., Boers, M., and van der Linden, S. (1993). Measures to assess ankylosing spondylitis: taxonomy, review and recommendations. *Journal of Rheumatology*, **20**, 1724–30.

Baldassano, R. N., Schreiber, S., Johnston, R. B., Jr., Fu, R. D., Muraki, T., and MacDermott, R. P. (1993). Crohn's disease monocytes are primed for accentuated release of toxic oxygen metabolites. *Gastroenterology*, **105**, 60–6.

Baldassare, A., Weiss T., Cheng, C. T., *et al.* (1981). Immunoprotein deposition in synovium tissue in Reiter's syndrome. *Annals of the Rheumatic Diseases*, **40**, 281–5.

Ball, J. (1971). Enthesopathy of rheumatoid and ankylosing spondylitis. *Annals of Rheumatic Diseases*, **30**, 213–23.

Bañares, A. A., Jover, J. A., Fernandez-Gutierrez B., Benitez del Castillo, J. M., Garcia, J., Gonzalez, F. *et al.* (1995). Bowel inflammation in anterior uveitis and spondylarthropathy. *Journal of Rheumatology*, **22**, 1112–7.

Bañares, A. A., Jover, J. A., Fernández-Gutiérrez, B., Benítez del Castillo, J. M., García, J., Vargas, E., and Hernández-García, C. (1997). Patterns of uveitis as a guide in making rheumatologic and immunologic diagnoses. *Arthritis and Rheumatism* **40**, 358–70.

Bardin, T., Enel, C., and Lathrop, G. M. (1990). Treatment of tetracycline and erythromycin of urethritides allows significant prevention of post-venereal arthritis flares in Reiter's syndrome patients. *Arthritis and Rheumatism*, **33**, S26 (Abstract).

Bardin, T., Enel, C., Cornelis, F., Salski, C., Jorgensen, C., Ward, R., and Lathrop, G. M. (1992). Antibiotic treatment of venereal disease and Reiter's syndrome in a Greenland population. *Arthritis and Rheumatism*, **35**, 190–4.

Bardin, T. and Lathrop, G. M. (1992). Postvenereal Reiter's syndrome in Greenland. *Rheumatic Disease Clinics of North America*, **18**, 81–93.

Bargen, J. A. (1929). Complications and sequelae of chronic ulcerative colitis. *Annals of Internal Medicine*, **3**, 335.

Barlon, R. J. and Schulz, E. J. (1991). Chronic subcorneal pustulosis with vasculitis, variant of generalized pustular psoriasis in Black South Africans. *British Journal of Dermatology*, **124**, 470–4.

Barlow, J. H. (Autumn/Winter 1994). Fatigue in ankylosing spondylitis: a personal perspective. *NASS Newsletter*, 5–8.

Barlow, J. H., Macey, S. J., and Struthers, G. R. (1992). Psychosocial factors and self-help in ankylosing spondylitis patients. *Clinical Rheumatology*, **11**, 220–5.

Bas, S., Griffais, R., Kvien, T. K., Glennås, A., Melby, K., and Vischer, T. L. (1995). Amplification of plasmid and chromosome chlamydia DNA in synovial fluid of patients with reactive arthritis and undifferentiated seronegative oligoarthropathies. *Arthritis and Rheumatism*, **38**, 1005–13.

Bas, S., Cunningham, T., Kvien, T. K., Glennås, A., Melby, K, and Vischer, T. L. (1996*a*). The value of isotype determination of serum antibodies against Chlamydia for the diagnosis of Chlamydia reactive arthritis. *British Journal of Rheumatology*, **35**, 542–7.

Bas, S., Cunningham, T., Kvien, T. K., Glennås, A., Melby, K, and Vischer, T. L. (1996*b*). Synovial fluid and serum antibodies against Chlamydia in different forms of arthritis: Intra-articular IgA production in Chlamydia sexually aquired reactive arthritis. *British Journal of Rheumatology*, **35**, 548–52.

Battafarano, D. F., West, S. G., Rak, K. M., Fortenbery, E. J., and Chatelois, A. E. (1993). Comparison of bone scan, computed tomography, and magnetic resonance imaging in the diagnosis of active sacroiliitis. *Seminars in Arthritis and Rheumatism*, **23**, 161–76.

Bazin, P. (1860). Lefons théoretiques et cliniques sur les affections cutanées de nature. *Arthritique et Arthreux*, pp. 154–61. Delahaye, Paris.

Beatty, P. R. and Stephens, R. S. (1994). CD8+ T lymphocyte-mediated lysis of Chlamydia-infected L cells using an endogenous antigen pathway. *Journal of Immunology*, **153**, 4588–95.

Beatty, W. L., Byrne, G. I., and Morrison, R. P. (1993). Morphological and antigenic characterization of interferon-y mediated persistent *Chlamydia trachomatis* infection *in vitro*. *Proceedings of the National Academy of Science, USA*, **85**, 4000–4.

Beatty, W. L., Morrison, R. P., and Byrne, G. I. (1994). Persistent chlamydiae: from cell culture to a paradigm for chlamydial pathogenesis. *Microbiological Reviews*, **58**, 686–99.

Beaudreuil, J., Hayem, G., Meyer, O., and Kahn, M. F. (1995). Arthrite réactionelle attribuée a Chlamydia pneumoniae: A propos d'un cas. *Revue de Rhumatisme*, **62**, 234.

Becker, G. J., Waldburger, M., Hughes, G. R. V., and Pepys M. B. (1980). Value of serum C- reactive protein measurement in the investigation of fever in systemic lupus erythematosus. *Annals of Rheumatic Diseases*, **39**, 50–2.

Beckingsale, A. B., Davies, J., Gibson, J. M. and Rosenthal, A. R. (1984). Acute anterior uveitis, ankylosing spondylitis, back pain and HLA-B27. *British Journal of Ophthalmology*, **68**, 741–5.

Bengtsson, A., Ahlstrand, C., Lindström, F. D., and Kihlström, E. (1983). Bacteriological findings in 25 patients with Reiter's syndrome (reactive arthritis). *Scandinavian Journal of Rheumatology*, **12**, 157–60.

Benjamin, R. and Parham, P. (1990). Guilt by association: HLA-B27 and ankylosing spondylitis. *Immunology Today*, **11**, 137–42.

Bennett, P. H. and Burch, T. A. (1968*a*). *The epidemiological diagnosis of ankylosing spondylitis in population studies of the rheumatoid disease* (ed. P. H. Bennett and P. H. N. Wood), pp. 301–11.

Bennett, P. H., and Burch T. A. (1968*b*). *Population studies of the rheumatic diseases*, pp. 456–7. Excerpta Medica Foundation, Amsterdam.

Bennett, P. H. and Burch, T. A. (1968*c*). The epidemiological diagnosis of ankylosing spondylitis. *Proceedings of the 3rd International Symposium of Population Studies of the Rheumatic Diseases*, New York 1966, *International Congress Series* No. 148 (ed. P. H. Bennett, and P. H. N. Wood), pp. 305–13. Exerpta Medical Foundation, New York.

Benoist, C. and Mathis, D. (1990). Regulation of major histocompatibility complex class-II genes: X, Y and other letters of the alphabet. *Annual Review of Immunology*, **8**, 681–715.

Benoist, M. (1995). Pierre Marie: pioneer investigator in anklyosing spondylitis. *Spine* **20**, 849–52.

Bergfeldt, L., Insulander, P., Lindblom, D., Möller, E., and Edhag, O. (1988). HLA-B27: an important genetic risk factor for lone aortic regurgitation and severe conduction system abnormalities. *American Journal of Medicine*, **85**, 12–18.

Beukelman, S. J., Quärles, V. U. H., *et al.*. (1990). Trial and error in producing ankylosing–spondylitis–selective artisera according to Andrew Geczy. *Scandinavian Journal of Rheumatology* (Suppl.), **87**, 74–9.

Beutler, A. M., Wittum-Hudson, J. A., Nanagara, R., Schumacher, H. R., and Hudson, A. P. (1994). Intracellular location of inapparently infecting Chlamydia in synovial tissue from patients with with Reiter's syndrome. *Immunological Research*, **13**, 163–71.

Beutler, A. M., Schumacher, H. R., and Wittum-Hudson, J. A. (1995). In situ hybridization for detection of inapparent infection with *Chlamydia trachomatis* in synovial tissue of a patient with Reiter's syndrome. *American Journal of Medical Science*, **310**, 206–13.

Beutler, A. M., Hudson, A. P., Whittum-Hudson, J. A., *et al.* (1997). *Chlamydia trachomatis* can persist in joint tissue after antibiotic treatment in chronic Reiter's syndrome/reactive arthritis. *Journal of Clinical Rheumatology* **3**, 125–30.

Beyeler, C., Armstrong, M., *et al.* (1996). Relationship between genotype for the cytochrome P450 CYP2D6 and susceptibility to ankylosing spondylitis and rheumatoid arthritis. *Annals of Rheumatic Diseases*, **55**, 66–8.

Bhopal, R. S. and Thomas, G. O. (1982). *Psittacosis* presenting with Reiter's syndrome. *British Medical Journal*, **294**, 1606.

Bianchi, G., Marchesini, G., Zoli, M., Falasconi, M. C., Lervese, T., Vecchi, F., *et al.* (1993). Thyroid involvement in chronic inflammatory rheumatological disorders. *Clinical Rheumatology*, **12**, 479–84.

Billison, F. A., De Dombal, F. T., Watkinson, G., and Goligher, J. C. (1967). Ocular complications of ulcerative colitis. *Gut*, **8**, 102–6.

Biondi Oriente, C., Scarpa, R., and Oriente, P. (1994). Prevalence and clinical features of juvenile psoriatic arthritis in 425 psoriatic patients. *Acta Dermatologica Venereologica Suppl.* (Stockholm), **186**, 109–10.

Birkbeck, M. Q., Buckler, W. S., Mason, R. M., and Tegner, W. S. (1951). Iritis as the presenting symptom in ankylosing spondylitis. *Lancet*, **2**, 802.

Bissoli, E. and Sansone, V. (1994). Sacroiliitis in seronegative arthritis. The anatomic-opathological aspects and imaging methods compared. *Radiology Medicine* (Torino), **88**, 198–208.

Bjarnason, I. and Peters, T. J. (1996). Influence of antirheumatic drugs on gut permeability and on the gut associated lymphoid tissue. *Baillière's Clinical Rheumatology*, **10** (in press).

Bjarnason, I., O'Moran, C., Levi, J., and Peters, T. J. (1983). Absorption of ^{51}Chromium-labeled ethylenediamine tetracetate in inflammatory bowel disease. *Gastroenterology*, **85**, 318–22.

Bjarnason, I., Williams, P., So, A., *et al.* (1984). Intestinal permeability and inflammation in rheumatoid arthritis, effects of non-steroidal anti-inflammatory drugs. *Lancet*, **2**, 1171–4.

Bjarnason, I., Zanelli, G., Smith, T., *et al.* (1987). Non-steroidal anti-inflammatory drug induced intestinal inflammation. *Gastroenterology*, **93**, 480–9.

Bjarnason, I., Fehilly, B., Smethurst, P., *et al.* (1991). The importance of local versus systemic effects of non-steroidal anti-inflammatory drugs to increase intestinal permeability in man. *Gut*, **32**, 275–7.

Bjarnason, I., Hayllar, J., Mc Pherson, A., and Russell, A. S. (1993). Side effects of nonsteroidal anti-inflammatory drugs on the small and large intestine. *Gastroenterology*, **104**, 1832–47.

Bjorkman, P. J., Saper, M. A., *et al.* (1987). Structure of the human class I histocompatibility antigen, HLA-A2. *Nature*, **329**, 506–12

Bjorkman, P. J., Saper, M. A., Samraoui, B., Bennett, W. S., Strominger, J. L., Wiley, D. C. (1987a). The foreign antigen binding site and T cell recognition regions of class I histocompatibility antigens. *Nature* **329**, 512–8.

Black, R., Jackson, R., Tsai, T., Medvesky, M., Shayegani, M., Feeley, J., *et al.* (1978). Epidemic *Yersinia enterocolitica* infection due to contaminated chocolate milk. *New England Journal of Medicine*, **298**, 76–9.

Black, R. L., O'Brien, W. M., Van Scott, E. J., and Auerbach, R. (1964). Methotrexate therapy in psoriatic arthritis. *Journal of the American Medical Association*, **189**, 743–7.

Blanche, P., Taelman, H., and Saraux, A. (1993). Acute arthritis and human immunodeficiency virus infection in Rwanda. *Journal of Rheumatology*, **20**, 2123–7.

Bliska, J. B., Galan, J. E., and Falkow, S. (1993). Signal transduction in the mammalian cell during bacterial attachment and entry. *Cell*, **73**, 903–20.

Blumberg, B. S., Bunin, J. J., Calkins, E., Pirani, C. L., and Zvaifler, N. J. (1964). ARA nomenclature and classification of arthritis and rheumatism (tentative). *Arthritis and Rheumatism*, **7**, 93–7.

Boers, M. and Tugwell, P. (1993). The validity of pooled outcome measures (indices) in rheumatoid arthritis clinical trials. *Journal of Rheumatology*, **20**, 568–74.

Bohn, E., Heesemann, J., Ehlers, S., and Autenrieth, I. B. (1994). Early gamma interferon mRNA expression is associated with resistance of mice against *Yersinia enterocolitica*. *Infection and Immunity*, **62**, 3027–32.

Boisgérault, F., Tieng, V., Stolzenberg, M. C., Dulphy, N., Khalil, I., Tamouza, R., Charron, D., Toubert, A. (1996). Differences in endogenous peptides presented by HLA-B*2705 and B*2703 allelic variants. Implications for susceptibility to spondylarthropathies. *Journal of Clinical Investigation* **98**, 2764–70.

Bombardier, C. and Tugwell, P. (1982). A methodological framework to develop and select indices for clinical trials: stastistical and judgmental approaches. *Journal of Rheumatology*, **9**, 753–7.

Boone, D. C., Azen, S. P., Lin, C., Spence, C., Baron, C., and Lee, L. (1978). Reliability of goniometric measurements. *Physical Therapy*, **58**, 1355–60.

Borg, A. A., Gray, J., and Dawes, P. T. (1992). Yersinia-related arthritis in the United Kingdom. A report of 12 cases and review of the literature. *Quarterly Journal of Medicine, New Series*, **84**, 575–82.

Borg, A. A., Nixon, N. B., Dawes, P. T., and Mattey, D. L. (1994). Increased IgA antibodies to cytokeratins in the spondyloarthropathies. *Annals of Rheumatic Diseases*, **53**, 391–5.

Bourdillon, C. (1888). *Psoriasis et arthropathies*. MD Thesis, Paris.

Bourne, J. T., Kumar, P., Huskisson, E., Mageed, R., Unsworth, D. S., and Wostulewski, J. A. (1985). Arthritis and celiac disease. *Annals of Rheumatic Diseases*, **44**, 592–8.

Bowling, A. (1995). *Measuring disease*. Open University Press, Buckinghamshire, England.

Bowness, P., Allen, R., and McMichael, A. J. (1995). HLA-B27-restricted peptide presentation to cytotoxic T cells in reactive arthritis. *Arthritis and Rheumatism*, **38**, S181.

Boyer, G. S., Lanier, A. P., and Templin, D. W. (1988). Prevalence rates of spondyloarthropathies, rheumatoid arthritis, and other rheumatic disorders in an Alaskan Inupiat Eskimo population. *Journal of Rheumatology*, **15**, 678–83.

Boyer, G. S., Templin, D. W., and Goring, W. P. (1993). Evaluation of the European spondylarthropathy study group preliminary classification criteria in Alaskan Eskimos. *Arthritis and Rheumatism*, **36**, 534–8.

Boyer, G. S., Templin, D. W., Cornoni-Huntley, J. C., *et al.* (1994). Prevalance of spondylarthropathies in Alaskan Eskimos. *Journal of Rheumatology*, **21**, 2292–7.

Boyson, J. E., Shufflebotham, C., Cadavid, L. F., *et al.* (1996). The MHC class I genes of the rhesus monkey: different evolutionary histories of MHC class I and II genes in primates. *Journal of Immunology*, **156**, 4656–65.

Brandes, M. E., Allen, M. E., Allen, J. B., Ogawa, Y-, and Wahl, S. M. (1991). Transforming growth factor (1 suppresses acute and chronic arthritis in experimental animals. *Journal of Clinical Investigation*, **87**, 1108–13.

Brandt, K. D., Carthcart, E. S., and Cohen, A. S. (1968). Studies of immune deposits in synovial membranes and corresponding synovial fluids. *Journal of Laboratory and Clinical Medicine*, **72**, 631–47.

Brandtzaeg, P. (1995). Autoimmunity and ulcerative colitis: Can two enigmas make sense together? *Gastroenterology*, **109**, 3–12.

Branigan, P. J., Gerard, H. C., Saaibi, D., *et al.* (1995). PCR screening of synovial tissue vs fluid from patients with Reiter's syndrome and other spondyloarthropathies for *Chlamydia trachomatis*. *Arthritis and Rheumatism*, **38**, (Suppl. 9) S348.

Braun, J. and Sieper, J. (1995). Comment on glossary for the rheumatic spinal diseases. *Annals of Rheumatic Diseases*, **55**, 76–8.

Braun, J. and Sieper, J. (1996). The sacroiliac joint in the spondyloarthropathies. *Current Opinion in Rheumatology*, 8, 275–87.

Braun, J., Bollow, M., Eggens, U., *et al. (1994a)*. Use of dynamic magnetic resonance imaging with fast imaging in the detection of early and advanced sacroilitis in spondylarthropathy patients. *Arthritis and Rheumatism*, **37**, 1039–45.

Braun, J., Grolms, M., and Sieper, J. (1994*b*). Three colour flow cytometric examination of CD4/CD45 subsets reveals no difference in peripheral blood and synovial fluid between patients with reactive arthritis and rheumatoid arthritis. *Clinical and Experimental Rheumatology*, **12**, 17–22.

Braun, J., Grolms, M., Distler, A., and Sieper, J. (1994*c*). The specific anti-bacterial proliferation of reactive arthritis synovial T cells is not due to their higher proportion of CD45RO+ cells compared to peripheral blood. *Journal of Rheumatology*, **21,** 1702–7.

Braun, J., Laitko, S., Treharne, J., Eggens, U., Wu, P., Distler, A., and Sieper, J. (1994*d*). *Chlamydia pneumomiae*-a new causative agent of reactive arthritis and undifferentiated oligoarthritis. *Annals of Rheumatic Diseases*, **53**, 100–5.

Braun, J., Bollow, M., Neure, L., *et al.* (1995*a*). Use of immunohistologic and in situ hybridisation techniques in the examination of sacroiliac joint biopsy specimens from patients with ankylosing spondylitis. *Arthritis and Rheumatism*, **38**, 499–505.

Braun, J., Bollow, M., Wu P., *et al.* (1995*b*). Further examination of sacroiliac biopsies of spondylarthropathy patients—investigation of the cytokine pattern and of bacterial DNA. *Arthritis and Rheumatism*, **38**, (Suppl. 9), S315.

Braun, J., Bollow, M., Seyrekbasan, F., and Sieper, J. (1996). Computed tomography guided corticoid injection of the sacroiliac joint in patients with sacroiliitis: Clinical outcome and followup by dynamic magnetic resonance imaging. *Journal of Rheumatology*, **23**, 659–64.

Braun, J., Bollow, M., Remlinger, G., *et al.* (1997). Prevalence of spondyloarthropathies in HLA-B27-positive and -negative blood donors. (in press)

Breban, M., Hammer, R. E., Richardson, J. A., and Taurog, J. D. (1993). Transfer of the inflammatory disease of HLA-B27 transgenic rats by bone marrow engraftment. *Journal of Experimental Medicine*, **178**, 1606–16.

Breban, M., Fernández-Sueiro, J. L., Simmons, W. A., *et al.*. (1996). T cells but not thymic exposure to HLA-B27 are required for the inflammatory disease of HLA-B27 transgenic rats. *Journal of Immunology*, **156**, 794–803.

Breitbart, A., Bauer, H., Krastel, H., Brado, B., and Pezzutto, A. (1993). Sulfasalazine in recurrent anterior uveitis: a new therapeutical strategy. *Arthritis and Rheumatism*, **36** (Supp.), S225.

Bremell, T., Bjelle, A., and Svedhem, A. (1991). Rheumatic symptoms following an outbreak of Campylobacter enteritis: a five year follow-up. *Annals of Rheumatic Diseases*, **50**, 934–8.

Brennan, F. R., Mikecz, K., Buzas, E. I. *et al.* (1995). Antigen-specific B cells present cartilage proteoglycan (aggrecan) to an autoreactive T cell hybridoma derived from a mouse with proteoglycan-induced arthritis. *Clinical and Experimental Immunology*, **101**, 414–21.

Breur-Vriesendorp, B. S., Dekker-Saeys, A.J., *et al.* (1987). Distribution of HLA-B27 subtypes in patients with ankylosing spondylitis: the disease is associated with a common determinant of the various B27 molecules. *Annals of Rheumatic Diseases*, **46**, 353–6.

Brewer, E.J., Bass, J., Baum, J., *et al.* (1977). Current proposed revision of JRA criteria. *Arthritis and Rheumatism*, **20**, 194–9.

Brewerton, D. A., Caffrey, M., Hart, F. D., James, D. C. O., Nicholls, A., and Sturrock, R. D. (1973*a*). Ankylosing spondylitis and HLA-27. *Lancet*, **1**, 904–7.

Brewerton, D.A., Caffrey, M., Nicholls, A., Walters, D., and James, D. C. O. (1973*b*). Acute anterior uveitis and HLA-B27. *Lancet*, **2**, 994–6.

Brewerton, D. A., Caffrey, M., Nicholls, A., Walters, D., and James, D. C. O. (1974). HLA-27 and arthropathies associated with ulcerative colitis and psoriasis. *Lancet*, **1**, 956–7.

Brewerton, D. A., Webley, M., *et al.* (1978). The alpha 1-antitrypsin phenotype MZ in acute anterior uveitis (letter). *Lancet*, **1**, 1103.

Brewerton, D. A., Webley, M., and Ward, A.M. (1985). Acute anterior uveitis and the fourteenth chromosome. *Advances in Inflammation Research*, **9**, 225–9.

Bristol-Rothstein, L. A. and Schwab, J. H. (1992). Bone-resorbing activity is expressed by rat macrophages in response to arthropathic streptococal cell wall polymers. *Inflammation*, **16**, 485–96.

Brooke, B. N., Dykes, P. W., and Walker, F. C. (1961). A study of liver disorder in ulcerative colitis. *Postgraduate Medical Journal*, **37**, 245–51.

Brooks, J. M., Murray, R. J., Thomas, W. A., Kurilla, M. G., Rickinson, A. B. (1993). Different HLA-B27 subtypes present the same immunodominant Epstein-Barr virus peptide. *Journal of Experimental Medicine* **178**, 879–87.

Brown, M. A., Pile, K. D., *et al.* (1995*a*). HLA Class II associations of ankylosing spondylitis. *British Journal of Rheumatology*, **34**, 146.

Brown, M. A., Pile, K. D., *et al.* (1995*b*). The HLA component of the genetic contribution to ankylosing spondylitis. *British Journal of Rheumatology*, **34**, 72.

Brown, M. A., Pile, K. D., Kennedy, L. G., *et al.* (1996*a*). HLA class I associations of ankylosing spondylitis in the white population in the United Kingdom. *Annals of Rheumatic Disease*, **55**, 268–70.

Brown, M. A., Jepson, A., Young, A., *et al.* (1996*b*). Spondyloarthritis in the Gambia—Evidence for a non-HLA B27 protective effect (Abstract). *British Journal of Rheumatology*, **35** (Suppl. 1). 113.

Brown, M. A., Bunce, M., *et al.* (1996*c*). HLA-B associations of B27 negative ankylosing spondylitis: comment on article by Yamaguchi *et al. Arthritis and Rheumatism*, **39**, 1768–9.

Brown, M. A., Jepson, A., *et al.* (1997*a*). Spondyloarthritis in The Gambia: Evidence for a non-HLA B27 protective effect. *Annals of Rheumatic Diseases*, **56**, 68–70.

Brown, M. A., Kennedy, L. G., MacGregor, A. J., Darke, C., Duncan, E., Shatford, J. L., Taylor, A., Calin, A., Wordsworth, P. (1997). Susceptibility to ankylosing spondylitis in twins: the role of genes, HLA, and the environment *Arthritis & Rheumatism*, **40**, 1823–8.

Brown, M., and Wordsworth, P. (1997*b*). Predisposing factors to spondyloarthropathies. *Current Opinion in Rheumatology*, **9**, 308–14.

Bruneau, C., Villiaumeocy, J., Avouac, B., *et al.* (1986). Seronegative spondyloarthropathies and IgA glomerulonephritis: A report of four cases and a review of the literature. *Seminars in Arthritis and Rheumatism*, **15**, 179–84.

Brunt, L.M., Portnoy, D. A., and Unanue, E. R. Presentation of Listeria monocytogenes to CD8+T cells requires secretion of hemolysin and intracellular bacterial growth. *Journal of Immunology*, **145**, 3540–46.

Buchanan, J.(1981). The social and economic disadvantages of ankylosing spondylitis. *National Ankylosing Spondylitis Society Symposium*, 41–8.

Buisseret, P. D., Pembrey, M. E., *et al.* (1977). Alpha 1-antitrypsin phenotypes in rheumatoid arthritis and ankylosing spondylitis (letter). *Lancet*, **2**, 1358–9.

Bulbul, R., Williams, W. V., and Schumacher, H. R., Jr. (1995). Psoriatic arthritis: Diverse and sometimes highly destructive. *Postgraduate Medicine*, **97**, 103–6.

Burgos-Vargas, R. (1991). Ankylosing spondylitis of juvenile onset. In *HLA-B27-positive spondylarthropathies* (ed. P. E. Lipsky, J. Taurog), pp. 161–73. Elsevier, New York.

Burgos-Vargas, R. and Clark, P. (1989). Axial involvement in the seronegative enthesopathy and arthropathy syndrome and its progression to ankylosing spondylitis. *Journal of Rheumatology*, **16**, 192–7.

Burgos-Vargas, R. and Granados-Arriola, J. (1990). Ankylosing spondylitis and related diseases in the Mexican Mestizo. *Spine: State of the Art Reviews*, **4**, 665–78.

Burgos-Vargas, R. and Petty, R. E. (1992). Juvenile ankylosing spondylitis. *Rheumatic Disease Clinics of North America*, **18**, 123–42.

Burgos-Vargas, R. and Vazquez-Mellado, J. (1989). El reconocimiento y diagnostico temprano de la espondilitis anquilosant juvenil: Anliasis clinico y estudio comparativo con la artritis rheumatoid juvenil. *Boletin Medico del Hospital Infantil de Mexico*, **45**, 500–11.

Burgos-Vargas, R. and Vasquez-Mellado, J. (1995). The early clinical recognition of juvenileonset ankylosing spondylitis and its differentiation from juvenile rheumatoid arthritis. *Arthritis and Rheumatism*, **38**, 835–44.

Burgos-Vargas, R., Naranjo, A., Castillo, J., and Katona, G. (1989). Ankylosing spondylitis in the Mexican mestizo: patterns of disease according to age at onset. *Journal of Rheumatology*, **16**, 186–91.

Burgos-Vargas, R., Castelazo-Duarte, G., Orozco, J. A., Gardu/no-Espinosa, J., Clark, P., and Sanabria, L. (1993). Chest expansion in healthy adolescents and patients with the seronegative enthesopathy and arthropathy syndrome or juvenile ankylosing spondylitis. *Journal of Rheumatology*, **20**, 1957–60.

Burgos-Vargas, R., Pacheco-Tena, C., and Vazquez-Mellado, J. (1997). Juvenile-onset spondyloarthropathies. *Rheumatic Disease Clinics of North America*, **23**, 569–98.

Burmester, G. R., Daser, A., Kamradt, T., *et al.* (1995). Immunology of reactive arthritis. *Annual Review of Immunology*, **13**, 229–50.

Burney, R. O., Pile, K. D., Gibson, K., *et al.* (1994). Analysis of the MHC class II encoded components of the HLA class I antigen processing pathway in ankylosing spondylitis. *Annals of Rheumatic Diseases*, **53**, 58–60.

Burns, T. M. and Calin, A. (1984). Undifferentiated spondylarthropathy. In *Spondylarthropathies* (ed. A. Calin), pp. 253–64. Grune and Stratton, Orlando, Florida.

Buxton, S. E., Benjamin, R. J., Clayberger, C., Parham, P., Krensky, A. M. (1992). Anchoring pockets in human histocompatibility complex leukocyte antigen (HLA) class I molecules: analysis of the conserved B ('45') pocket of HLA-B27. *Journal of Experimental Medicine* **175**, 809–20.

Buzas, E. I., Brennan, F. R., Mikecz, K., *et al.* (1995). A proteoglycan (aggrecan)-specific T cell hybridoma induces arthritis in BALB/c mice. *Journal of Immunology*, **155**, 2679–87.

Byrne, G. I. (1988). Host cell relationships. In *Microbiology of chlamydia* (ed. A. L. Barron), pp. 135–50. CRC Press, Boca Raton.

Byron, N. A., Campbell, M. A., Hobbs, J. R., *et al.* (1979). T and B lymphocytes in patients with acute anterior uveitis and ankylosing spondylitis, and in their household contacts. *Lancet*, **2**, 601–3.

Bywaters, A. G. L. (1984). Pathology of the spondylarthropathies. In *Spondylarthropathies* (ed. A. Calin), pp. 43–68. Grune and Stratton., Orlando, Florida.

Bywaters, A. G. L. and Ansell, B. M. (1958). Arthritis associated with ulcerative colitis. *Annals of Rheumatic Diseases*, **17**, 169–83.

Cabral, D. A., Oen, K. G., and Petty, R. E. (1992). SEA syndrome revisted: a longterm followup of children with a syndrome of seronegative enthesopathy and arthropathy. *Journal of Rheumatology*, **19**, 1282–5.

Cabral, D. A., Petty, R. E., Malleson, P. N., Ensworth S., McCormick, A.Q., and Shroeder, M.-L. (1994). Visual prognosis in children with chronic anterior uveitis and arthritis. *Journal of Rheumatology*, **21**, 2370–5.

Caffrey, M. F. P. and James, D. C. O. (1973). Human lymphocyte antigen association in ankylosing spondylitis. *Nature*, **242**, 121.

Cain, T. K. and Rank, R. G. (1995). Local Th1-like responses are induced by intravaginal infection of mice with the mouse pneumonitis biovar of *Chlamydia trachomatis. Infection and Immunity*, **63**, 1784–9.

Calin, A. (1979). Keratodermia blennorrhagica and mucocutaneous manifestations of Reiter's syndrome. *Annals of Rheumatic Diseases*, **38** (Suppl 1), 68–72.

Calin, A. (1984) Reiter's syndrome. In *Spondylarthropathies* (ed. A. Calin), pp. 119–50. Grune and Stratton, Orlando, Florida.

Calin, A. (1984). *Spondylarthropathies*. Grune and Stratton, Orlando, Florida.

Calin, A. (1985). Ankylosing spondylitis. In *Textbook of rheumatology*, (2nd edn). (ed. W. N. Kelly, E. D. Harris, S. Ruddy, and C. B. Sledge), pp. 993–1005. WB Saunders, Philadelphia.

Calin, A. (1986). A placebo-controlled cross-over study of azathioprine in Reiter's syndrome. *Annals of the Rheumatic Diseases*, **45**, 653–5.

Calin, A. (1989). Ankylosing spondylitis. In *Textbook of rheumatology* (3rd edn), (ed. W. N. Kelly, E. D. Harris, S. Ruddy, and C. B. Sledge), pp. 1021–1137. WB Saunders, Philadelphia.

Calin, A. (1993*a*). Spondylarthritis, undifferentiated spondylarthritis and overlap. In *Oxford textbook of rheumatology*, Chapter 5.5.1 (ed. P. Maddison, D. A. Isenberg, P. Woo, D. N. Glass), pp. 661–74. Oxford University Press.

Calin, A. (1993*b*). Ankylosing spondylitis. In *Oxford textbook of rheumatology*, Chapter 5.5.3 (ed. P. Maddison, D. A. Isenberg, P. Woo, and D. N. Glass). Oxford University Press 681–90

Calin, A. (1995). The individual with ankylosing spondylitis: define disease status and the impact of the illness. *British Journal of Rheumatology*, **34**, 663–72.

Calin, A. (1996). Radiology and spondylarthritis. In *Modern imaging techniques* (ed. H. A. Bird and M. Dougados) pp. 445–76. Bailliere Tindall, London.

Calin, A. and Elswood, J. (1989*a*). Relative role of genetic and environmental factors in disease expresion: sib-pair analysis in ankylosing spondylitis. *Arthritis and Rheumatism*, **32**, 77–81.

Calin, A. and Elswood, J. (1989*b*). The outcome of 138 total hip replacements and 12 revisions in ankylosing spondylitis: high success rate after a mean follow-up of 7.5 years. *Journal of Rheumatology*, **16**, 955–8.

Calin, A. and Elswood, J. (1989*c*). Retrospective case-control analysis of 376 irradiated patients with ankylosing spondylitis. *Journal of Rheumatology*, **16**, 1443–5.

Calin, A. and Fries, J. F. (1975*a*). Striking prevalence of ankylosing spondylitis in 'healthy' W27 positive males and females. A controlled study. *New England Journal of Medicine*, **293**, 835–9.

Calin, A. and Fries, J. F. (1975*b*). Epidemic Reiter's syndrome: genetics and environment. *Arthritis and Rheumatism* **18**, 390.

Calin, A. and Fries, J. F. (1976). An 'experimental' epidemic of Reiter's syndrome revisited: follow-up evidence on genetic and environmental factors. *Annals of Internal Medicine*, **84**, 564–6.

Calin, A. and Fries, J. F. (1978). *Ankylosing spondylitis: discussions in patient management*. Medical Examination Publishing Company, New York.

Calin, A., Porta, J., Fries, J. F., and Schurman, D. J. (1977). Clinical history as a screening test for ankylosing spondyltis. *Journal of the American Medical Association*, **237**, 2613–14

Calin, A., Marder, A., Becks, E., *et al.* (1983). Genetic differences between B27 positive patients with ankylosing spondylitis and B27 positive healthy controls. *Arthritis and Rheumatism*, **26**, 1460–4. (1,4)

Calin, A., Marder, A., Marks, S., *et al.* (1984). Familial aggregation of Reiter's syndrome and ankylosing spondylitis: a comparative study. *Journal of Rheumatology*, **11**, 672–7.

Calin, A., Goulding, N., and Brewerton, D. (1987). Post salmonella vaccination reactive arthropathy. *Arthritis and Rheumatism* **30**, 1197.

Calin, A., Elswood, J., Rigg, S., and Skevington, S. M. (1988). Ankylosing spondylitis—an analytical review of 1500 patients: the changing pattern of disease. *Journal of Rheumatology*, **15**, 1234–8.

Calin, A., Edmunds, L., and Kennedy, L. G. (1993). Fatigue in ankylosing spondylitis—why is it ignored? *Journal of Rheumatology*, **20**, 991–5.

Calin, A., Garrett, S. L., Whitelock, H. C., *et al.* (1994). A new approach to defining functional ability in ankylosing spondylitis: the development of the Bath Ankylosing Spondylitis Functional Index. *Journal of Rheumatology*, **21**, 2281–5.

Callahan, L. F. and Pincus, T. (1995). Mortality in the rheumatic diseases. *Arthritis Care and Research*, **8**, 229–41.

Canvin, J. M. G., MacPherson, B. C. M. and Sturrock, R. D. (1995). High prevalence of apical pulmonary fibrosis in ankylosing spondylitis by high resolution computerised tomography. *British Journal of Rheumatology*, **34** (Abstracts supplement 1), abstract number 223.

Cappuccio, A. L., Patton, D. L., Kuo, C. C., and Campbell, L. A. (1994). Detection of *Chlamydia trachomatis* deoxyribonucleic acid in monkey models (*Macaca nemestrina*) of salpingitis by in situ hybridization: implications for pathogenesis. *American Journal of Obstetrics and Gynecology*, **171**, 102–10.

Carbone, L. D., Cooper, C., Michet, C. J., *et al.* (1992). Ankylosing spondylitis in Rochester, Minnesota, 1935–1989. *Arthritis and Rheumatism*, **35**, 1476–82.

Careless, D. J. and Inman, R. D. (1995). Acute anterior uveitis: clinical and experimental aspects. *Seminars in Arthritis and Rheumatism*, **24**, 432–41.

Carette, S., Graham, D., Little, H., Rubenstein, J., and Rosen, P. (1983). The natural disease course of ankylosing spondylitis. *Arthritis and Rheumatism*, **26**, 186–90.

Carr, W. P. (1983). Acute-phase proteins. *Clinics in Rheumatic Diseases*, **9**, 227–39.

Carreno, B., Winter, C. C., Taurog, J. D., Hansen, T. H., Biddison, W. E. (1993). Residues in pockets B and F of HLA-B27 are critical in the presentation of an influenza A nucleo protein peptide and influence the stability of peptide/MHC complexes. *International Immunology* **5**, 353–60.

Carter, E. T., McKenna, C. H., Brian, D. D., and Kurland, L. T. (1979). Epidemiology of ankylosing spondylitis in Rochester, Minnesota, 1935–1973. *Arthritis and Rheumatism*, **22**, 365–70.

Casini-Raggi, V., Kam, L., Chong, Y. J., Fiocchi, C., Pizarro, T. T., and Cominelli, F. (1995). Mucosal imbalance of IL-1 and IL-1 receptor antagonist in inflammatory bowel disease. A novel mechanism of chronic intestinal inflammation. *Journal of Immunology*, **154**, 2434–40.

Casserly, I. P., Fenlon, H. M., Breatnach, E. and Sant, S. M. (1997). Lung findings on high-resolution computed tomography in idiopathic ankylosing spondylitis: correlation with clinical findings, pulmonary function testing and plain radiography. *British Journal of Rheumatology*, **36**, 677–82.

Cassidy, J. T. and Petty, R. E. (1990). Spondyloarthropathies. *Textbook of pediatric rheumatology* (ed. J. T. Cassidy and R. E. Petty), pp. 221–59. WB Saunders Company, Philadelphia.

Cassidy, J. T. and Petty, R. E. (1995). Spondyloarthropathies. *Textbook of pediatric rheumatology* (ed. J. T. Cassidy and R. E. Petty), pp. 224–59, WB Saunders Company, Philadelphia.

Cedoz, J. -P., Wendlin, D., and Viel, J. -F. (1995). The B7 cross-reactive group and spondyloarthropathies: an epidemiological approach. *Journal of Rheumatology*, **22**, 1884–90.

Cerundolo, V. and Braud, V. (1996). Cell biology of MHC class I molecules. In *HLA and MHC, genes, molecules and function* (ed. M. Browning and A. McMichael), pp. 193–223. Bios Scientific Publishers, Oxford.

Chakravarty, K. and Scott, D. G. I. (1992). Oligoarthritis—a presenting feature of ocult coeliac disease. *British Journal of Rheumatology*, **31**, 349–50.

Chamberlain, M. A. (1981). Socio-economic effects of ankylosing spondylitis. *International Rehabilitation Medicine*, **3**, 94–9.

Chen, H., Gabrilovich, D., *et al.* (1996). A functionally defective allele of TAP1 results in loss of MHC class I antigen presentation in a human lung cancer. *Nature Genetics*, **13**, 210–14.

Chetty, C., Klapper, D. G., and Schwab, J. H. (1982). Soluble peptidoglycan–polysaccharide fragments of the bacterial cell wall induce acute inflammation. *Infection and Immunity*, **38**, 1010–19.

Chicz, R. M., Urban, R. G., Gorga, J. C., Vignali, D. A. A., Lane, W. S., Strominger, J. L. (1993). Specificity and promiscuity among naturally processed peptides bound to HLA-DR alleles. *Journal of Experimental Medicine*, **178**, 27–47.

Chung, Y.-M., Yeh, T.-S., and Liu, J.-H. (1988). Endogenous uveitis in Chinese—an analysis of 240 cases in a uveitis clinic. *Japanese Journal of Ophthalmology*, **32**, 64–9.

Clegg, D. O. and Reda, D. J. (1995). Comparison of sulphasalazine and placebo for the treatment of axial, oligoarticular and polyarticular manifestations of the seronegative spondylarthropathies. *Arthritis and Rheumatism*, **38**, abstr 1176.

Clegg, D. O., Zone, J. J., Samuelson, C. O., and Ward, J. R. (1985). Circulating immune complexes containing secretory IgA in jejunoileal bypass disease. *Annals of Rheumatic Diseases*, **44**, 239–44.

Clegg, D. O., Reda, D. J., Weisman, M. H., *et al.* (1996). Comparison of sulfasalazine and placebo in the treatment of ankylosing spondylitis, psoriatic arthritis, and reactive arthritis (Reiter's syndrome). *Arthritis and Rheumatism*, **39**, 2004–27. (3 articles)

Cohen, L. M., Mittal, K. K., Schmid, F. R., *et al.* (1976). Increased risk for spondylitis stigmata in apparently healthy HL-AW27 men. *Annals of Internal Medicine*, **84**, 1.

Colbert, R. A., Rowland-Jones, S. L., *et al.* (1993). Allele-specific B pocket transplant in class I major histocompatibility complex protein changes requirement for anchor residue at P2 of peptide. *Proceedings of the National Academy of Science. USA*, **90**, 6879–83.

Colbert, R. A., Rowland-Jones, S. L., *et al.* (1994). Differences in peptide presentation between B27 subtypes: the importance of the P1 side chain in maintaining high affinity peptide binding to B*2703. *Immunity*, **1**, 121–30.

Cole, B. C., Washburn, L. R., and Taylor-Robinson, D. (1986). Mycoplasma-induced arthritis. In: *The mycoplasmas. Vol. IV Mycoplasma pathogenicity*, (ed. M. F. Razin and M. F. Bariele), pp. 107–60. Academic Press, New York.

Collado, A., Gratacós, J., Ebringer, A., *et al.* (1994). Serum IgA anti-klebsiella antibodies in ankylosing spondylitis patients from Catalonia. *Scandinavian Journal of Rheumatology*, **23**, 119–23.

Collins, E. J., Garboczi, D. N., and Wiley, D. C. (1994). Three-dimensional structure of a peptide extending from one end of a class I MHC binding site. *Nature*, **371**, 626–9.

Cong, Y., Brandwein, S. L., Lazenby, A., *et al.* (1996). Th1 CD4+ T cell reactivity to enteric bacteria antigens in colitis C3H/HeJ Bir mice. *Gastroenterology*, **110**, A887.

Convit, J. (1962). Investigation of the incidence of psoriasis among Latin American Indians. In *Proceedings of the XII Congress of Dermatology*, p. 196. Excerpta Medica Foundation, Amsterdam.

Cooper, R., Fraser, S. M., Sturrock, R. D., and Gemmell, C. G. (1988). Raised titres of anti-klebsiella IgA in ankylosing spondylitis, rheumatoid arthritis, and inflammatory bowel disease. *British Medical Journal*, **296**, 1432–4.

Coulton, B. L., Thomson, K., Symmons, D. P. M., and Popert, A. J. (1989). Outcome in patients hospitalised for psoriatic arthritis. *Clinical Rheumatology*, **8**, 261–5.

Court-Brown, W. M. and Doll, R. (1965). Mortality from cancer and other causes after radiotherapy for ankylosing spondylitis. *British Medical Journal*, **2**, 1327–32.

Cowling, P., Ebringer, R., Cawdell, D., Ishii, M., and Ebringer, A. (1980) C-reactive protein, ESR, and klebsiella in ankylosing spondylitis. *Annals of Rheumatic Diseases*, **39**, 45–9.

Creamer, P., Edmonds, J., Sullivan, J., and Matthews, S. (1992). Measurement of HLA class I expression in ankylosing spondylitis. *Annals of Rheumatic Diseases*, **51**, 1138–42.

Creemers, M. C. W., van't Hof, M. A., Franssen, M. J. A. M., van de Putte, L. B. A., Gribnau, F. W. J., and van Riel, P. L. C. M. (1994*a*). A Dutch version of the functional index for ankylosing spondylitis: development and validation in a long-term study. *British Journal of Rheumatology*, **33**, 842–6.

Creemers, M. C. W., van Riel, P. L., Franssen, M. J., Van de Putte, L. B. A., and Gribnau, F. W. (1994*b*). Second line treatment in seronegative spondylarthropathies. *Seminars in Arthritis and Rheumatism*, **24**, 71–81.

Creemers, M. C. W., Franssen, M. J., van de Putte, L. B., Gribnau, F. W., and van Riel, P. L. (1995). Methotrexate in severe ankylosing spondylitis: an open study. *Journal of Rheumatology*, **22**, 1104–7.

Cronbach, L. J. (1951). Coefficient alpha and the internal structure of tests. *Psychometrika* **16**, 297–334.

Csonka, G. W. (1958). The course of Reiter's syndrome. *British Medical Journal*, **1**, 1088–90.

Csonka, G. W. (1960). Recurrent attacks in Reiter's disease. *Arthritis and Rheumatism*, **3**, 164–9.

Cuéllar, M. L. and Espinoza, L. R. (1995). Psoriatic arthritis: Current developments. *Journal of the Florida Medical Association*, **82**, 338–42.

Cuéllar, M. L. and Espinoza, L. R. (1996). Management of spondyloarthropathies. *Current Opinion in Rheumatology*, **8** 288–95.

Cuéllar, M. L., Citera, G., and Espinoza, L. R. (1994*a*). Treatment of psoriatic arthritis. *Baillière's Clinical Rheumatology*, **8**, 483–98.

Cuéllar, M. L., Silveira, L. H., and Espinoza, L. R. (1994*b*). Psoriatic arthritis. *Current Opinion in Rheumatology*, **6**, 378–84.

Cunnane, G., Brophy, D. P., Gibney, R. G., and FitzGerald, O. (1996). Diagnosis and treatment of heel pain in chronic inflammatory arthritis using ultrasound. *Seminars in Arthritis and Rheumatism*, **25**, 383–9.

Cutolo, M. (1997). Do sex hormones modulate the synovial macrophages in rheumatoid artheritis? *Annals of Rheumatic Diseases*, **56**, 281–6.

Cuvelier, C., Barbatis, C., Mielants, H., De Vos, M., Roels, H., and Veys, E. M. (1987). The histopathology of intestinal inflammation related to reactive arthritis. *Gut*, **2**, 394–401.

Czeizel, A. E. (1992). Familial aggregation of Crohn's disease and ankylosing spondylitis in a mother and her son. *Journal of Clinical Gastroentroenterology*, **14**, 349–57.

Daar, A. S., Fuggle, S. V., Fabre, J. W., Ting, A., and Morris, P. J. (1984). The detailed distribution of HLA-A, B, C antigens in normal human organs. *Transplantation*, **38**, 287–92.

D'Alessandro, L. P., Forster, D. J., and Rao, N. A. (1991). Anterior uveitis and hypopyon. *American Journal of Ophthalmology*, **112**, 317–21.

Daltroy, L. H., Larson, M. G., Roberts, W. N., and Liang, M. H. (1990). A modification of the health assessment questionnaire for the spondyloarthropathies. *Journal of Rheumatology*, **17**, 946–50.

D'amato, M., Fiorillo, M., *et al.* (1995). Relevance of residue 116 of HLA-B27 in determining susceptibility to ankylosing spondylitis. *European Journal of Immunology*, **25**, 3199–201.

Darville, T. and Laffoon, K. K. (1996). Examination of immune responses in chlamydia-resistant and susceptible mouse strains reveals a differential production of tumor necrosis factor (Abst). *Journal of Investigative Medicine*, **44**, 72A.

Davenport, M. P. (1995). The promiscuous B27 hypothesis (letter). *Lancet*, **346**, 500–1.

Davenport, M. P., Godkin, A., Friede, T., Stevanovic, S., Willis, A. C., Hill, A. V. S., Rammensee, H. G. (1997). A distinctive peptide binding motif for HLA-DRB1*0407, an HLA-DR4 subtype not associated with rheumatoid arthritis. *Immunogenetics* **45**, 229–32.

Davies, J. L., Kawaguchi, Y., *et al.* (1994). A genome-wide search for human type I diabetes susceptibility genes. *Nature*, **371**, 130–7.

Davis, P. Thomson, A. B., and Lentle, B. C. (1978). Quantitative sacroiliac scintigraphy in patients with Crohn's disease. *Arthritis and Rheumatism*, **21**, 234–7.

Davis, P., and Stein, M. (1991). Human immunodeficiency virus-related connective tissue diseases: a Zimbabwean perspective. *Rheumatic Disease Clinics of North America*, **17**, 89–97.

De Ancos, E., Pittet, N., and Herbort, C. P. (1994). Quantitative measurement of inflammation in HLA-B27 acute anterior uveitis using the Kowa FC-100 laser flare-cell meter. *Klinische* Monatsblatter fur Augenheilkinde, **204**, 330–3.

Deane, K., Jeacock, R., Hassell, A., Pearce, J., and Gaston, J. S. H. (1994). Identification of two target antigens recognized by synovial fluid T cells in Chlamydia-induced reactive arthritis. *Arthritis and Rheumatism*, **37**, S367.

Dekker-Saeys, A. J. and Keat, A. C. S., (1990). Follow-up study of ankylosing spondylitis over a period of 12 years. *Scandinavian Journal of Rheumatology*, **19** (Suppl. 57), 120–1.

DeKoning, J., Heesemann, J., Hoogkamp-Korstanje, J. A. A., Festen, J. M., Houtman, P. M., and Oijen, P. L. M. (1989). Yersinia in intestinal biopsy specimens from patients with seronegative spondylarthropathy: correlation with specific serum IgA antibodies. *Journal of Infectious Diseases*, **159**, 109–112.

DeLa Cadena, R. A., Stadnicki, A., Sartor, R. B., Kettner, C. A., Adam, A., and Colman, R. C. (1995). Inhibition of plasma kallikrein blocks the development of acute peptidoglycan-induced arthritis and anemia in the Lewis rat. *FASEB Journal*, **9**, 446–52.

DeLa Salle, H., Hanau, D., *et al.* (1994). Homozygous human TAP peptide transporter mutation in HLA class I deficiency [published erratum appears in *Science* (Dec 2, 1994); **266**, 1464]. *Science*, **265**, 237–41.

Della Santa, L., Grimaldi, G., Pellegrini, V., Migliaccio, P., and Pampana, A. (1994). Lung infections in children. IV. Pneumonia due to *Chlamydia pneumoniae*. *Minerva Pediatrica*, **46**, 269–73.

del Porto, P., D'Amato, M., Fiorillo, M. T., *et al.* (1994). Identification of a novel HLA-B27 subtype by restriction analysis of a cytotoxic gamma delta T cell clone. *Journal of Immunology*, **153**, 3093–100.

Dequeker, J., Jamar, R., and Walravens, M. (1980). HLA-B27, arthritis and *Yersinia enterocolitica* infection. *Journal of Rheumatology*, **7**, 706–10.

Derhaag, P. J. F. M., de Waal, L. P., Linssen, A., and Feltkamp, E. W. (1988*a*). Acute anterior uveitis and HLA-B27 subtypes. *Investigative Ophthalmology and Visual Science*, **29**, 1137–40.

Derhaag, P. J. F. M., Linssen, A., Broekema, N., de Waal, L. P., and Feltkamp, T. E. W. (1988*b*). A familial study of the inheritance of HLA-B27-positive acute anterior uveitis. *American Journal of Ophthalmology*, **105**, 603–6.

De Vos, M., Mielants, H., Cuvelier, C., Elewaut, A., and Veys, E. M. (1996). Long-term evolution of gut inflammation in patients with spondylarthropathy. *Journal of Gastroenterology*, (in press).

Dick, A. P., Grayson, M. J., Carpenter, R. C., and Petrie, A. (1964). Controlled trial of Sulphasalazine in the treatment of ulcerative colitis. *Gut*, **5**, 437–42.

Disla, E., Rhim, H. R., Reddy, A., and Taranta, A. (1994). Improvement in CD4 lymphocyte count in HIV-Reiter's syndrome after treatment with sulfasalazine. *Journal of Rheumatolology*, **21**, 662–4.

Dissanayake, A. S. and Truelove, S. C. (1973). A controlled trial of long-term maintenance treatment of ulcerative colitis with Sulphasalazine. *Gut*, **14**, 923–6.

Dobbins, W. D. (1987). HLA-antigens in Whipple's disease. *Arthritis and Rheumatism*, **30**, 102–5.

Dobbins, W. O. and Kawanishi, H. (1981). Bacillary characteristics in Whipple's disease. An electronmicroscopy study. *Gastroenterology*, **80**, 1465–75.

Doherty, P., Mitchell, M. J., MacMillan, L., Mosher, D., Barnes, D. C., and Hanly, J. G. (1992). Magnetic resonance imaging in the detection of sacroiliitis. *Journal of Rheumatology*, **19**, 393–401.

Dorwat, B., Gall, E. P., Schumacher, H. R., and Krauser, R. E. (1978). Chrysotherapy in psoriatic arthropathy. *Arthritis and Rheumatism*, **21**, 513–5.

Dougados, M., Boumier, P., and Amor, B. (1986). Sulphasalazine in ankylosing spondylitis: a double blind controlled study in 60 patients. *British Medical Journal*, **293**, 911–14.

Dougados, M., Gueguen, A., Nakache, J-P., Nguyen, M., Mery, C., and Amor B. (1988). Evaluation of a functional index and an articular index in ankylosing spondylitis. *Journal of Rheumatology*, **15**, 302–7.

Dougados, M., Gueguen, A., Nakache, J-P., Nguyen, M., and Amor B. (1990). Evaluation of a functional index for patients with ankylosing spondylitis. *Journal of Rheumatology*, **17**, 1254–5.

Dougados, M., van der Linden, S., Juhlin, R., *et al.* (1991*a*). The European Spondylarthropathy Study Group preliminary criteria for the classification of spondylarthropathy. *Arthritis and Rheumatism*, **34**, 1218–27.

Dougados, M., Berenbaum, F., Maetzel, A., and Amor, B. (1991*b*). Use of Sulfasalazine for the prevention of attacks of acute anterior uveitis associated with spondylarthropathy. *Arthritis and Rheumatism*, **34** (Suppl), abstr. D190, S195.

Dougados, M., van der Linden, S., Leirisalo-Repo, M., *et al.* (1995a) Sulfasalazine in the treatment of spondylarthropathy. A randomized, multicenter, double-blind, placebo-controlled study. *Arthritis and Rheumatism*, **38**, 618–27.

Doury, P., Eulry, F., and Pattin, S. (1983). Aspets cliniques des arthrites rèactionnelles á chlamydia. *Revue de Rhumatologie*, **50**, 753–7.

Duchmann, R., Kaiser, I., Hermann, E., Mayet, W., Ewe, K., and Meyer zum Büschenfelde, K.-H. (1995). Tolerance exists towards resident intestinal flora but is broken in active inflammatory bowel disease (IBD). *Clinical and Experimental Immunology* **102**, 448–55.

Duchmann, R., Schmitt, E., Knolle, P., Meyer zum Büschenfelde, K.-H., and Neurath, M. (1996). Tolerance towards resident intestinal flora in mice is abrogated in experimental colitis and restored by treatment with interleukin-10 or antibodies to interleukin-12. *European Journal of Immunology* **26**, 934–8.

Duchmann, R., May, E., Ackermann, B., Goergen, B., Meyer zum Büschenfelde, K.-H., and Märker-Hermann, E. (1996). HLA-B27 restricted cytotoxic T lymphocyte responses to arthritogenic enterobacteria or self antigens are dominated by closely related TCRBV gene segments. *Scandinavian Journal of Immunology*, **43**, 101–8.

Duffy, C. M., Duffy, K. N. W, Gladman, D. D., *et al.* (1992). The utility of the arthritis impact measurement scales for patients with psoriatic arthritis. *Journal of Rheumatology*, **19**, 1727–32.

Dunlop, E. M. C., Harper, I. A., and Jones, B. R. (1968). Seronegative polyarthritis: the Bedonia (Chlamydia) group of agents and Reiter's disease. *Annals of the Rheumatic Diseases*, **27**, 234–40.

Eastmond, C. J., Willshaw, H. E., Burgess, S. E., Shinebaum, R., Cooke, E. M., and Wright, V. (1980). Frequency of faecal *Klebsiella aerogenes* in patients with ankylosing spondylitis and controls with respect to individual features of the disease. *Annals of the Rheumatic Diseases*, **39**, 118–23.

Eastmond, C. J., Rennie, J. A. N., and Reid, T. M. S. (1983). An outbreak of campylobacter enteritis—a rheumatological followup survey. *Journal of Rheumatology*, **10**, 107–8.

Ebringer, A. (1992). Ankylosing spondylitis is caused by Klebsiella: Evidence from immunogenetic, microbiologic, and serologic studies. *Rheumatic Disease Clinics of North America*, **18**, 105–21.

Ebringer, A. (1995). HLA-B27: twenty years on. *Rheumatology in Europe*, **24**, 83–4.

Ebringer, R. W., Cooke, D., Cawdell, D. R., Cowling, P., and Ebringer, A. (1977). Ankylosing spondylitis: Klebsiella and HLA B27. *Rheumatology and Rehabilitation*, **16**, 190–6.

Ebringer, R. W., Cawdell, D. R., Cowling, P., and Ebringer, A. (1978). Sequential studies in ankylosing spondylitis. Association of *Klebsiella pneumoniae* with active disease. *Annals of the Rheumatic Diseases*, **37**, 146–51.

Ebringer, R. W., Cawdell, D., and Ebringer, A. (1979). *Klebsiella pneumoniae* and acute anterior uveitis in ankylosing spondylitis. *British Medical Journal*, **i** 383.

Ebringer, A., and Wilson, C. (1996). The use of a low starch diet in the treatment of patients suffering from ankylosing spondylitis. *Clinical Rheumatology* **15**, 62–6.

Eden, K., Rosenberg, M., Stoopler, M., *et al.* (1977). Waterborne gastrointestinal illness at a ski resort. Isolation of *Yersinia enterocolitica* from drinking water. *Public Health Reports*, **92**, 245–50.

Edmunds, L., Elswood, J., Kennedy, L. G. and Calin, A. (1991*a*). Primary ankylosing spondylitis, psoriatic and enteropathic spondylarthropathy: a controlled analysis. *Journal of Rheumatology*, **18**, 696–8.

Edmunds, L., Elswood, J., and Calin, A. (1991*b*). New light on uveitis in ankylosing spondylitis. *Journal of Rheumatology*, **18**, 50–2.

Edwards, L. and Hansen, R.C. (1992). Reiter's syndrome of the vulva. The psoriasis spectrum. *Archives of Dermatology*, **128**, 811–14.

Ehlers, N., Kissmeyer-Nielsen, F., Kjerbye, K. E., and Lamm, L. U. (1974). HLA-B27 in acute and chronic uveitis (letter). *Lancet*, **1**, 99.

Eibschutz, B., Baird, S. M., Weisman, M. H., *et al.* (1995). Oral 2-chlorodeoxyadenosine in psoriatic arthritis. A preliminary report. *Arthritis and Rheumatism*, **38**, 1604–9.

Elliott, T., Smith, M., *et al.* (1993). Peptide selection by class I molecules of the major histocompatibility complex. *Current Biology*, **3**, 854–66.

Elst, P., Sybesma, T., van der Stadt, R. J., *et al.* (1984). Sexual problems in rheumatoid arthritis and anlylosing spodylitis *Arthritis and Rheumatism*, **27**

Ely, P. H. (1980). The bowel bypass syndrome: A response to bacterial peptidoglycans. *Journal of American Academic Dermatology* **2** 473–87.

Emery, A. E. H. and Lawrence, J. S. (1967). Genetics of ankylosing spondylitis. *Journal of Medical Genetics*, **4** 239–45.

Engleman, E. P., Schachter, J., Gilbert, R. J., Smith, D. E., and Meyer, K. F. (1969). Bedsonia and Reiter's syndrome: a progress report (abstract). *Arthritis and Rheumatism*, **12**, 292.

Enlow, R. W., Bias, W. B., and Arnett, F. C. (1980). The spondylitis of inflammatory bowel disease. Evidence for a non-HLA linked axial arthropathy. *Arthritis and Rheumatism*, **23**, 1359–65.

Erard, F. and LeGros, G. (1994). Th2-like CD8 T cells: Their role in protection against infectious diseases. *Parasitology Today*, **10**, 313–15.

Erdesz, S., Shubin, S. V., Shoch, B. P., *et al.* (1994). Spondylarthropathies in circumpolar populations of Chukotka (Eskimos and Chukchi): Epidemiology and clinical characteristics. *Journal of Rheumatology*, **21**, 1101–4.

Erlacher, L., Wintersberger, W., Menschik, M., *et al.* (1995). Reactive arthritis: Urogenital swab culture is the only useful diagnostic method for the detection of the arthritogenic infection in extra-articularly asymptomatic patients with undifferentiated oligoarthritis. *British Journal of Rheumatology*, **34**, 838–42.

Escalante, A., Weaver, W. J., and Beardmore, T. D. (1995). An estimate of the prevalence of reactive systemic amyloidosis in ankylosing spondylitis (Letter). *Journal of Rheumatology*, **22**, 2192–3.

Espinoza, L. R. (1985). Psoriatic arthritis: Further epidemiological and genetic considerations. In *Psoriatic Arthritis* (ed. L. H. Gerber and L. R. Espinoza), pp. 9–32. Grune and Stratton, Orlando, Florida.

Espinoza, L. R., Vasey, F. B., Oh, J. H., Dove, F., and (Osterland, C. K. (1978). Association between HLA-Bw38 and peripheral psoriatic arthritis. *Arthritis and Rheumatism*, **21**, 72–5.

Espinoza, L. R., Berman, A., Vasey, F. B., Cahalin, K., Nelson, R., and Germain, B. F. (1988). Psoriatic arthritis and acquired immunodeficiency syndrome. *Arthritis and Rheumatism*, **31**, 1034–40.

Espinoza, L. R., Cuéllar, M. L., and Silveira, L. H. (1992*a*). Psoriatic arthritis. *Current Opinion in Rheumatology*, **4**, 470–8.

Espinoza, L. R., Zakranoui, L., Espinoza, C. G., *et al* (1992*b*). Psoriatic arthritis: Clinical response and side effects to methotrexate therapy. *Journal of Rheumatology*, **19**, 872–7.

Espinoza, L. R., Aguilar, J. L., Espinoza, C. G., Cuéllar, M. L., Scopelitis, E., and Silveira, L. H. (1994*a*). Fibroblast function in psoriatic arthritis I. Alteration of cell kinetics and growth factor responses. *Journal of Rheumatology*, **21**, 1502–6.

Espinoza, L. R., Espinoza, C. G., Cuéllar, M. L., Scopelitis, E., Silveira, L. H., and Grotendorst, G. R. (1994*b*). Fibroblast function in psoriatic arthritis. II. Increased expression of B platelet derived growth factor (PDGF) receptor and increased production of growth factor and cytokines. *Journal of Rheumatology*, **21**, 1507–11.

EULAR (European League Against Rheumatism) (1977). Nomenclature and classification of arthritis in children. *Bulletin No. 4* Basel, National Zeitung AG.

Falgarone, G., Blanchard, H., Riot, B., *et al.* (1996). Yersinia infection of HLA-B27 transgenic rats induces a specific cytotoxic CD8+ T cell mediated response restricted by rat class I MHC but not by B27. *Arthritis and Rheumatism*, in press (abstract).

Falk, K., Rotzchke, O., *et al.* (1991). Allele-specific motifs revealed by sequencing of self-peptides eluted from MHC molecules. *Nature*, **351**, 290–6.

Farmer, R. C., Hawk, W., and Turnbull, R. B. (1975). Clinical patterns in Crohn's disease. A statistical study of 615 cases. *Gastroenterology*, **68**, 627–35.

Farr, M., Kitas, G. D., and Waterhouse, L. (1990). Sulphasalazine in psoriatic arthritis. A double-blind placebo-controlled study. *British Journal of Rheumatology*, **29**, 46–9.

Fausa, O., Schrumpf E., and Elgjo, K. (1991). Relationship of inflammatory bowel disease and primary sclerosing cholangitis. *Seminars in Liver Diseases*, **11**, 31–9.

Faustman, D., Li, X., Lin, H. Y., *et al.* (1991). Linkage of faulty major histocompatibility complex class I to autoimmune diabetes. *Science*, **254**, 1756–61.

Feige, U., Schulmeister, A., Mollenhauer, J., Brune, K., and Bang, H. (1994). A constitute 65 kDa chondrocyte protein as a target antigen in adjutant arthritis in Lewis rats. *Autoimmunity*, **17**, 233–9.

Feldtkeller, E. (1997). *Morbus Bechterew—Leitfaden für Patienten*. 3rd edition, pp. 107. Novartis Pharma Verlag, Wehr.

Feldtkeller, E. (1997). Zur Situation der Morbus-Bechterew-Patienten. Teil I: Diagnose und Symptome. *Bechterew-Brief*, **69** (June), 3–18.

Feldtkeller, E. (1997). Zur Situation der Morbus-Bechterew-Patienten. Teil II: Schwere der Erkrankung und private Situation. *Bechterew-Brief*, **70** (September), 3–17.

Feltelius, N. and Hällgren, R. (1986). Sulphasalazine in ankylosing spondylitis. *Annals of the Rheumatic Diseases*, **45**, 396–9.

Feltelius, N., Hvatum, M., Brandtzaeg, P., Knutson, L., and Hällgren, R. (1994). Increased jejunal secretory IgA and IgM in ankylosing spondylitis: normalization after treatment with sulfasalazine. *Journal of Rheumatology*, **21**, 2076–81.

Feltkamp, T. E. W. (1985). HLA-B27, acute anterior uveitis, and ankylosing spondylitis. *Advances in Inflammation Research*, **9**, 211–16.

Feltkamp, T. E. W., Khan, M. A., and Lopez de Castro, J. A. (1996). The pathogenetic role of HLA-B27. *Immunology Today*, **17**, 5–7.

Ferraz, M. G., Tugwell, P., Goldsmith, C. H., and Atra, E. (1990). Meta-analysis of Sulphasalazine in ankylosing spondylitis. *Journal of Rheumatology*, **17**, 1482–6.

Feurle, G. E. (1985). Association of Whipple's disease with HLA-B27. *Lancet*, **1**, 1336.

Fielder, M., Pirt, S. J., Tarpey, I., *et al.* (1995). Molecular mimicry and ankylosing spondylitis: possible role of novel sequence in pullulanase of *Klebsiella pneumoniae*. *FEBS Letters*, **369**, 243–8.

Finch, M., Rodey, G., Lawrence, D., and Blake, P. (1986). Epidemic Reiter's syndrome following an outbreak of Shigellosis. *European Journal of Epidemiology*, **2**, 26–9.

Finch, W. (1989). Arthritis and the gut. *Postgraduate Medicine*, **86**, 229–30.

Fink, C. W. (1995). Proposal for the development of classification criteria for idiopathic arthritides of childhood. *Journal of Rheumatology*, **22**, 1566–9.

Fiorillo, M. T., Greco, G., and Sorrentino, R. (1995). The Asp116-His116 substitution in a novel HLA-B27 subtype influences the acceptance of the peptide C-terminal anchor. *Immunogenetics* **41**, 38–9.

Fiorillo, M. T., Meadows, L., D'Amato, M., Shabanowitz, J., Hunt, D. F., Appella, E., and Sorrentino, R. (1997). Susceptibility to ankylosing spondylitis correlates with the C-terminal residue of peptides presented by various HLA-B27 subtypes. *European Journal of Immunology* **27**, 368–73.

Fleming, J., Russel, H., Wiesnek, D., and Shorter, R. G. (1988). Whipple's disease: clinical, biological and histopathologic features and assessment of treatment in 29 patients. *Mayo Clinic Proceedings*, **63**, 539–51.

Ford, D. K., and Schulzer, M. (1994). Synovial lymphocytes indicate 'bacterial' agents may cause some cases of rheumatoid arthritis. *Journal of Rheumatology*, **21**, 1447–9.

Ford, D. K., daRoza, D. M., and Shah, P. (1981*a*). Cell-mediated immune responses to synovial mononuclear cells to sexually transmitted, enteric and mumps antigens in patients with Reiter's syndrome, rheumatoid arthritis and ankylosing spondylitis. *Journal of Rheumatology*, **8**, 220–32.

Ford, D. K., DaRoza, D., and Schulzer, M. (1981*b*). Lymphocytes from the site of disease but not the blood lymphocytes indicate the cause of arthritis. *Annals of the Rheumatic Diseases*, **44**, 701–10.

Forster, S. M., Seifert, M. H., Keat, A. C., *et al.* (1988). Inflammatory joint disease and human immunodeficiency virus infection. *British Medical Journal*, **296**, 1625–7.

Foster, C. S. and Sainz de la Maza, M. (1994). *The Sclera*. Springer Verlag, New York.

Fox, R., Calin, A., Gerber, R. C., and Gibson, D. (1979). The chronicity of symptoms and disability in Reiter's syndrome: an analysis of 131 consecutive patients. *Annals of Internal Medicine*, **91**, 190–3.

Francois, R. J., Eulderink, F., and By water, E. G. L. (1995). Commented glossary for rheumatic spinal diseases, based on pathology. *Annals of Rheumatic Diseases*, **54**, 615–25.

Frangoulis, B., Reboul, M., Rocca, A., and Pla, M. (1993). Cross-reactivity among evolutionarily distant major histocompatibility complex class I molecules (HLA-B27 and H-$2K^k$) revealed by xenoreactive T lymphocytes. *European Journal of Immunology*, **23**, 338–42.

Fraser, S. M., Hopkins, R., Hunter, J. A., Neumann, V., Capell, H. A., and Bird, H. A. (1993). Sulphasalazine in the management of psoriatic arthritis. *British Journal of Rheumatology*, **32**, 923–5.

Fremont, D. H., Matsumura, M., Stura, E. A., Peterson, P. A., Wilson, I. A. (1992). Crystal structure of two viral peptides in complex with murine MHC class I H-$2K^b$. *Science* **257**, 919–27.

Friede, T., Gnau, V., Jung, G., Keilholz, W., Stevanovic, S., Rammensee, H. G. (1996). Natural ligand motifs of closely related HLA-DR4 molecules predict features of rheumatoid arthritis associated peptides. *Biochimica et Biophysica Acta* **1316**, 85–101.

Fries, J. F., Spitz, P., Kraines, R. G., and Holman, H. R. (1980). Measurement of patient outcome in arthritis. *Arthritis and Rheumatism*, **23**, 137–45.

Fries, J. F., Singh, G., Bloch, D. A., *et al.* (1989). The natural history of ankylosing spondylitis: is the disease really changing? *Journal of Rheumatology*, **16**, 860–3.

Fruci, D., Butler, R. H., Greco, G., Rovero, P., Pazmany, L., Vigneti, E., Tosi, R., Tanigaki, N. (1995). Differences in peptide-binding specificity of two ankylosing spondylitis-associated HLA-B27 subtypes. *Immunogenetics* **42**, 123–8.

Fuzakawa, T., Wang, J., Huang, F., *et al.* (1994). Testing the importance of each residue in an HLA-B27-binding peptide using monoclonal antibodies. *Journal of Immunology* **152**, 1190–6.

Gaede, K. I. and Heesemann, J. (1995). Arthritogenicity of genetically manipulated *Yersinia enterocolitica* serotype O8 for Lewis rats. *Infection and Immunity*, **63**, 714–19.

Gall, V. (1994). Exercise in the spondyloarthropathies. *Arthritis Care and Research* **7**, 215–20.

Galocha, B., Lamas, J. R., Villadangos, J. A., Albar, J. P., López de Castro, J. A. (1996). Binding of peptides naturally presented by HLA-B27 to the differentially disease-associated B*2704 and B*2706 subtypes, and to mutants mimicking their polymorphism. *Tissue Antigens* **48**, 509–18.

Gao, X. M., Wordsworth, P., and McMichael, A. (1994). Collagen-specific cytotoxic T lymphocyte responses in patients with ankylosing spondylitis and reactive arthritis. *European Journal of Immunology*, **24**, 1665–70.

Gao, X.-M., Wordsworth, P., McMichael, A. J., Kyaw, M. M., Seifert, M., Rees, D., and Dougan. G. (1996). Homocysteine modification of HLA antigens and its immunological consequences *European Journal of Immunology* **26**, 1443–50.

García, F., Galocha, B., Villadangos, J. A., Lamas, J. R., Albar, J. P., Marina, A., López de Castro, J. A. (1997). HLA-B27 (B*2701) specificity for peptides lacking Arg2 is determined by polymorphism outside the B pocket. *Tissue Antigens*, **49**, 580–7.

García, F., Marina, A., Albar, J. P., López de Castro, J. A. (1997a). HLA-B27 presents a peptide from a polymorphic region of its own molecule with homology to proteins from arthritogenic bacteria. *Tissue Antigens* **49**, 23–8.

García, F., Marina, A., López de Castro, J. A. (1997b). Lack of carboxyl-terminal tyrosine distinguishes the B*2706-bound peptide repertoire from those of B*2704 and other HLA-B27 subtypes associated with ankylosing spondylitis. *Tissue Antigens* **49**, 215–21.

García, F., Rognan, D., Lamas, J. R., Marina. A., López de Castro, J. A. An HLA-B27 polymorphism (B*2710) that is critical for T-cell recognition has limited effects on peptide specificity. *Tissue Antigens*, in press.

Garcia-Morteo, O., Maldonado-Cocco, J. A., Suarez-Almazor, M. E., and Garay, E. (1983). Ankylosing spondylitis of juvenile onset: comparison with adult onset disease. *Scandinavian Journal of Rheumatology*, **12**, 246–8.

Gardiner, K. R., Halliday, M. I., Barclay, G. R., *et al.* R. J., *et al.* (1995*a*). Significnce of systemic endotoxaemia in inflammatory bowel disease. *Gut*, **36**, 897–901.

Gardiner, K. R., Anderson, N. H., Rowlands, B. J., and Barbul, A. (1995*b*). Colitis and colonic mucosal barrier dysfunction. *Gut*, **37**, 530–5.

Gäre, A., Fasth, A., Anderson, J., *et al.* (1987). Incidence and prevalence of juvenile chronic arthritis: a population survey. *Annals of Rheumatic Diseases*, **46**, 277–81.

Garrett, S. (Spring/Summer 1994). *NASS Newsletter*, 3–5.

Garrett, S. L., Jenkinson, T. R., Kennedy, L. G., Whitelock, H. C., Gaisford, P., and Calin, A. (1994). A new approach to defining disease status in ankylosing spondylitis: the Bath Ankylosing Spondylitis Disease Activity Index. *Journal of Rheumatology*, **21**, 2286–91.

Garrett, T. P. J., Saper, J. A., *et al.* (1989). Specificity pockets for the side chains of peptide antigens in HLA-Aw68. *Nature*, **342**, 692–6

Garrido, F., Cabrera, T., Concha, A., Glew, S., Ruiz-Cabello, F., and Stern, P. L. (1993). Natural history of HLA expression during tumour development. *Immunology Today*, **14**, 491–9.

Gaston, J. S. H., Life, P. F., Granfors, K., *et al.* (1989). Synovial T lymphocyte recognition of organisms that trigger reactive arthritis. *Clinical and Experimental Immunology*, **76**, 348–53.

Gaston, J. S. H., Deane, K. H., Jecock, R. M., and Pearce, J. H. (1996). Identification of 2 *Chlamydia trachomatis* antigens recognized by synovial fluid T cells from patients with Chlamydia induced reactive arthritis. *Journal of Rheumatology*, **23**, 130–6.

Geczy, A. F., McGuigan, L. E., Sullivan, J. S., and Edmonds, J. (1986). Cytotoxic T lymphocytes against associated determinants in ankylosing spondylitis. *Journal of Experimental Medicine*, **164**, 932–7.

Gedalia, A., Barash, J., Press, J., and Buskila, D. (1993). Sulphasalazine in the treatment of pauciarticular onset juvenile chronic arthritis. *Clinical Rheumatology*, **12**, 511–14.

Genc, M. and Mardh, P. A. (1991). Direct antigen detection tests in the diagnosis of chlamydial infections. In *Chlamydial infections of the genital respiratory tracts and allied conditions* (ed. P. A. Mardh, P. Saikku), pp. 112–21. Gummerus Kirjapaino Oy, Jyvaskyla, Finland.

Genc, M. and Mardh, P. A. (1996). A cost-effectiveness analysis of screening and treatment for *Chlamydia trachomatis* infection in asymptomatic women. *Annals of Internal Medicine*, **124**, 1–7.

Genth, E., Peuckert, H., Brude, E., *et al.* (1978). HLA-B27 positive oligoarthritis. *Zeitschrift für Rheumatologie*, **37**, 313–15.

Gérard, H. C., Branigan, P. J., Schumacher, H. R., and Hudson, A. P. (1995*a*). Inapparently infecting *Chlamydia trachomatis* in the synovia of Reiter's syndrome/reactive arthritis patients are viable. *Arthritis and Rheumatism* **38** (Suppl. 9), R24.

Gérard, H. C., Branigan, P. J., Schumacher, H. J., and Hudson, A. P. (1995*b*). Screening of synovial tissue from reactive arthritis (ReA) patients for the presence of *Chlamydia pneumoniae*. *Arthritis and Rheumatism*, **38** (Suppl.), S394.

Gerber, L. H., Murray, C. L., Perlman, S. G., and Mann, D. (1982). Human lymphocyte antigens characterizing psoriatic arthritis and its subtypes. *Journal of Rheumatology*, **9**, 703–7.

Germain, R. N. (1994). MHC-dependent antigen processing and peptide presentation: providing ligands for T lymphocyte activation. *Cell*, **76**, 287–99.

Gewanter, H. L., Roghmann, K. J., and Baum, J. (1983). The prevalence of juvenile arthritis. *Arthritis and Rheumatism*, **26**, 599–603.

Ginsburg, W. W., Cohen, M. D., Miller, G. M., and Bartleson, J. D. (1997). Posterior vertebral body erosion by arachnoid diverticula in canda equina syndrome: An unusual manifestation of ankylosing spondylitis. *Journal of Rheumatology*, **24**, 1417–20.

Giordano, N., Battisti, E., Senasi, M., and Gennari, C. (1996). A problematic case of chlamdia pericarditis and sicca syndrome. *Clinical Rheumatology*, **15**, 99.

Gladman, D. D. (1992). Psoriatic arthritis: Recent advances in pathogenesis and treatment. *Rheumatic Diseases Clinics of North America*, **18**, 247–56.

Gladman, D. D. (1994). Natural history of psoriatic arthritis. *Baillière's Clinical Rheumatology*, **8**, 379–94.

Gladman, D. D. (1995). Psoriatic arthritis. In *Classification and assessment of rheumatic disease: Part 1 Baillière's clinical rheumatology. International practice and research.* vol. 9 (ed. A. J. Silman and D. P. N. symmons), pp. 319–29. Baillière Tindall, London.

Gladman, D. D. and Espinoza, L. R. (1992). International symposium on psoriatic arthritis. *Journal of Rheumatology*, **19**, 290–1.

Gladman, D. D. and Farewell, V. T. (1995). The role of HLA antigens as indicators of disease progression in psoriatic arthritis. Multivariate relative risk model. *Arthritis and Rheumatism*, **38**, 845–50.

Gladman, D. D., Anhorn, K. A. B., Schachter, R. K., and Mervat, H. (1986). HLA antigens in psoriatic arthritis. *Journal of Rheumatology*, **13**, 586–92.

Gladman, D. D., Schuckett, R., Russell, M. L., Thorne, J. C., and Schachter, R. K. (1987). Psoriatic arthritis (PsA)—an analysis of 220 patients. *Quarterly Journal of Medicine*, **62**, 127–41.

Gladman, D. D., Farewell, V. T., Buskila, D., *et al.* (1990*a*). Reliability of measurement of active and damaged joints in psoriatic arthritis. *Journal of Rheumatology*, **17**, 62–4.

Gladman, D. D., Stafford-Brady, F., Chang, C. H., Lewandowski, K., and Russell, M. L. (1990*b*). Longitudinal study of clinical and radiological progression of psoriatic arthritis. *Journal of Rheumatology*, **17**, 809–12.

Gladman, D. D., Blake, R., Brubacher, B., and Farewell, V. T. (1992). Chloroquine therapy in psoriatic arthritis. *Journal of Rheumatology*, **19**, 1724–6.

Gladman, D. D., Brubacher, B., Buskila, D., Langevitz, P., and Farewell, V. T. (1993). Differences in the expression of spondyloarthropathy; A comparison between ankylosing spondylitis and psoriatic arthritis. *Clinical and Investigative Medicine*, **16** 1–7.

Gladman, D. D., Farewell, V. T., and Nadeau, C. (1995). Clinical indicators of progression in psoriatic arthritis: multivariate relative risk model. *Journal of Rheumatology*, **22**, 675–9.

Glant, T. T. and Mikecz, K. (1991). Antiproteoglycan antibodies in experimental spondylarthritis. In *Monoclonal antibodies, cytokines, and arthritis* (ed. T. F. Kresina), Marcel Dekker, New York.

Glant, T. T., Mikecz, K., Arzoumanian, A., and Poole, A. R., (1987). Proteoglycan-induced arthritis in BALB/c mice. Clinical features and histopathology. *Arthritis and Rheumatism*, **30**, 201–12.

Glant, T. T., Fulop, C., Cs-Szabo, G., Buzas, E., Ragasa, D., and Mikecz, K. (1995). Mapping of arthritogenic/autoimmune epitopes of cartilage aggrecans in proteoglycan-induced arthritis. *Scandinavian Journal of Rheumatology—Supplement*, **101**, 43–9.

Glennås, A., Kvien, T. K., Melby, K., *et al.* (1994). Reactive arthritis: a favourable 2 year course and outcome, independent of triggering agent and HLA-B27. *Journal of Rheumatology*, **21**, 2274–80.

Gofton, J. P. (1980). Epidemiology, tissue type antigen and Bechterew's syndrome (ankylosing spondylitis) in various ethnical populations. *Scandinavian Journal of Rheumatology*, **9** (Suppl. 32) 166–8.

Gofton, J. P., Chalmers, A., Price, G. E., and Reeve, C. E. (1975). HLA 27 and ankylosing spondylitis in B. C. Indians. *Journal of Rheumatology*, **2**, 314–18.

Goie The, H. S., Steven, M. M., van der Linden, S. M., and Cats, A. (1985). Evaluation of diagnostic criteria for ankylosing spondylitis: a comparison of the Rome, New York and modified New York criteria in patients with a positive clinical history screening test for ankylosing spondylitis. *British Journal of Rheumatology*, **24**, 242–9.

Goldsmith, C. H., Smythe, H. A., and Helewa, A. (1993). Interpretation and power of a pooled index. *Journal of Rheumatology*, **20**, 575–8.

Gonzalez-Roces, S., Alvarez, M. V., Gonzalez, S. *et al.* (1997). HLA-B27 polymorphism and worldwide susceptibility to ankylosing spondylitis. *Tissue Antigens*, **49**, 116–23.

Good, A. E. (1974). Reiter's disease: A review with special attention to cardiovascular and neurological sequelae. *Seminars in Arthritis and Rheumatism*, **3**, 253–86.

Gordon, F. B., Quan, A. L., Steinman, T. I., and Phillips, R. N. (1973). Chlamydial isolates from Reiter's syndrome. *British Journal of Venereal Disease*, **49**, 376–80.

Gran, J. T. and Husby, G. (1990). Ankylosing spondylitis in women. *Seminars in Arthritis and Rheumatism*, **19**, 303–12.

Gran, J. T. and Husby, G. (1993). The epidemiology of ankylosing spondylitis. *Seminars in Arthritis and Rheumatism*, **22**, 319–34.

Gran, J. T., Hjetland, R., and Andreassen, A. H. (1993). Pneumonia, myocarditis and reactive arthritis due to *Chlamydia pneumoniae*. *Scandinavian Journal of Rheumatology*, **22**, 43–4.

Granfors, K. (1992). Do bacterial antigens cause reactive arthritis? *Rheumatic Disease Clinics of North America*, **18**, 37–48.

Granfors, K. and Toivanen, A. (1986). IgA-anti-yersinia antibodies in yersinia triggered reactive arthritis. *Annals of the Rheumatic Diseases*, **45**, 561–5.

Granfors, K., Isomäki, H., von Essen, R., Maatela, J., Kalliomäki, L. J., and Toivanen, A. (1983). Yersinia antibodies in inflammatory joint diseases. *Clinical and Experimental Rheumatology*, **1**, 215–18.

Granfors, K., Jalkanen, S., von Essen, R., *et al.* (1989*a*). Yersinia antigens in synovial-fluid cells from patients with reactive arthritis. *New England Journal of Medicine*, **320**, 216–21.

Granfors, K., Ogasawara, M., Hill, J. L., Lahesmaa-Rantala, R., Toivanen, A., and Yu, D. T. Y. (1989*b*). Analysis of IgA antibodies to lipopolysaccharide in Yersinia-triggered reactive arthritis. *Journal of Infectious Diseases* **159**, 1142–7.

Granfors, K., Jalkanen, S., Lindberg, A. A., Maki-Ikola, O., Von Essen, R., Lahesmaa-Rantala, R. (1990). Salmonella lipopolysaccharides in synovial cells from patients with reactive arthritis. *Lancet*, **335**, 6985–8.

Granfors, K., Jalkanen, S., Toivanen, P., Koski, J., and Lindberg, A. A. (1992). Bacterial lipopolysaccharide in synovial fluid cells in Shigella triggered reactive arthritis. *Journal of Rheumatology*, **19**, 500.

Granfors, K., Laitio, P., Virtala, M., and Salmi, M. (1995*a*). HLA-B27 influences survival of salmonella in monocytic cell line U-937. *Arthritis and Rheumatism*, **38**, S394.

Granfors, K., Mäki-Ikola, O., and Leirisalo-Repo, M. (1995*b*). Association of gut inflammation with the increased serum *Klebsiella pneumoniae*-specific antibody levels in patients with axial type of ankylosing spondylitis. *Arthritis and Rheumatism*, **38**, S348.

Gratacos, J., Orellana, C., Sanmarti, R. *et al.* (1997). Secondary amyloidosis in ankylosing spondylitis: a systemic survey of 137 patients using abdominal fat aspiration. *Journal of Rheumatology*, **24**, 912–5.

Gravallese, E. M. and Kantrowitz, F. G. (1988). Arthritic manifestations of inflammatory bowel disease. *American Journal of Gastroenterology*, **83**, 703–9.

Grayston, J. Th. (1989). *Chlamydia pneumoniae*, Strain TWAR. *Chest*, **95**, 664–9.

Grayston, J. Th. (1992). *Chlamydia pneumoniae*, Strain TWAR pneumoniae. *Annual Review of Medicine*, **43**, 317–23.

Greenstein, A. J., Janowitz, H. D., and Sachar, D. B. (1976). The extra-intestinal complications of Crohn's disease and ulcerative colitis: a study of 700 patients. *Medicine*, **55**, 401–12.

Griffin, T. A., Yuan, J., Friede, T., Stevanovic, S., Ariyoshi, K., Rowland-Jones, S. L., Rammensee, H.-G., Colbert, R. A. (1997). Naturally occurring A pocket polymorphism in HLA-B*2703 increases the dependence on an accessory anchor residue at P1 for optimal binding of nonamer peptides. *Journal of Immunology*, in press.

Grillet, B., De Clerck, L., Dequeker, J., Rutgeerts, P., and Geboes, K. (1987). Systematic ileocolonoscopy and bowel biopsy in spondylarthropathy. *British Journal of Rheumatology*, **26**, 338–40.

Gripenberg-Lerche, C., Skurnik, M., Zhang, L., Söderström, K.-O., and Toivanen, P. (1994). Role of YadA in arthritogenicity of *Yersinia enterocolitica* serotype O:8: experimental studies with rats. *Infection and Immunity*, **62**, 5568–75.

Gripenberg-Lerche, C., Skurnik, M., and Toivanen, P. (1995). Role of YadA mediated collagen binding in arthritogenicity of *Yersinia enterocolitica* serotype O:8: experimental studies with rats. *Infection and Immunity*, **63**, 3222–6.

Groenhagen-Riska, C., Saikku, P., Riska, H., Froeseth, B., and Grayston, J. T. (1988). Antibodies to TWAR—a novel type of Chlamydia—in sarcoidosis. In *Sarcoidosis and other granulomatous disorders* (ed. C. Grassi, *et al.*), pp. 297–301. Elsevier Science Publishers, Amsterdam.

Grönberg, A., Fryden, A., and Kihlström, E. (1989). Humoral immune response to individual *Yersinia enterocolitica* antigens in patients with and without reactive arthritis. *Clinical and Experimental Immunology*, **76**, 361–5.

Grosskurth, H., Mosha, F., Todd, J., *et al.* (1995). Impact of improved treatment of sexually transmitted diseases on HIV infection in rural Tanzania: randomised controlled trial. *Lancet*, **346**, 530–6.

Gubner, R., August, S., and Ginberg, V. (1951). Therapeutic suppression of tissue reactivity. II. Effect of aminopterin in rheumatoid arthritis and psoriasis. *American Journal of Medical Sciences*, **221**, 176–82.

Guerra, J. and Resnick, D. (1984). Radiographic and scintigraphic abnormalities in seronegative spondylarthropathies and juvenile chronic arthritis. In *Spondylarthropathies* (ed. A. Calin), pp. 339–81. Grune and Stratton, Orlando, FL.

Guerrant, R. L., Hughes, J. M., Lima, N. L., and Crane, J. (1990). Diarrhea in developed and developing countries: magniture, special settings, and etiologies. *Reviews of Infectious Diseases*, **12**, (Suppl. 1), S41–50.

Guo, H.-C., Madden, D. R., Silver, M. L., Jardetzky, T. S., Gorga, J. C., Strominger, J. L., Wiley, D. C. (1993). Comparison of the P2 specificity pocket in three human histocompatibility antigens, HLA-A*6801, HLA-A*0201, and HLA-B*2705. *Proceedings of the National Academy of Science, USA* **90**, 8053–7.

Gupta, A. K., Grober, J. S., Hamilton, T. A., *et al.* (1995). Sulfasalazine therapy for psoriatic arthritis: a doubb-blind, placebo-controlled trial. *Journal of Rheumatology*, **22**, 894–8. (ch 14)

Gutierrez-Ureña, S. and Espinoza, L. R. (1995). Methotrexate: the agent of choice for chronic inflammatory disorders. A perspective ten years later. *Clinical and Experimental Rheumatology*, **13**, 281–4.

Gutierrez-Ureña, S., Molina, J. F., Garcia, C., Cuéllar, M. L., and Espinoza, L. R. (1996). Pancytopenia secondary to methotrexate therapy in rheumatoid arthritis. *Arthritis and Rheumatism*, **39**, 272–6.

Haarr, M. (1960). Rheumatic iridocyclitis. *Acta Ophthalmologica*, **38**, 37–45.

Häfner, R. (1987). Die juvenile spondyarthritis. Retrospektive untersuchung an 71 Patienten. *Monatsschrift Kinderheilkunde*, **135**, 41–6.

Hahn, D. L. (1995). Treatment of chlamydia penumoniae infection in adult asthma: a before–after trial. *Journal of Family Practice*, **41**, 345–51.

Hahn, D. L., Dodge, R. W., and Golubjatnikov, R. (1991). Association of *Chlamydia pneumoniae* (strain TWAR) infection with wheezing, asthmatic bronchitis, adult-onset asthma. *Journal of the American Medical Association*, **206**, 225–30.

Håkansson, U., Löw, B., Eitrem, R., and Winblad, S. (1975). HL-A27 and reactive arthritis in an outbreak of salmonellosis. *Tissue Antigens*, **6**, 366–7.

Hakim, F. T., Cranley, R., Brown, K. S., Eanes, E. D., Harne, L., and Oppenheim, J. J. (1984). Hereditary joint disorder in progressive ankylosis (*ank/ank*) mice. I. Association of calcium hydroxyapatite deposition with inflammatory arthropathy. *Arthritis and Rheumatism*, **27**, 1411–20.

Hakim, F. T., Brown, K. S., and Oppenheim, J. J. (1986). Hereditary joint disorder in progressive ankylosis (*ank/ank*) mice. II. Effect of high-dose hydrocortisone treatment on inflammation and intraarticular calcium hydroxyapatite deposits. *Arthritis and Rheumatism*, **29**, 114–23.

Hakkinen, A., Hakkinen, K., and Hannonen, P. (1994). Effects of strength training in neuromuscular function and disease activity in patients with recent-onset-inflammatory arthritis. *Scandinavian Journal of Rheumatology*, **23**, 237–42.

Halla, J. T., Bliznal, J., and Hardin, J. G. (1988). Involvement of the cranio-cervical junction in Reiter's snydrome. *Journal of Rheumatology*, **15**, 1722–5.

Haller, E. M., Langmann, G., Langmann, A., and Lerchner, H. (1991). Persistence of *Chlamydia trachomatis* in patients with chronic therapy refractory conjunctivitis. *Fortschritte der Opthalmologie*, **88**, 248–51.

Halstensen, T. S., Das, K. M., and Brandzaeg, P. (1993). Epithelial deposits of immunoglobulin G1 and activated complement colocalise with the M(r) 40 kD putative autoantigen in ulcerative colitis. *Gut*, **34**, 650–7.

Hammer, M. and Zeidler, H. (1994). 'Inflammation or sepsis' is not the actual question in reactive arthritis. *British Journal of Rheumatology*, **33**, 199–200.

Hammer, M., Zeidler, H., Klimsa, S., and Heesemann, J. (1990*a*). *Yersinia enterocolitica* in the synovial membrane of patients with yersinia-induced arthritis. *Arthritis and Rheumatism*, **33**, 1795–800.

Hammer, R. E., Maika, S. D., Richardson, J. A., Tang, J.-P., and Taurog, J. D. (1990*b*). Spontaneous inflammatory disease in transgenic rats expressing HLA-B27 and human beta-2 microglobulin: An animal model of HLA-B27-associated human disorders. *Cell*, **63**, 1099–12.

Hammer, M., Nettelnbreker, E., Hopf, S., Schmitz, E., Pörschke, K., and Zeidler, H. (1992). Chlamydial rRNA in the joints of patients with chlamydia-induced arthritis and undifferentiated arthritis. *Clinical and Experimental Rheumatology*, **10**, 63–6.

Hammer, R. E., Richardson, J. A., Simmons, W. A., White, A. L., Breban, M., and Taurog, J. D. (1995). High prevalence of colorectal cancer in HLA-B27 transgenic F344 rats with chronic inflammatory bowel disease. *Journal of Investigative Medicine*, **43**, 262–8.

Hancock, J. A. H. (1960). Surface manifestations of Reiter's disease in the male. *British Journal of Venereal Disease*, **36**, 36–9.

Hanly, J. G., Russell, M. L., and Gladman, D. D. (1988). Psoriatic spondyloarthropathy: a long term prospective study. *Annals of Rheumatic Diseases*, **47**, 386–93.

Hannu, T. J. and Leirisalo-Repo, M. (1988). Clinical picture of reactive salmonella arthritis. *Journal of Rheumatology*, **15**, 1668–71.

Hasegawa, T., Ogawa, A., Sugahara, Y. *et al.* (1997). Novel HLA-B27 allele (B*2711) encoding on antigen reacting with both B27- and B40-specific antisera. *Tissue Antigens*, **49**, 649–52.

Haslock, I. (1973). Arthritis and Crohn's disease—A family study. *Annals of Rheumatic Diseases*, **32**, 479–86.

Hassell, A. B., Reynolds, D. J., Deacon, M., Gaston, J. S., and Pearce, J. H. (1993). Identification of T-cell stimulatory antigens of *Chlamydia trachomatis* using synovial fluid derived T-cell clones. *Immunology*, **79**, 513–19.

Hassell, A. B., Life, P. F., Viner, N. J., and Gaston, J. S. (1994). A longitudinal study of peripheral blood mononuclear cell proliferative responses to bacterial antigens in reactive arthritis. *British Journal of Rheumatology*, **33**, 210–14.

Hawkins, J. C. F., Farr, M., and Morris, J. (1976). Detection by electromicroscopy of rod shaped organisms in synovial membrane from a patient with the arthritis of Whipple's disease. *Annals of Rheumatic Diseases*, **35**, 502–9.

Hayden, J. B. and Davey, M. P. (1994). An RA associated MHC molecule (DRB1 0404) naturally selects different peptides than a non-RA associated molecule. *Arthritis and Rheumatism*, **37**, S282.

Hayllar, J., Smith, T., Mac Pherson, A., Price, A. B., Gumpel, M., and Bjarnason, I. (1994). Non-steroidal anti-inflammatory drug-induced small intestinal inflammation and blood loss. *Arthritis and Rheumatism*, **37**, 1146–50.

Hazelton, R., Cope, J., Seymour, G., Douglas, W., and Cross, S. (1985). A report of three cases of Yersinia reactive arthritis. *Australia and New Zealand Journal of Medicine*, **15**, 331–5.

Heesemann, J. and Gruter, L. (1987). Genetic evidence that the outer membrane protein YOP1 of *Yersinia enterocolitica* mediates adherence and phagocytosis resistance to human epithelial cells. *FEMS Microbiology Letters*, **40**, 37.

Heesemann, J., Gaede, K., and Autenrieth, I. B. (1993). Experimental *Yersinia enterocolitica* infection in rodents: A model for human yersiniosis. *APMIS*, **101**, 417–29.

Helliwell, P. S., Marchesoni, A., Peters, M., Barker, M., and Wright, V. (1991*a*). Re-evaluation of osteoarticular manifestations of psoriasis. *British Journal of Rheumatology*, **30**, 339–45.

Helliwell, P. S., Marchesoni, A., Peters, M., Platt, R., and Wright, V. (1991*b*). Cytidine deaminase activity, C reactive protein, histidine, and erythrocyte sedimentation rate as measures of disease activity in psoriatic arthritis. *Annals of the Rheumatic Diseases*, **50**, 362–5.

Hench, P. S. (1935). Acute and chronic arthritis. In *Nelson's looseleaf of surgery I* (ed. G. Whipple), pp. 104. Thomas Nelson Sons, New York.

Henderley, D. E., Genstler, A. J., Smith, R. E., and Rao, N. A. (1987). Changing patterns of uveitis. *American Journal of Ophthalmology*, **103**, 131–6.

Hermann, E. (1993). T cells in reactive arthritis. *APMIS*, **101**, 177–86.

Hermann, E., Yu, D. T. Y., Meyer zum Büschenfelde, K.-H., and Fleischer, B. (1993). HLA-B27-restricted CD8 T cells derived from synovial fluids of patients with reactive arthritis and ankylosing spondylitis. *Lancet*, **342**, 646–50.

Hermann, E., Fleischer, B., and Meyer zum Büschenfelde, K. H. (1994). Bacteria-specific cytotoxic CD8+ T cells: A missing link in the pathogenesis of the HLA-B27-associated spondylarthropathies. *Annals of Medicine*, **26**, 365–9.

Hermann, E., Sucke, B., Droste, U., and Meyer zum Büschenfelde, K.-H. (1995). Klebsiella pneumoniae-reactive T cells in blood and synovial fluid of patients with ankylosing spondylitis. *Arthritis and Rheumatism*, **38**, 1277–82.

Hermans, P. J., Fievez, M. L., Descamps, C. L., and Aupaix, M. A. (1984). Granulomatous synovitis and Crohn's disease. *Journal of Rheumatology*, **11**, 710–12.

Herrlinger, J. D. and Asmussen, J.-U. (1992). Long term prognosis in Yersinia arthritis: clinical and serological findings. *Annals of the Rheumatic Diseases*, **51**, 1332–4.

Hicken, G. L., Kitaoka, H. B., and Valente, R. M. (1994). Foot and ankle surgery in patients with psoriasis. *Clinical Orthopedics*, **300**, 201–6.

Highton, J. and Poole, E. (1993). Sexually acquired reactive arthritis: inflammation or sepsis? *British Journal of Rheumatology*, **32**, 649–52.

Hildebrand, W., Domena, J., Shen, S., *et al.* (1994). The HLA-B7Qui antigen is encoded by a new subtype of HLA-B27 (B*2708). *Tissue Antigens*, **44**, 47–51.

Hill, A., Elvin, J., *et al.* (1992). Molecular analysis of the association of HLA-B53 and resistance to severe malaria. *Nature*, **360**, 434–419.

Hill, A. V., Allsopp, C. E., *et al.* (1991). HLA class I typing by PCR: HLA-B27 and an African B27 subtype. *Lancet*, **337**, 640–2.

Hill, J. L. and Yu, D. T. Y. (1987). Development of an experimental animal model for reactive arthritis induced by *Yersinia enterocolitica* infection. *Infection and Immunity*, **55**, 721–6.

Hill, J. L. and Yu, D. T. Y. (1988). Experimental animal models and reactive arthritis. In *Reactive arthritis* (ed. A. Toivanen and P. Toivanen), CRC Press, Boca Raton, FL.

Hilt, W. Wolf, D. (1996). Proteasomes: destruction as a programme. *Trends in Biochemical Sciences*, **21**, 96–102.

Hoak, E. W., Spitters, C., Reichart, C. A., Neumann, T. M., and Quinn, T. C. (1994). Use of cell culture and rapid diagnostic assay for *Chlamydia trachomatis* screening. *Journal of the American Medical Association*, **212**, 867–70.

Hobson, C. H., Butt, T. J., Ferry, D. M., Hunter, H., Chadwick, V. S., and Broom, M. F. (1988). Enterohepatic circulation of bacterial chemotactic peptide in rats with experimental colitis. *Gastroenterology*, **94**, 1006–13.

Hochberg, M. C. (1995). Classification criteria for childhood arthritic diseases. *Journal of Rheumatology*, **22**, 1445–6.

Hodgson, H. J., Potter, B. J., and Jewell, D. P. (1977). Immune complexes in ulcerative colitis and Crohn's disease. *Clinical and Experimental Immunology*, **29**, 187–96.

Hogervorst, E. J., Wagenaar, J. P., Boog, C. J., van der Zee, R., van Embden, J. D., and van Eden, W. (1992). Adjuvant arthritis and immunity to the mycobacterial 65 kDa heat shock protein. *International Immunology*, **4**, 719–27.

Holgate, M. C. (1975). The age of onset of psoriasis and the relationship to parental psoriasis. *British Journal of Dermatology*, **92**, 443–8.

Hollander, D., Wadheim, C., Brettholz, E., *et al.* (1986). Increased intestinal permeability in patients with Crohn's disease and their relatives. *Annals of Internal Medicine*, **105**, 883–5.

Hollingsworth, P. N., Cheah, P. S., Dawkins, R. L., Owen, E. T., Calin, A., and Wood, P. H. N. (1983). Observer variation in grading sacroiliac radiographs in HLA-B27 positive individuals. *Journal of Rheumatology*, **10**, 247–54.

Hoogkamp-Korstanje, J. A. A. (1987). Antibiotics in *Yersinia enterocolitica* infections. *Journal of Antimicrobial Chemotherapy*, **20**, 123–31.

Hoogkamp-Korstanje, J. A. A., de Koning, J., and Heesemann, J. (1988). Persistence of *Yersinia enterocolitica* in man. *Infection*, **16**, 81–8.

Hoogkamp-Korstanje, J. A. A., de Koning. J., Heesemann, J., Festen, J. J. M., Houtman, P. M., and van Oyen, P. L. M. (1992). Influence of antibiotics on IgA and IgG response and persistence of *Yersinia enterocolitica* in patients with Yersinia-associated spondylarthropathy. *Infection*, **20**, 53–7.

Hooten, T. M., Batteiger, B. E., Judson, F. N., *et al.* (1992). Ofloxacin vs. doxycycline for treatment of cervical infection with *Chlamydia trachomatis. Antimicrobial Agents and Chemotherapy*, **36**, 1144–6.

Hoppenfeld, S. (1976). *Physical examination of the spine and extremities*, pp. 261–2. Appleton–Century- Crofts, New York.

Horowitz, S., Horowitz, J., Taylor-Robinson, D., *et al.* (1994). *Ureaplasma urealyticum* in Reiter's syndrome. *Journal of Rheumatology*, **21**, 877–82.

Huckins, D., Felson, D. T., and Holick, M. (1990). Treatment of psoriatic arthritis with oral 1,25-dihydroxyvitamin D3: a pilot study. *Arthritis and Rheumatism*, **33**, 1723–7.

Hudson, A. P., Whittum-Hudson, J. A., Ganeshamurthy, A., *et al.* (1990). A molecular hybridization study of ocular chlamydial infection in cynomolgus monkeys. *Investigations in Opthalmolology and Vision Science*, **31**, 448.

Huet, S., Nixon, D. F., Rothbard, J. B., Townsend, A., Ellis, S. A., McMichael, A. J. (1990). Structural homologies between two HLA B27-restricted peptides suggest residues important for interaction with HLA B27. *International Immunology* **2**, 311–6.

Hughes, R. A. and Keat, A. C. (1994). Reiter's syndrome and reactive arthritis: A current view. *Seminars in Arthritis and Rheumatism*, **24**, 190–210.

Hugot, J. P., Laurent-Puig, P., Gower-Rousseau, C., *et al.* (1996). Mapping of a suceptibility locus for Crohn's disease on chromosome 16. *Nature*, **379**, 821–3.

Hülsemann, J. L. and Zeidler, H. (1995). Undifferentiated arthritis in an early synovitis out-patient clinic. *Clinical and Experimental Rheumatology*, **13**, 37–43.

Hülsemann, J. L., Zeidler, H., and Krech, T. (1989). Diagnostische Charakteristika früher Arthritiden and Spondylarthropathien. *Aktuelle Rheumatologie*, **14**, 115–18.

Hunt, D. F., Henderson, R. A., Shabanowitz, J., Sakaguchi, K., Michel, H., Sevilir, N., Cox, A. L., Appella, E., Engelhard, V. H. (1992). Characterization of peptides bound to the class I MHC molecule HLA-A2.1 by mass spectrometry. *Science* **255**, 1261–3.

Hunter, T., Hardin, G. K., Kaprove, R. W., and Schroeder, M. L. (1981). Fecal carriage of Klebsiella and Enterobacter species in patients with active ankylosing spondylitis. *Arthritis and Rheumatism*, **24**, 106–8.

Huskisson, E. C. and Hart, F. D. (1972). Pain threshold and arthritis. *British Medical Journal*, **4**, 193–5.

Hussein, A., Abdul-Khaliq, H., and vonder Hardt, H. (1989). Atypical spondyloarthropathies in children: proposed diagnostic criteria. *European Journal of Pediatrics*, **148**, 513–7.

Husted, J. A., Gladman, D. D., Long, J. A., and Farewell, V. T. (1995). A modified version of the Health Assessment Questionnaire (HAQ) for psoriatic arthritis. *Clinical and Experimental Rheumatology*, **13**, 439–43.

Hyla, J. F., Franck, W. A., and Davis, J. S. (1976). Lack of association of HLA B27 with radiographic sacroiliitis in inflammatory bowel disease. *Journal of Rheumatology*, **3**, 196–200.

Ikawa, T. and Yu, D. T. Y. (1995). Bacterial invasion has profound effect on HLA-B27. *Arthritis and Rheumatism*, **38**, S201.

Iliopoulos, A., Karras, D., loakimidis, D., *et al.* (1995). Change in the epidemiology of Reiter's syndrome (reactive arthritis) in the post-AIDS era? An analysis of cases appearing in the Greek army. *Journal of Rheumatology*, **22**, 252–4.

Ingram, J. T. (1964). The uniqueness of psoriasis. *Lancet*, **1**, 121–3.

Inman, R. D. and Scofield, R. (1994). Etiopathogenesis of ankylosing spondylitis and reactive arthritis. *Current Opinion in Rheumatology*, **6**, 360–70.

Inman, R. D., Johnston, M. E. A., Hodge, M., Falk, J., and Helewa, A. (1988). Postdysenteric reactive arthritis. A clinical and immunogenetic study following an outbreak of salmonellosis. *Arthritis and Rheumatism*, **31**, 1377–83.

Inman, R. D., Chiu B., Johnston, M. E. A., Vas, S., and Falk, J. (1989). HLA class I-related impairment in IL-2 production and lymphocyte response to microbial antigens in reactive arthritis. *Journal of Immunology*, **142**, 4256–60.

Isaacs, K. L., Sartor, R. B., and Haskill, J. S. (1992). Cytokine mRNA profiles in inflammatory bowel disease mucosa detected by PCR amplification. *Gastroenterology*, **103**, 1587–95.

Isdale, A. and Wright, V. (1989). Seronegative arthritis and the bowel. *Baillière's Clinical Rheumatology*, **3**, 285–301.

Ishikawa, H., Ohono, O., Yamasaki, K., Ikutas, S., and Hirohata, K. (1986). Arthritis presumably caused by Chlamydia in Reiter's syndrome. *Journal of Bone and Joint Surgery*, **68**, 777–9.

Islam, S. M. M., Numaga, J., Fujino, Y., *et al.* (1995). HLA-DR8 and acute anterior uveitis in ankylosing spondylitis. *Arthritis and Rheumatism*, **38**, 547–50.

Ismail, N. and Inman, R. D. (1994). YadA accounts for HLA-B27 modulation of *Yersinia enterocolitica* invasion of transfected L cells. *Arthritis and Rheumatism* **37**, S204.

Ismail, N., Chamberlain, J., and Inman, R. D. (1994). Persistence and dissemination of *Yersinia enterocolitica* O:8 after intragastric challenge in B27-transgenic mice. *Arthritis and Rheumatism*, **37**, S211 (abstract).

Isomäki, H., Raunio, J., and von Essen, R. (1979). Incidence of inflammatory rheumatic diseases in Finland. *Scandinavian Journal of Rheumatology*, **8**, 188–92.

Jardetzky, T. S., Lane, W. S., Robinson, R. A., Madden, D. R., and Wiley, D. C. (1991). Identification of self peptides bound to purified HLA-B27. *Nature*, **353**, 326–9.

Jenkinson, T., Armas, J., Evison, G., Cohen, M., Lovell, C., and McHugh, N. J. (1994*a*). The cervical spine in psoriatic arthritis: a clinical and radiological study. *British Journal of Rheumatology*, **33**, 255–9.

Jenkinson, T. R., Mallorie, P. A., Whitelock, H. C., Kennedy, L. G., Garrett, S. L., and Calin, A. (1994*b*). Defining spinal mobility in ankylosing spondylitis. The Bath Ankylosing Spondylitis Disease Activity Index. *Journal of Rheumatology*, **21**, 1694–8.

Jevtic, V., Watt, I., Rozman, B., Kos-Golja, M., Demsar, F., and Jarh, O. (1995). Distinctive radiological features of small hand joints in rheumatoid arthritis and seronegative spondyloarthritis demonstrated by contrast-enhanced (Gd-DTPA) magnetic resonance imaging. *Skeletal Radiology*, **24**, 351–5.

Jiménez-Balderas, F. J. (1989). Cuadroclinico de la espondilitis anquilosante en el caucásico y en el mestizo mexicano. *Revista Mexicana de Rheumatologia*, **4**, 7–21.

Job-Lusanre, C. and Menkes, C. J. (1993). Sulphasalazine treatment for juvenile arthorpathy. *Revue du Rhumatisme*, **60**, 489–93.

Joly, E., Deverson, E. V., Coadwell, J. W., Gunther, E., Howard, J. C., and Butcher, G. W. (1994). The distribution of Tap2 alleles among laboratory rat RT1 haplotypes. *Immunogenetics*, **40**, 45–53.

Jones, S. (Autumn/Winter 1994). Life-assurance investigation results. *NASS Newsletter*, 5–6.

Jones, S. D., Porter, J., Garrett, S. L., Kennedy, L. G., Whitelock, H., and Calin, A. (1995). A new scoring system for the Bath Ankylosing Spondylitis Metrology Index (BASMI). *Journal of Rheumatology*, **22**, 1609.

Jones, S. D., Calin, A., and Steiner, A. (1996*a*). An update on the Bath Ankylosing spondylitis Disease Activity and Functional Indices (BASDAI, BASFI): excellent Cronbach's alpha scores. *Journal of Rheumatology*, **23**, 407.

Jones, S. D., Steiner, A., Garrett, S. L., and Calin, A. (1996*b*). The Bath Ankylosing Spondylitis Patient Global Score (BAS-G). *British Journal of Rheumatology*, **35**, 66–71.

Jones, S. M., Armas, J. B., Cohen, M. G., Lovell, C. R., Evison, G., and McHugh, N. J. (1994). Psoriatic arthritis outcome of disease subsets and relationship of joint disease to nail and skin disease. *British Journal of Rheumatology*, **33**, 834–9.

Joos, R., Veys, E. M., Mielants, H., Van Werveke, S., and Goemaere, S. (1991). Sulphasalazine treatment in juvenile chronic arthritis: an open study. *Journal of Rheumatology*, **18**, 880–4.

Julkunen, H. and Korpi, J. (1984). Ankylosing spondylitis in three Finnish population samples. *Scandinavian Journal of Rheumatology*, **52**, (Suppl.), 16–8.

Kahn, M.-F. and Khan, M. A. (1994). SAPHO syndrome. *Baillières Clinical Rheumatology*, **8** 333–62.

Kaipianen-Seppanen, O. (1996). Incidence of psoriatic arthritis in Finland. *British Journal of Rheumatology*, **35**, 1289–91.

Kaipianen-Seppanen, O. and Savolainen, A. (1996). Incidence of chronic juvenile rheumatic diseases in Finland during 1980–1990. *Clinical and Experimental Rheumatology*, **14**, 441–4.

Kalinke, U., Arnold, B., and Hammerling, G. J. (1990). Strong xenogeneic HLA response in transgenic mice after introducing an alpha 3 domain into HLA B27. *Nature*, **348**, 642–4.

Kalliomäki, J. L. and Leino, R. (1979). Follow-up studies of joint complications in yersiniosis. *Acta medica Scandinavica*, **205**, 521–5.

Kammer, G. M., Soter, N. A., Gibson, D. J., and Schur, P. H. (1979). Psoriatic arthritis: a clinical, immunologic and HLA study of 100 patients. *Seminars in Arthritis and Rheumatism*, **9**, 75–9.

Kandil, H. M., Saberi, A. A., Bender, D., Argenzio, R. A., and Sartor, R. B. (1994). Interaction between prostaglandin E-2 and interleukin 1a (Ila) in experimental rat colitis. *Gastroenterology*, **106**, A708.

Kanga, U., Mehra, N. K., Larrea, C. L., Lardy, N. M., Kumar, A., Feltkamp, T. E. W. (1996). Seronegative spondylarthropathies and HLA-B27 subtypes: A study in Asian Indians. *Clinical Rheumatology* **15** (supplement 1), 13–8.

Kapasi, K. and Inman, R. D. (1992). HLA-B27 expression modulates gram-negative bacterial invasion into transfected L cells. *Journal of Immunology*, **148**, 3554–9.

Kapasi, K. and Inman, R. D. (1994). ME1 epitope of HLA-B27 confers class I-mediated modulation of Gram-negative bacterial invasion. *Journal of Immunology*, **153**, 833–40.

Kapperud, G., Namork, E., Skurnik, M., and Nesbakken, T. (1987). Plasmid-mediated surface fibrillae of *Yersinia pseudotuberculosis* and *Yersinia enterocolitica*; relationship to the outer membrane protein YOP1 and possible importance for pathogenesis. *Infection and Immunity*, **55**, 2247–54.

Karaman-Kraljevic, K., Stambuk, V., Stambuk, N., and Kastelan, A. (1990). A prospective study of the etiology of uveitis. *Current Eye Research*, **9** (Suppl.), 13–16.

Kaslow, R. A., Ryder, R. W., and Calin, A. (1979). Search for Reiter's Syndrome following and outbreak of *Shigella sonnei* dysentery. *Journal of Rheumatology*, **6**, 562–6.

Kaslow, R. A., Simon, D., Calin, A., *et al.* (1981). Reiter's disease following epidemic Shigellosis. *Journal of Rheumatology*, **8**, 969–73.

Kaufman, H. J. and Taubin, H. L. (1987). NSAID activate quiescent inflammatory bowel disease. *Annals of Internal Medicine*, **107**, 513–16.

Kaufmann, S. H. E. (1990). Heat shock proteins and the immune response. *Immunology Today*, **11**, 129–36.

Kaufmann, S. H. E. (1993). Immunity to intracellular bacteria. In *Fundamental immunology* (ed. W. E. Paul), pp 1251–86. Raven Press, New York

Kawaguchi, G., Kato, N., *et al.* (1993). Structural analysis of HLA-B40 epitopes. *Human Immunology*, **36**, 193–8.

Kean, W. F., Anastassiades, T. P., and Ford, P. M. (1980). Aortic incompetence in HLA-B27 positive juvenile arthritis. *Annals of the Rheumatic Diseases*, **39**, 294–5.

Keat, A. C. (1987). *Chlamydia trachomatis*: Reiter's syndrome and reactive arthritis. In *Chlamydial infections* (ed. P. Reeve), pp. 96–119. Springer, New York.

Keat, A. C., Maini, R. N., Nkwazi, C., Pegrum, G. D., Ridgway, G. L., and Scott, J. T. (1978). Role of *Chlamydia trachomatis* and HLA B27 in sexually-acquired reactive arthritis. *British Medical Journal*, **1**, 605–7.

Keat, A. C., Thomas, B. J., Taylor-Robinson, D., Pegrum, G. D., Maini, R. N., and Scott, J. T. (1980). Evidence of *Chlamydia trachomatis* infection in sexually acquired reactive arthritis. *Annals of Rheumatic Diseases*, **39**, 431–7.

Keat, A. C., Thomas, B. J., and Taylor-Robinson, D. (1983). Chlamydial infection in the aetiology of arthritis. *British Medical Bulletin*, **39**, 168–74.

Keat, A. C., Thomas, B. J., Dixey, J., Osborn, M. F., Sonnex, C., and Taylor-Robinson, D. (1987). *Chlamydia trachomatis* and reactive arthritis—the missing link. *Lancet*, **1**, 72–4.

Keat, A. E. (1983). Reiter's syndrome and reactive arthritis in perspective. *New England Journal of Medicine*, **309**, 1606–15.

Kellgren, J. H. (1962). Diagnostic criteria for population studies. *Bulletin of Rheumatic Diseases*, **3**, 291–2.

Kellgren, J. H., Jeffrey, M. R., and Ball, J. (eds) (1963). *The epidemiology of chronic rheumatism*. Volume 1. Blackwell Scientific Publications, Oxford.

Kellner, H. and Granfors, K. (1995). Reactive arthritis: Mechanisms and drug therapy. *Clinical Immunotherapeutics*, **4**, 338–45.

Kendall, M. J., Lawrence, D. S., Shuttleworth, G. R., and Whitfield, A. G. W. (1973). Haematology and biochemistry of ankylosing spondylitis. *British Medical Journal*, **1**, 235–7.

Kennedy, L. G., Edmunds, L., and Calin, A. (1993*a*). The natural history of ankylosing spondylitis. Does it burn out? *Journal of Rheumatology*, **20**, 688–92.

Kennedy, L. G., Will, R., and Calin, A. (1993*b*). Sex ratio in the spondylarthropathies and its relationship to phenotypic expression, mode of inheritance and age at onset. *Journal of Rheumatology*, **20**, 1900–4.

Kennedy, L. G., Jenkinson, T. R., Mallorie, P. A., Whitelock, H. C., Garrett, S. L., and Calin, A. (1995). Ankylosing spondylitis: the correlation between a new metrology index and radiology. *British Journal of Rheumatology*, **34**, 767–70.

Kenney, J. A. (1971). Psoriasis in the American black. In *Psoriasis. Proceedings of the international symposium* (ed. E. M. Farber and A. J. Cox), pp. 49–52. Stanford University Press, Stanford.

Khalil, A., Khare, S., Luthra, H., and David, C. (1997). HLA-B27 transgenic mice lacking CD4 gene have decreased incidence of spontaneous inflammatory disease. *Arthritis and Rheumatism*, in press (abstract).

Khan, M. A. (1982). Axial arthropathy in Whipple's disease. *Journal of Rheumatology*, **9**, 928–9.

Khan, M. A. (1983). B7-CREG and ankylosing spondylitis. *British Journal of Rheumatology*, **22** (Suppl. 2), 129–32.

Khan, M. A. (1984). Ankylosing spondylitis. In *Spondylarthropathies* (ed. A. Calin), pp. 69–117. Grune and Stratton, New York.

Khan, M. A. (1985). Spondyloarthropathies in non-Caucasian populations of the world. In *The spondyloarthropathies (Advances in inflammation research*), Vol. 9. (ed M. Ziff and S. B. Cohen), pp. 91–9. Raven Press, New York.

Khan, M. A. (1987). HLA and ankylosing spondylitis. In *Ankylosing spondylitis: new clinical applications in rheumatology*, Vol. 1. (ed. J. J. Calabro and C. Dick), pp. 23–44. MTP Press, Lancaster.

Khan, M. A. (ed.) (1990). Ankylosing spondylitis and related spondyloarthropathies. *Spine: State of the Art Reviews*, Vol. 4. Hanley & Belfus, Philadelphia.

Khan, M. A. (ed.) (1992). Spondyloarthropathies. *Rheumatic Disease Clinics of North America*, **18**, 1–276.

Khan, M. A. (1993). Ankylosing spondylitis. In *Primer on the rheumatic diseases* (10th edn) (ed. H. R. Schumacher Jr.), pp. 154–8. Arthritis Foundation, Atlanta.

Khan, M. A. (1995). HLA-B27 and its subtypes in world populations. *Current Opinion in Rheumatology*, **7**, 263–69.

Khan, M. A. (1996*a*). Editorial review: Spondyloarthropathies/ Spondyloarthritides. *Current Opinion in Rheumatology*, **9**, 267–8.

Khan, M. A. (1996*b*). Epidemiology of HLA-B27 and arthritis. *Clinical Rheumatology*, **15**, (Suppl. 1), 10–12.

Khan, M. A. (1996*c*). Ankylosing spondylitis: Clinical features. In *Rheumatology* (2nd edn), (ed. J. H. Klippel and P. A. Dieppe), pp. 6.16.1–10. Mosby-Wolfe, London.

Khan, M. A. (1996*d*). Prevalence of HLA-B27 in world populations. In *HLA-B27 in the development of spondyloarthropathies* (ed. C. Lopez-Larrea), pp. 95–112. R. C. Landes Company, Austin, TX.

Khan, M. A. (1997). Spondyloarthropathies: Editorial review. *Current Opinion in Rheumatology*, **9**, 281–3.

Khan, M. A., Lai, J-H., Chou, C. T. *et al.* (1993). Spinal fractures in ankylosing spondylitis. *Journal of Musculoskeletal Medicine*, **10**, 45–57.

Khan, M. A., and Kellner, H. (1992). Immunogenetics of spondyloarthropathies. *Rheumatic Disease Clinics of North America*, **18**, 837–64.

Khan, M. A. and Khan, M. K. (1982). Diagnostic value of HLA-B27 testing in ankylosing spondylitis and Reiter's syndrome. *Annals of Internal Medicine*, **96**, 70–6.

Khan, M. A. and Kushner, I. (1984). Diagnosis of ankylosing spondylitis. In *Progress in clinical rheumatology*, Vol. 1 (ed. A. S. Cohen), pp. 145–78. Grune and Stratton, Orlando.

Khan, M. A. and van der Linden, S. M. (1990*a*). Undifferentiated spondylarthropathies (Vol. 3). In *Ankylosing spondylitis and related spondyloarthropathies* (ed. M. A. Khan), pp. 657–64.

Khan, M. A. and van der Linden, S. M. (1990*b*). Ankylosing spondylitis and other spondyloarthropathies. *Rheumatic Disease Clinics of North America*, **16**, 551–79.

Khan, M. A. and van der Linden S. M. (1990*c*). A wider spectrum of spondyloarthropathies. *Seminars in Arthritis and Rheumatology*, **20**, 107–13.

Khan, M. A. and Wilber, R. G. (1996). Back and neck pain. In *Current practice of medicine*, Vol. 2 (ed. R. C. Bone), pp. VI:8.1–14. Churchill Livingstone-Current Medicine, Philadelphia.

Khan, M. A. Kushner, I., *et al.* (1978). A subgroup of ankylosing spondylitis associated with HLA-B7 in American blacks. *Arthritis and Rheumatism*, **21**, 528–30.

Khan, M. A., Kushner, I., and Braun, W. E. (1980). Genetic heterogeneity in primary ankylosing spondylitis. *Journal of Rheumatology*, **7**, 383–6.

Khan, M. A., Khan, M. K., and Kushner, I. (1981). Survival among patients with ankylosing spondylitis: a life-table analysis. *Journal of Rheumatology*, **8**, 86–90.

Khare, S. D., Luthra, H. S., and David, C. S. (1995*a*). Spontaneous inflammatory arthritis in transgenic mice expressing HLA-B27 and human $\beta 2$ m in the absence of mouse $\beta 2$m. *Arthritis and Rheumatism*, **38** (Suppl), S398. (Abstract)

Khare, S. D., Luthra, H. S., and David, C. C. (1995*b*). Spontaneous inflammatory arthritis in HLA B27 transgenic mice lacking b2-microglobulin: a model of human spondylarthropathies. *Journal of Experimental Medicine*, **182**, 1153–8.

Kidd, B. L., Wilson, P. J., Evans, P. R., and Cawley, M. I. D. (1995). Familial aggregation of undifferentiated spondyloarthropathy associated with HLA-B7. *Annals of Rheumatic Diseases*, **54**, 125–7.

Kijlstra, A., Linssen, A., and Ockhuizen, T. (1984). Association of Gm allotypes with the occurrence of ankylosing spondylitis in HLA-B27-positive anterior uveitis. *American Journal of Ophthalmology*, **98**, 732–5.

Kimura M. (1994). Experimental study on the mechanisms of chlamydia pneumoniae respiratory infection in mice with former chlamydial exposure. *Journal of Japanese Association for Infectious Disease*, **68**, 50–8.

Kingsley, G. and Panayi, G. S. (1992). Antigenic responses in reactive arthritis. *Rheumatic Disease Clinics of North America*, **18**, 49–66.

Kingsley, G. and Sieper, J. (1993). Current perspectives in reactive arthritis. *Immunology Today*, **14**, 1–5.

Kinne, R. W., Schmidt-Weber, C. B., Hoppe, R., *et al.* (1995). Long-term amelioration of rat adjuvant arthritis following systemic elimination of macrophages by clodronate-containing liposomes. *Arthritis and Rheumatism*, **38**, 1777–90.

Kippers, V. and Parker, A. W. (1987). Toe-touch test. A measure of its validity. *Physical Therapy*, **67**, 1680–4.

Kirsner, J. B. (1973). Genetic aspects of inflammatory bowel disease. *Clinical Gastroenterology*, **2**, 557–62.

Kirwan, J., Edwards, E., Huitfeldt, B., Thompson, P., and Currey, H. (1993). The course of established ankylosing spondylitis and the effects of sulphasalazine over 3 years. *British Journal of Rheumatology*, **32**, 729–33.

Kits, G., Thompson, H., and Allan, R. N. (1979). Finger clubbing in inflammatory bowel disease: its prevalence and pathogenesis. *British Medical Journal*, **2**, 825.

Klasen, I. S., Melief, M. J., Swaak, T. J. G., Severijnen, A. J., and Hazenberg, M. P. (1993). Responses of synovial fluid and peripheral blood mononuclear cells to bacterial antigens and autologous antigen presenting cells. *Annals of Rheuamtic Diseases*, **52**, 127–32.

Klasen, I. S., Melief, M. J., van Halteren, A. G. S., *et al.* (1994). The presence of peptidoglycan-polysaccharide complexes in the bowel wall and the cellular responses to these complexes in Crohn's disease. *Clinical Immunology and Immunopathology*, **71**, 303–8.

Klinkhoff, A. V., Gertner, E., Chalmers, A., *et al.* (1989). Pilot study of etretinate in psoriatic arthritis. *Journal of Rheumatology*, **16**, 789–91.

Kloppenburg M., Breedveld, F. C., Terwiel, J. P., Mallee, C., and Dukmans, A. C. (1994). Minocycline in active rheumatoid arthritis: a double blind, placebo-controlled trial. *Arthritis and Rheumatism*, **37**, 629–36.

Köhler, L., Nettelnbrecker, E., Ott, N., Drommer, W., and Zeidler, H. (1994). Persistent, non-productive infection of human peripheral blood monocytes with Chlamydia trachomatis is due to an arrest of the growth cycle at an early stage of the chlamydial development. In *Chlamydial infections. Proceedings of the eighth international symposium on human chlamydial infections*, (ed. J. Orfila *et al.*), pp. 427–30. Societa editrice eoculapio, Italy.

Köhler, L., Bonk, C., Nettelnbreker, E., Wollenhaupt, J., and Zeidler, H. (1995). Persistence of Chlamydia trachomatis in human monocytes is not due to the induction of indol-2,3-diaminooxygenase. *Arthritis and Rheumatism*, **38**, (Suppl), S380.

Kool, J., Ruselerk-van Embden, J. G. H., van Lieshout, L. M. C., *et al.* (1991). Arthritis induction in rats by soluble peptidoglycan–polysaccharide complexes present in human intestinal contents. *Arthritis and Rheumatics*, **34**, 1611–16.

Koski, P., Rhen, M., Kantele, J., and Vaara, M. (1989). Isolation, cloning, and primary structure of a cationic 16-kDa outer membrane protein of *Salmonella typhimurium*. *Journal of Biological Chemistry*, **264**, 18973–80.

Kotake, S., Schumacher, H. R., Kanik, K. S., *et al.* (1995). Type 1 and Type 2 cytokine profiles in synovium from early synovitis patients. *Arthritis and Rheumatism*, **38**, (Suppl 9), S395.

Kotake, S., Schumacher, H. R. Jr., Yarboro C. H., *et al.* (1997). *In vivo* gene expression of type 1 and type 2 cytokines in synovial tissues from patients in early stages of rheumatoid, reative, and undifferentiated arthritis. *Proceedings of the Association of American Physicians* **109**, 286–302.

Kousa, M., Saikku, P., Richmond, S., and Lassus, A. (1978). Frequent association of chlamydial infection with Reiter's syndrome. *Sexually Transmitted Diseases*, **5**, 57–61.

Kovalev, IuN. (1991). The chrysotherapy of patients with Reiter's disease. *Terapevticheskii Arkhiv*, **63**, 123–5.

Kraus, E., and Eisenmenger-Weber, S. (1945). Evaluation of posture based on structural and functional measurements. *Physical Therapy*, **25**, 267–71.

Kriegsmann, J., Franklin, B. N., Gay, R. E., Taurog, J. D., Hammer, R. E., and Gay, S. (1995). Fusion of vertebral bodies and the sacroiliac joint by cartilaginous tissue in HLA-B27 transgenic rats. *Arthritis and Rheumatism*, **38**, S 202 (abstract).

Krimpenfort, P., Rudenko, G., Hochstenbach, F., Guessow, D., Berns, A., and Ploegh, H. (1987). Crosses of two independently derived transgenic mice demonstrate functional complementation of the genes encoding heavy (HLA-B27) and light (beta 2-microglobulin) chains of HLA class I antigens. *EMBO Journal*, **6**, 1673–6.

Krug, H. E., Mahowald, M. L., and Clark, C. (1989). Progressive ankylosis (ank/ank) in mice: an animal model of spondyloarthropathy. III. Proliferative spleen cell response to T cell mitogens. *Clinical and Experimental Immunology*, **78**, 97–101.

Krug, H. E., Wietgrefe, M. M., Ytterberg, S. R., Taurog, J. D., and Mahowald, M. L. (1996). Murine progressive ankylosis is not immunologically mediated. *Journal of Rheumatololgy*, (In press).

Krüger, K. and Schattenkirchner, M. (1983). Die reaktive Arthritis—Klinik und Verlauf. *Wiener klinische Wochenschrift*, **95**, 884–9.

Kulka, J. P. (1962). The lesions of Reiter's syndrome. *Arthritis and Rheumatism*, **5**, 195–201.

Kunnamo, I., Kallio, P., and Pelkonen, P. (1986). Incidence of arthritis in urban Finnish children. *Arthritis and Rheumatism*, **29**, 1232–8.

Kuo, C.-C. (1988). Host response. In *Microbiology of chlamydia* (ed. A. L. Barron), pp. 193–208, CRC Press, Boca Raton.

Kuo, C.-C., Shor, A., Campbell, L. A., *et al.* (1993). Demonstration of chlamydia pneumoniae in atherosclerotic lesions of coronary arteries. *Journal of Infectious Disease*, **167**, 841–9.

Kuo, C.-C., Grayston, J. T., Campbell, L. A., *et al.* (1995). *Chlamydia pneumoniae* (TWAR) in coronary arteries of young adults (15–34 years old). *Proceedings of the National Academy of Science, USA*, **92**, 6911–14.

Kuon, W., Lauster, R., Böttcher, U., *et al.* (1997). Recognition of Chlamydial antigen by HLA-B27 restricted cytotoxic T cells in HLA-B*2705 transgenic CBA mice. *Arthritis and Rheumatism*, **40**, 945–54.

Kvien T. K., Glennås, A., Melby, K., *et al.* (1994). Reactive arthritis: incidence, triggering agents and clinical presentation. *Journal of Rheumatology*, **21**, 115–22.

Lahesmaa, R., Skurnik, M., Vaara, M., *et al.* (1991). Molecular mimickry between HLA B27 and Yersinia, Salmonella, Shigella and Klebsiella within the same region of HLA α1-helix. *Clinical and Experimental Immunology*, **86**, 399–404.

Lahesmaa, R., Skurnik, M., Granfors, K., *et al.* (1992*a*). Molecular mimicry in the pathogenesis of spondylarthropathies. A critical appraisal of cross-reactivity between microbial antigens and HLA-B27. *British Journal of Rheumatology*, **31**, 221–8.

Lahesmaa, R., Yssel, H., Batsford, S., *et al.* (1992*b*). *Yersinia enterocolitica* activates a T helper type 1-like cell subset in reactive arthritis. *Journal of Immunology*, **148**, 3079–85.

Lahesmaa, R., Skurnik, M., and Toivanen, P. (1993). Molecular mimicry: any role in the pathogenesis of spondyloarthropathies? *Immunologic Research*, **12**, 193–208.

Lahesmaa, R., Soderberg, C., Bliska, J., *et al.* (1995). Pathogen antigen- and superantigen-reactive synovial fluid T cells in reactive arthritis. *Journal of Infectious Diseases*, **172**, 1290–7.

Lahesmaa-Rantala, R., Granfors, K., Isomäki, H., and Toivanen, A. (1987*a*). Yersinia specific immune complexes in the synovial fluid of patients with Yersinia-triggered reactive arthritis. *Annals of the Rheumatic Diseases*, **46**, 510–14.

Lahesmaa-Rantala, R., Granfors, K., Kekomäki, R., and Toivanen, A. (1987*b*). Circulating yersinia specific immune complexes after acute yersiniosis: a follow up study of patients with and without reactive arthritis. *Annals of the Rheumatic Diseases*, **46**, 121–6.

Laitio, P., M. Virtala, M. Salmi, L. J. Pelliniemi, D. T. Y. Yu, and K. Granfors. (1997). HLA-B27 modulates intracellular survival of Salmonella enteritidis in human monocytic cells. *European Journal of Immunology*, **27**, 1331–8.

Laivoranta, S., Ilonen, J., *et al.* (1995). HLA frequencies in HLA-B27 negative patients with reactive arthritis. *Clinical and Experimental Rheumatology*, **13**, 637–40.

Lally, E. V. and Ho, G. (1985). A review of methotrexate therapy in Reiter's syndrome. *Seminars in Arthritis and Rheumatism*, **15**, 139–41.

Lambert, J. R. and Wright, V. (1976). Eye inflammation in psoriatic arthritis. *Annals of Rheumatic Disease*, **35**, 354–6.

Lancet (1987). Assessing disease activity in ankylosing spondylitis. *Lancet*, **i**, 1072.

Landers, D. V., Sung, M. L., Bottles, K., and Schachter, J. (1993). Does addition of anti-inflammatory agents to antimicrobial therapy reduce infertility after murine chlamydial salpingitis. *Sexually Transmitted Diseases*, **20**, 121–5.

Langman, M. S., Morgan, L., and Worrall, A. (1985). Use of anti-inflammatory drugs by patients with small or large bowel perforation and haemorrhage. *British Medical Journal*, **290**, 347–9.

Lanham, J. G. and Doyle, D. V. (1984). Reactive arthritis following psittacosis. *British Journal of Rheumatology*, **23**, 225–6.

Lassus, A. (1975). Circinate erosive balanitis. *Annals of Rheumatic Diseases*, **34** (Suppl.), 55.

Lauhio, A., Lähdevirta, J., Janes, R., Kontiainen, S., and Repo, H. (1988). Reactive arthritis associated with *Shigella sonnei* infection. *Arthritis and Rheumatism*, **31**, 1190–3.

Lauhio, A., Leirisalo-Repo, M., Lähdevirta, J., Saikku, P., and Repo, H. (1991). Double-blind, placebo-controlled study of three-month treatment with lymecycline in reactive arthritis, with special reference to chlamydia arthritis. *Arthritis and Rheumatism*, **34**, 6–14.

Lauhio, A., Sorsa, T., Lindy, O., *et al.* (1992). The anticollagenolytic potential of lymecycline in the long-term treatment of reactive arthritis. *Arthritis and Rheumatism*, **35**, 195–8.

Laurent, M. R. and Panayi, G. S. (1983). Acute-phase proteins and serum immunoglobulins in ankylosing spondylitis. *Annals of Rheumatic Disease*, **42**, 524–8.

Laurent, M. R., Buchanan, W. M., and Bellamy, N. (1991). Methods of assessment used in ankylosing spondylitis clinic trials: a review. *British Journal of Rheumatology*, **30**, 326–9.

Lavaroni, G., Kokelj, F., Pauluzzi, P., and Trevisan, G. (1994). The nails in psoriatic arthritis. *Acta Dermatologica Venereologica Suppl.* (Stockholm), **186**, 113.

Lawley, T. J., James, S. P., and Jones, E. A. (1980). Circulating immune complexes: Their detection and potential significance in some hepatobiliary and intestinal diseases. *Gastroenterology*, **76**, 626–41.

Lawlor, D. A., Warren, E., Taylor, P., and Parham, P. (1991). Gorilla class I major histocompatibility complex alleles: comparison to human and chimpanzee class I. *Journal of Experimental Medicine*, **174**, 1491–509.

Lawrence, J. (1977). *Rheumatisms in populations*. William Heinemann Medical Books, London.

Lawrence, R. C., Hochberg, M. C., Kelsey, J. L., *et al.* (1989). Estimates of the prevalence of selected arthritic and musculoskeletal diseases in the United States. *Journal of Rheumatology*, **16** (Suppl 4), 427–41.

Lee, F. I., Bellary, S. V., and Francis, C. (1990). Increased occurrence of psoriasis in patients with Crohn's disease and their relatives. *American Journal of Gastroenterology*, **85**, 962–3.

Lehtinen, M. and Paavonen, J. (1994). Heat-shock proteins in the immunopathogenesis of chlamydial pelvic inflammatory disease. In *Chlamydial infections. Proceedings of the eighth international symposium on human chlamydial infections* (ed. J. Orfila *et al.*.), pp. 599–610. Societa editrice eoculapio, Italy.

Lehtinen, A., Taavitsainen, M., and Leirisalo-Repo, M. (1994). Sonographic analysis in low extremities of patients with spondyloarthropathy. *Clinical and Experimental Rheumatology*, **12**, 143–8.

Lehtinen, A., Leirisalo-Repo, M. and Taavitsainen, M. (1995). Persistence of enthesopathic changes in patients with spondyloarthropathy during a 6-month followup. *Clinical and Experimental Rheumatology*, **13**, 733–6.

Lehtonen, L., Kortekangas, P., Oksman, P., Eerola, E., Aro, H., and Toivanen, A. (1994). Synovial fluid muramic acid in acute inflammatory arthritis. *British Journal of Rheumatology*, **33**, 1127–30.

Leino, R. and Kalliomäki, J. L. (1974). Yersiniosis as an internal disease. *Annals of Internal Medicine*, **81**, 458–61.

Leino, R., Vuento, R., Koskimies, S., Viander, M., and Toivanen, A. (1983). Depressed lymphocyte transformation by Yersinia and *Escherichia coli* in Yersinia arthritis. *Annals of the Rheumatic Diseases*, **42**, 176–81.

Leirisalo-Repo, M. (1993). Are antibiotics of any use in reactive arthritis? *APMIS*, **101**, 575–81.

Leirisalo-Repo, M. (1994). Long-term prognosis of reactive Salmonella arthritis. *Arthritis and Rheumatism*, **37**, S236.

Leirisalo-Repo, M. (1995). Treatment of reactive arthritis. *Rheumatology in Europe*, **24**, 20–2.

Leirisalo-Repo, M. and Repo, H. (1992). Gut and spondyloarthropathies. *Rheumatic Diseases Clinics of North America*, **18**, 23–35.

Leirisalo-Repo, M. and Suoranta, H. (1988). Ten-year follow-up study of patients with Yersina-arthritis. *Arthritis and Rheumatism* **31**, 533–7.

Leirisalo-Repo, M., Skylv, G., Kousa, M., *et al.* (1982). Follow-up study on patients with Reiter's disease and with reactive arthritis, with special reference to HLA-B27. *Arthritis and Rheumatism*, **25**, 249–59.

Leirisalo-Repo, M., Skylv, G., and Kousa, M. (1987). Follow-up of Reiter's disease and reactive arthritis. Factors influencing the natural course and the prognosis. *Clinical Rheumatology*, **6** (Suppl. 2), 73–82.

Leirisalo-Repo, M., Helenius, P., and Laasila, M. (1994*a*). Prognostic factors in reactive arthritis. *Scandinavian Journal of Rheumatology* (Suppl.), **98**, Abstr. 159.

Leirisalo-Repo, M., Turunen, U., Stenman, S., Helenius, P., and Seppälä, K. (1994*b*). High frequency of silent inflammatory bowel disease in spondyloarthropathy. *Arthritis and Rheumatism*, **37**, 23–31.

Leirisalo-Repo, M., Helenius, P., and Turunen, U. (1995). Evolution of inflammatory bowel disease in spondylarthropathy. *Arthritis and Rheumatism*, **39**, 9, Abstr. 308, S203.

Leroux, J.-Y., Poole, A. R., Webber, C., and Banerjee, S. (1992). Characterization of proteoglycan-reactive T cell lines and hybridomas from mice with proteoglycan-induced arthritis. *Journal of Immunology* **148**, 2090–6.

Leroux, J.-Y., Guerassimov, A., Cartman, A., *et al.* (1996). Immunity to the G1 globular domain of the cartilage proteoglycan aggrecan can induce inflammatory erosive polyarthritis and spondylitis in BALB/c mice but immunity to G1 is inhibited by covalently bound keratan sulfate in vitro and in vivo. *Journal of Clinical Investigation* **97**, 621–32.

Levine, A. J. B. (1994). Arthropathies and complications of inflammatory bowel disease. In *Inflammatory bowel disease: from bench to the bedside* (ed. S. R. Targan and F. Shanahan), pp. 668–81. Williams and Wilkins, Baltimore, MD.

Levy, J., Paulus, H., Eugene, V., *et al.* (1972). A double-blind controlled evaluation of azathioprine treatment in rheumatoid arthritis and psoriatic arthritis. *Arthritis and Rheumatism*, **15**, 116–17.

Li, F., Bulbul, R., Schumacher, H. R., *et al.* (1996). Molecular detection of bacterial DNA in venereal-associated arthritis. *Arthritis and Rheumatism*, **39**, 950–8.

Li, Q., Peng, B., Whitcup, S. M., Jang, S. U., and Chan, C.-C. (1995). Endotoxin induced uveitis in the mouse: Susceptibility and genetic control. *Experimental Eye Research*, **61**, 629–32.

Liblau, R. S., Singer, S. M., and McDevitt, H. O. (1995). Th1 and Th2 CD4+ T cells in the pathogenesis of organ-specific autoimmune diseases. *Immunology Today*, **16**, 34–8.

Lichtman, S. N. and Sartor, R. B. (1994). Extraintestinal manifestations of inflammatory bowel disease: Clinical aspects and natural history. In *Inflammatory bowel disease: from bench to bedside* (ed. S. R. Targan and F. Shanahan), pp. 317–35. Williams and Wilkins, Baltimore, MD.

Lichtman, S. N., Sartor, R. B., Keku, J., and Schwab, J. H. (1990). Hepatic inflammation in rats with experimental small intestinal bacterial overgrowth. *Gastroenterology*, **98**, 414–23.

Lichtman, S. N., Keku, J., and Schwab, J. H. (1991). Evidence for peptidoglycan absorption in rats with experimental small bowel bacterial overgrowth. *Infection and Immunity*, **59**, 555–62.

Lichtman, S. N., Okoruwa, E. E., Keku, J., Schwab, J. H., and Sartor, R. B. (1992). Degradation of endogenous bacterial cell wall polymers by the muralytic enzyme mutanolysin prevents hepatobiliary injury in genetically susceptible rats with experimental intestinal bacterial overgrowth. *Journal of Clinical Investigation*, **90**, 1313–22.

Lichtman, S. N., Bachmann, S., Schwab, J. H., Sartor, R. B., and LeMasters, J. J. (1993). Bacterial cell wall polymers (peptidoglycan–polysaccharide) cause reactivation of arthritis. *Infection and Immunity*, **61**, 4645–53.

Lichtman, S. N., Wang, J., Sartor, R. B., *et al.* (1995). Reactivation of arthritis induced by small bowel bacterial overgrowth in rats: role of cytokines, bacteria, and bacterial polymers. *Infection and Immunity*, **63**, 2295–301.

Lichtman, S. N., Zhang, C., Wang, J., Schwab, J. H., and Winfield, J. B. (1996). T cells play a role in reactivation of arthritis by small bowel bacterial overgrowth. *Clinical and Experimental Immunology*, in press.

Lin, W. Y., Wang, S. J., Lang, J. L., *et al.* (1995). Bone scintigraphy in evaluation of heel pain in Reiter's disease: Compared with radiography and clinical examination. *Scandinavian Journal of Rheumatology*, **24**, 18–21.

Lindholm, H. and Visakorpi, R. (1991). Late complications after a *Yersinia enterocolitica* epidemic: a follow up study. *Annals of the Rheumatic Diseases*, **50**, 694–6.

Lindsley, C. B. (1977). Arthritis in inflammatory bowel disease in children. *Arthritis and Rheumatism*, **20** (Suppl.), 411–13.

Lindsley, C. B. and Schaller, J. G. (1974). Arthritis associated with inflammatory bowel disease in children. *Journal of Pediatrics*, **84**, 16–20.

Linschoten, N. J. and Krachkow, K. A. (1993). Psoriatic arthritis of the knee treated with synovectomy. *Orthopedics*, **16**, 1268–70.

Linssen, A. and Feltkamp, T. E. W. (1988). B27-positive disease versus B27-negative disease. *Annals of Rheumatic Diseases* **47**, 431–9.

Linssen, A. and Meenken, C. (1995). Outcomes of HLA-B27-positive and HLA-B27-negative acute anterior uveitis. *American Journal of Ophthalmology* **120**, 351–61.

Linssen, A., Rothova, A., Valkenburg, H. A., *et al.* (1991). The lifetime cumulative incidence of acute anterior uveitis in a normal population and its relation to ankylosing spondylitis and histocompatibility antigen HLA-B27. *Investigative Ophthalmology and Visual Science*, **32**, 2568–78.

Little, H., Harvie, J. N., and Lester, R. S. (1975). Psoriatic arthritis in severe psoriasis. *Canadian Medical Association Journal*, **112**, 317–19.

Liu, Y., van Kruiningen, H. J., West, A. B., Cartun, R. W., Cortot, A., and Colombel, J. F. (1995). Immunocytochemical evidence of *Listeria*, *Escherichia coli*, and *Streptococcus* antigens in Crohn's disease. *Gastroenterology*, **108**, 1396–404.

Locht, H., Kihlström, E., and Lindström, F. (1993). Reactive arthritis after salmonella among medical doctors—study of an outbreak. *Journal of Rheumatology*, **20**, 845–8.

Logroscino, C. A. (1981). Modifacazioni ultra strutturali della membrana synoviale mel morbo di Reiter. *Arch Putti Chir. Organi Mov*, **31**, 245–52.

Lohmuller, J. L., Pemerton, J. H., Dozols, R. R., Listrup, D., and Van-Heerden, J. (1990). Pouchitis and extra-intestinal manifestations of inflammatory bowel disease after ileal pouch anal anastomosis. *Annals of Surgery*, **211**, 622–5.

López, D., García-Hoyo, R., López de Castro, J. A. (1994). Clonal analysis of alloreactive T cell responses against the closely related B*2705 and B*2703 subtypes. Implications for HLA-B27 association to spondyloarthropathy. *Journal of Immunology* **152**, 5557–71.

Lopez de Castro, J. A. (1989). HLA-B27 and HLA-A2 subtypes: structure, evolution and function. *Immunology Today*, **10**, 239–46.

Lopez de Castro, J. A. (1995). Structural polymorphism and function of HLA-B27. *Current Opinion in Rheumatology*, **7**, 270–8.

Lopez-Larrea, C., Sujirachato, K., Mehra, N. K. *et al.* (1995). HLA-B27 subtypes in Asian patients with ankylosing spondylitis. Evidence for new associations. *Tissue Antigens*, **45**, 169–76.

Lopez-Larrea, C., Gonzales-Roces, S., and Alvarez, V. (1996). HLA-B27 structure, function and disease association. *Current Opinion in Rheumatology*, **8**, 296–308.

Louthrenoo, W. (1993). Successful treatment of severe Reiter's syndrome associated with human immunodeficiency virus infection with etretinate. Report of 2 cases. *Journal of Rheumatology*, **20**, 1243–6.

Ludwig, B., Bohl, J., and Haferkamp, G. (1981). Central nervous system involvement in Whipple's disease. *Neuroradiology*, **21**, 289–93.

Lügering, N., Kcharzik, T., Domschke, W., and Stoll, R. (1996). Crohn's disease patients suffering from joint complications show a selective depletion of T-cell receptor variable gene segments. *Gastroenterology*, **110**, A952.

Lynch, J. M., Lotner, G. Z., Betz, S. J., and Henson, P. M. (1979). The release of a platelet-activating factor by stimulated rabbit neutrophils. *Journal of Immunology*, **123**, 1219–26.

Lyons, J. L. and Rosenbaum, J. T. (1995). Uveitis associated with inflammatory bowel disease usually differs markedly from uveitis with spondyloarthropathy. *Investigative Ophthalmology and Visual Science*, (Suppl.), (in press). (Abstract)

Mackiewicz, A., Khan, M. A., Reynolds, T. L. *et al.* (1989). Serum IgA and acute phase proteins in ankylosing spondylitis. *Annals of Rheumatic Diseases*, **48**, 99–103.

MacLean, L. (1992). HLA-B27 subtypes: implications for the spondyloarthropathies. *Annals of the Rheumatic Diseases* **51**, 929–31.

Macrae, I. F. and Wright, V. (1969). Measurement of back movement. *Annals of Rheumatic Diseases*, **28**, 584–9.

Madden, D. R., Gorga, J. C., Strominger, J. L., Wiley, D. C. (1991). The structure of HLA-B27 reveals nonamer 'self-peptides' bound in an extended conformation. *Nature* **353**, 321–5.

Madden, D. R., Gorga, J. C., *et al.* (1992). The three-dimensional structure of HLA-B27 at 2.1 Å resolution suggests a general mechanism for tight peptide binding to MHC. *Cell*, **70**, 1035–48.

Magid, D., Douglas, J. M., and Schwartz, S. (1996). Doxycycline compared with azithromycin for treating women with genital chlamydia trachomatis infections: an incremental cost-effectiveness analysis. *Annals of Internal Medicine*, **124**, 389–99.

Magro, C. M., Crowson, A. N., and Peeling, R. (1995). Vasculitis as the basis of cutaneous lesions in Reiter's disease. *Human Pathology*, **26**, 633–8.

Mahowald, M. L., Krug, H., and Taurog, J. (1988). Progressive ankylosis in mice. An animal model of spondylarthropathy. I. Clinical and radiographic findings. *Arthritis and Rheumatism*, **31**, 1390–9.

Mahowald, M. L., Krug, H., and Halverson, P. (1989). Progressive ankylosis (*ank/ank*) in mice: an animal model of spondyloarthropathy. II. Light and electron microscopic findings. *Journal of Rheumatology*, **16**, 60–6.

Mäki-Ikola, O. and Granfors, K. (1992*a*). Salmonella-triggered reactive arthritis. *Lancet*, **339**, 1096–8.

Mäki-Ikola, O. and Granfors, K. (1992*b*). Salmonella-triggered reactive arthritis. *Scandinavian Journal of Rheumatology*, **21**, 265–70.

Mäki-Ikola, O., Viljanen, M. K., Tiitinen, S., Toivanen, P., and Granfors, K. (1991). Antibodies to arthritis-associated microbes in inflammatory joint diseases. *Rheumatology International*, **10**, 231–4.

Mäki-Ikola, O., Yli-Kerttula, U., Saario, R., Toivanen, P., and Granfors, K. (1992). Salmonella-specific antibodies in serum and synovial fluid in reactive arthritis. *British Journal of Rheumatology*, **31**, 25–9.

Mäki-Ikola, O., Arvilommi, H., Gaston, J. S. H., and Granfors, K. (1993). Salmonella antibodies in healthy populations in Finland and the UK—how many Salmonella-triggered reactive arthritides are there? *British Journal of Rheumatology*, **32**, 262–3.

Mäki-Ikola, O., Lahesmaa, R., Heesemann, J., *et al.* (1994*a*). Yersinia-specific antibodies in serum and synovial fluid in patients with Yersinia triggered reactive arthritis. *Annals of the Rheumatic Diseases*, **53**, 535–9.

Mäki-Ikola, O., Lehtinen, K., Nissilä, M., and Granfors, K. (1994*b*). IgM, IgA and IgG class serum antibodies against *Klebsiella pneumoniae* and *Escherichia coli* lipopolysaccharides in patients with ankylosing spondylitis. *British Journal of Rheumatology*, **33**, 1025–9.

Mäki-Ikola, O., Lehtinen, K., Toivanen, P., and Granfors, K. (1995*a*). Antibodies to *Klebsiella pneumoniae*, *Escherichia coli* and *Proteus mirabilis* in the sera of ankylosing spondylitis patients with/without iritis and enthesitis. *British Journal of Rheumatology*, **34**, 418–20.

Mäki-Ikola, O., Nissilä, M., Lehtinen, K., Leirisalo-Repo, M., and Granfors, K. (1995*b*). IgA1 and IgA2 subclass antibodies against *Klebsiella pneumoniae* in the sera of patients with peripheral and axial types of ankylosing spondylitis. *Annals of the Rheumatic Diseases*, **54**, 631–5.

Mäki-Ikola, O., Nissilä, M., Lehtinen, K., Leirisalo-Repo, M., Toivanen, P., and Granfors, K. (1995*c*). Antibodies to *Klebsiella pneumoniae*, *Escherichia coli* and *Proteus mirabilis* in the sera of patients with axial and peripheral form of ankylosing spondylitis. *British Journal of Rheumatology*, **34**, 413–17.

Mäki-Ikola, O., Mertsola, J., Granfors, K. *et al.* (1997). No endotoxin detected in plasma of patients with ankylosing spondylitis. *Annals of the Rheumatic Diseases*, **56**, 279.

Maksymowych, W. P. and Russell, A. S. (1995). Polymorphism in the LMP2 gene influences the relative risk for acute anterior uveitis in unselected patients with ankylosing spondylitis. *Clinical and Investigative Medicine—Medicine Clinique et Experimentale*, **18**, 42–6.

Maksymowych, W. P., Wessler, A., Schmitt-Egenolf, *et al.* (1994). Polymorphism in an HLA linked proteasome gene influences phenotypic expression of disease in HLA-positive individuals. *Journal of Rheumatology*, **21**, 665–9.

Maksymowych, W. P., Suarez-Almazor, M., Chou, C.-T., and Russell, A. S. (1995*a*). Polymorphism in the LMP2 gene influences susceptibility to extraspinal disease in HLA-B27 positive individuals with ankylosing spondylitis. *Annals of Rheumatic Diseases*, **54**, 321–4.

Maksymowych, W. P., Chou, C. T., and Russell, A. S. (1995*b*). Matching prevalence of peripheral arthritis and acute anterior uveitis in individuals with ankylosing spondylitis. *Annals of the Rheumatic Diseases*, **54**, 128–30.

Maksymowych, W. P., Tao, S., Li, Y., Wing, M., and Russell, A. S. (1995*c*). Allelic variation at the TAP 1 locus influences disease phenotype in HLA-B27 positive individuals with ankylosing spondylitis. *Tissue Antigens*, **45**, 328–32.

Malchow, H., Ewe, K., Brands, J. W., *et al.* (1984). European Cooperative Disease Study (ECDS): results of drug treatment. *Gastroenterology*, **86**, 249–66.

Mallas, E. C., Mc Intosh, P., Asquith, P., *et al.* (1976). Histocompatibility antigens in inflammatory bowel disease: their clinical significance and their association with arthropathy with special reference to HLA-B27. *Gut*, **17**, 906–10.

Malleson, P. N., Fung, M. Y., and Rosenberg, A. M. (1996). The incidence of pediatric rheumatic diseases: results from the Canadian Pediatric Rheumatology Association Disease Registry. *Journal of Rheumatology*, **23**, 1975–80.

Malleson, P. N., and Petty, R. E. (1997). Clinical and therapeutic aspects of juvenile-onset spondyloarthropathies. *Current Opinion in Rheumatology*, **9**, 291–4.

Mallya, R. K., de Beer, F. C., Berry, H., Hamilton, E. D. B., Mace, E. E. W., and Pepys, M. B. (1982). Correlation of clinical parameters of disease activity in rheumatoid arthritis with serum concentration of C-reactive protein and erythrocyte sedimentation rate. *Journal of Rheumatology*, **9**, 224–8.

Mander, M., Simpson, J. M., McLellan, A., Walker, D., Goodacre, J. A., and Dick, W. C. (1987). Studies with an enthesis index as a method of clinical assessment in ankylosing spondylitis. *Annals of Rheumatic Disease*, **46**, 197–202.

Manor, E. and Sarow, J. (1986). Fate of *Chlamydia trachomatis* in human monocytes and monocyte-derived macrophages. *Infection and Immunity*, **54**, 90–5.

Marcos, C. Y., Fernandez-Viña, M. A., Lazaro, A. M., Nulf, C. J., and Stastny, P. (1996). Nucleotide sequence of novel subtypes of HLA-B27, B55 and B57. *Human Immunology* **51** (supplement), 43 (abstract).

Mark, D. B. and McCulley, J. B. (1982). Reiter's keratitis. *Archives of Ophthalmology*, **100**, 781–4.

Marks, J. (1988). Cyclosporin A treatment of severe psoriasis. *British Journal of Dermatology*, **115**, 745–6.

Marks, S. H., Barnett, M., and Calin, A. (1982). A case-control study of juvenile- and adult-onset ankylosing spondylitis. *Journal of Rheumatology*, **9**, 737–41.

Marsal, L., Winblad, S., and Wollheim, F. A. (1981). *Yersinia enterocolitica* arthritis in southern Sweden: a four-year follow-up study. *British Medical Journal*, **283**, 101–3.

Marsh SGE. (1997). Nomenclature for factors of the HLA system, update April 1997. *Tissue Antigens* **50**, 207.

Martin, D. H., Pollack, H., Kuo, C.-C., *et al.* (1984). *Chlamydia trachomatis* infections in men with Reiter's syndrome. *Annals of Internal Medicine*, **100**, 207–13.

Martinez-Gonzales, O., Cantero-Hinojosa, J., Paule-Sastre, P., Gomez-Magan, J. C., and Salvatierra-Rios, D. (1994). Intestinal permeability in patients with ankylosing spondylitis and their healthy relatives. *British Journal of Rheumatology*, **33**, 644–7.

Mascia, M. T., Manzini, C. U., and Manzini, E. (1992). Chlamydia-induced arthritis. Immunofluorescent antibody studies of the synovial fluid from 4 patients (letter). *Clinical and Experimental Rheumatology*, **10**, 425–6.

Matsukawa, A., Ohkawara, S., Maeda, T., Takagi, K., and Yoshinaga, M. (1993). Production of IL-1 and IL-1 receptor antagonist and the pathological significance in lipopoly-saccharide-induced arthritis in rabbits. *Clinical and Experimental Immunology*, **93**, 206–11.

Matsumura, M., Fremont, D. H., *et al.* (1992). Emerging principles for the recognition of peptide antigens by MHC class I molecules. *Science*, **257**, 927–34.

Mattila, L., Leirisalo-Repo, M., Koskimies, S., Granfors, K., and Siitonen, A. (1994). Reactive arthritis following an outbreak of Salmonella infection in Finland. *British Journal of Rheumatology*, **33**, 1136–41.

Matzinger, P. (1994). Memories are made of this? *Nature*, **369**, 605–6.

Mau, W., Zeidler, H., Mau, R., Majewski, A., Freyschmidt, J., Stangel, W., Deicher, H. (1988). Clinical features and prognosis of patients with possible ankylosing spondylitis. Results of a 10-year followup. *Journal of Rheumatology*, **15**, 1109–14.

Mayberry, J. F., Ballantyne, K. C., Hardcastle, J. D., Maugham, C., and Pye, G. (1989). Epidemiological study of asymptomatic inflammatory bowel disease: the identification of cases during a screening programme for colorectal cancer. *Gut*, **30**, 481–3.

Mayer, L. and Janowitz, H. (1983). Extraintestinal manifestations of inflammatory bowel and disease. In *Inflammatory bowel disease* (ed. R. Allan, M. Keighley, S. Alexander-Williams, and C. Hawkins), pp. 501–11. Churchill Livingstone, London.

McCall, R. D., Haskill, S., Zimmermann, E. M., Lund, P. K., Thompson, R. C., and Sartor, R. B. (1994). Tissue IL-1 and IL-1 receptor antagonist expression in rat strains variably susceptible to granulomatous enterocolitis. *Gastroenterology*, **106**, 960–72.

McCannel, C. A., Holland, G. N., Helm, C. J., *et al.* (1996). Causes of uveitis in the general practice of ophthalmology. *American Journal of Ophthalmology*, **121**, 35–46.

McConkey, B., Crockson, R. A., and Crockson, A. R. (1972). The assessment of rheumatoid arthritis. A study based on the measurement of the acute phase reactions. *Quarterly Journal of Medicine*, **14**, 115–25.

McCormack, W. M., Alpert, S., McComb, D. E., *et al.* (1979). Fifteen month follow up study of women infected with *Chlamydia trachomatis*. *New England Journal of Medicine*, **300**, 123–5.

McEniff, N., Eustace, S., McCarthry, C., O'Malley, M., O'Morain, C. A., and Hamilton, S. (1995). Asymptomatic sacroiliitis in inflammatory bowel disease. *Clinical Imaging*, **19**, 258–62.

McEwen, G., Lingg, C., and Kirsner, J.B. (1962). Arthritis accompanying ulcerative colitis. *American Journal of Medicine*, **33**, 923–41.

McEwen, C., DiTata, D., Lingg, C. *et al.* (1971). Ankylosing spondylitis and spondylitis accompanying ulcerative colitis, regional enteritis, psoriasis and Reiter's disease: a comparative study. *Arthritis and Rheumatism*, **14**, 291–318.

McHugh, N., Laurent, M.,*et al.* (1987). Psoriatic arthritis: clinical subgroups and histocompatability antigens. *Annals of Rheumatic Diseases*, **46**, 184–18.

MacLean, I.L., Lowdell, M.W., *et al.* (1992). Absence of a specific effect of free radicals on HLA-B27. *Annals of Rheumatic Diseases*, **51**, 963–4.

MacLean, I.L., Iqball, S., *et al.* (1993). HLA-B27 subtypes in the spondarthropathies. *Clinic of Experimental Immunology*, **91**, 214–19.

MacLean, I.L., Hammer, R.E., and Taurog, J.D. (1994). Cytokine and T cell receptor Vb mRNA profiles in the inflammatory disease of HLA-B27 transgenic rats. *Arthritis and Rheumatism*, **37**, S223 (abstract).

MacLean, L., Hammer, R.E., and Taurog, J.D. (1995). Contrasting cytokine profiles in colitis and synovitis of HLA-B27 transgenic rats. *Arthritis and Rheumatism*, **38**, S315 (abstract).

Meenan, R.F., Gertman, P.M., and Mason, J.H. (1980). Measuring health status in arthritis: the arthritis impact measurement scales. *Arthritis and Rheumatism*, **23**, 146–52.

Merilahti-Palo, R., Söderström, K.-O., Lahesmaa-Rantala, R., Granfors, K., and Toivanen, A. (1991). Bacterial antigens in synovial biopsy specimens in yersinia triggered reactive arthritis. *Annals of the Rheumatic Diseases*, **50**, 87–90.

Mertz, A. K. H., Batsford, S. R., Curschellas, E., Kist, M. J., and Gondolf, K. B. (1991). Cationic Yersinia antigen-induced chronic allergic arthritis in rats: a model for reactive arthritis in humans. *Journal of Clinical Investigations*, **87**, 632–42.

Mertz, A., Daser, A., Skurnik, M., *et al.* (1994). The evolutionary conserved ribosomal protein L23 and the cationic urease β subunit of *Yersinia enterocolitica* 0:3 belong to the immunodominant antigens in Yersinia-triggered reactive arthritis: Implications for autoimmunity. *Molecular Medicine*, **1**, 44–55.

Mertz, A. K. H., Ugrinovic, S., Lauster, R., *et al.* (1997). Characterization of the synovial T cell response to various recombinant Yersinia antigens in Yersinia-triggered reactive arthritis: the hsp60 drives the major immune response. *Arthritis and Rheumatism* (in press).

Mielants, H. and Veys, E.M. (1990). The gut in the spondylarthropathies. *Journal of Rheumatology*, **17**, 7–10.

Mielants, H. and Veys, E.M. (1995). The gut and reactive arthritis. *Rheumatology in Europe*, **24**, 9–11.

Mielants, H., Veys, E.M., and Joos, R. (1986*a*). Sulphasalazine (Salazopyrin) in the treatment of enterogenic reactive synovitis and ankylosing spondylitis with peripheral arthritis. *Clinical Rheumatology*, **5**, 80–3.

Mielants, H., Veys, E.M., Joos, R., Cuvelier, C., and De Vos, M. (1986*b*). Familial aggregation in seronegative spondylarthropathies of enterogenic origin: a family study. *Journal of Rheumatology*, **13**, 126–8.

Mielants, H., Veys, E.M., Joos, R., Cuvelier, C., and De Vos, M. (1987*a*). Repeat ileocolonoscopy in reactive arthritis. *Journal of Rheumatology*, **14**, 456–8.

Mielants, H., Veys, E.M., Joos, R., Noens, L., Cuvelier, C., and De Vos, M. (1987*b*). HLA-antigens in seronegative spondylarthropathies. Reactive arthritis and arthritis in ankylosing spondylitis: relation to gut inflammation. *Journal of Rheumatology*, **14**, 466–71.

Mielants, H., Veys, E. M., Joos, R., Cuvelier, C., De Vos, M., and Proot, F. (1987*c*). Late onset pauci-articular juvenile chronic arthritis in relation to gut inflammation. *Journal of Rheumatology*, **14**, 459–65.

Mielants, H., Veys, E. M., Cuvelier, C., and De Vos, M. (1988). Ileocolonoscopic findings in seronegative spondyloarthropathies. *British Journal of Rheumatology*, **27** (Suppl II), 95–105.

Mielants, H., Veys, E. M., Goethals K., Vanderstraeten, C., Ackerman, C., and Goemaere, S. (1990*a*). Destructive hip lesions in seronegative spondylarthropathies. Relation to gut inflammation. *Journal of Rheumatology*, **17**, 335–40.

Mielants, H., Veys, E. M., Goethals K., Vanderstraeten, C., and Ackerman, C. (1990*b*). Destructive lesions of small joints in seronegative spondylarthropathies. Relation to gut inflammation. *Clinical and Experimental Rheumatology*, **8**, 23–7.

Mielants, H., Veys, E.M., and Joos, R. (1990*c*). Sulphasalazine in the treatment of enterogenic reactive arthritis and ankylosing spondylitis with peripheral arthritis. *Clinical Rheumatology*, **5**, 80–6.

Mielants, H., Veys, E. M., Verbraeken, H., De Vos, M., and Cuvelier, C. (1990*d*). HLA-B27 positive idiopathic acute anterior uveitis: a unique manifestation of subclinical gut inflammation. *Journal of Rheumatology*, **17**, 841–2.

Mielants, H., Veys, E.M., Goemaere, S., Goethals, K., Cuvelier, C., and De Vos, M. (1991*a*). Gut inflammation in the spondylarthropathies: clinical, radiological, biological and genetic features in relation to the type of histology. A prospective study. *Journal of Rheumatology*, **18**, 1542–51.

Mielants, H., Goemaere, S., De Vos, M., *et al.* (1991*b*). Intestinal mucosal permeability in inflammatory rheumatic diseases. I. Role of anti-inflammatory drugs. *Journal of Rheumatology*, **18**, 389–93.

Mielants, H., De Vos, M., Goemaere, S., *et al.* (1991*c*). Intestinal mucosal permeability in inflammatory rheumatic diseases. II. Role of disease. *Journal of Rheumatology*, **18**, 394–400.

Mielants, H., Veys, E.M., Goemaere, S., Cuvelier, C., and De Vos, M. (1993*a*). A prospective study of patients with spondylarthropathy with special reference to HLA-B27 and gut histology. *Journal of Rheumatology*, **20**, 1353–8.

Mielants, H., Veys, E. M., Maertens, M., *et al.* (1993*b*). Prevalence of inflammatory rheumatic diseases in an adolescent urban student population, age 12 to 18, in Belgium. *Clinical and Experimental Rheumatology*, **11**, 563–7.

Mielants, H., Veys, E.M., Cuvelier, C., De Vos, M., Goemaere, S., and Maertens, M. (1993*c*). Gut inflammation in children with late onset pauci-articular juvenile chronic arthritis and evolution to adult spondylarthropathy: a prospective study. *Journal of Rheumatology*, **20**, 1567–72.

Mielants, H., Veys, E. M., De Vos, M., *et al.* (1995*a*). The evolution of spondylarthropathies in relation to gut histology. I. Clinical aspects. *Journal of Rheumatology*, **22**, 2266–72.

Mielants, H., Veys, E.M., Cuvelier, C., *et al.* (1995*b*). The evolution of spondylarthropathies in relation to gut histology. II. Histological aspects. *Journal of Rheumatology*, **22**, 2273–8.

Mielants, H., Veys, E. M., Cuvelier, C., *et al.* (1995*c*). The evolution of spondyloarthropathies in relation to gut histology. III. Relation between gut and joint. *Journal of Rheumatology*, **22**, 2279–84.

Mielants, H., Veys, E. M., Cuvelier, C., and de Vos, M. (1996). Course of gut inflammation in spondylarthropathies and therapeutic consequences. *Baillière's Clinical Rheumatology*, **10**, 147–64.

Mijiyawa, M. (1993). Spondyloarthropathies in patients attending the Rheumatology Unit of Lome Hospital. *Journal of Rheumatology*, **20**, 1167–9.

Mikecz, K., Glant, T. T., and Poole, A. R. (1987). Immunity to cartilage proteoglycans in BALB/c mice with progressive polyarthritis and ankylosing spondylitis induced by injection of human cartilage proteoglycan. *Arthritis and Rheumatism*, **30**, 306–18.

Mikecz, K., Glant, T. T., Baron, M., and Poole, A. R. (1988). Isolation of proteoglycan-specific T lymphocytes from patients with ankylosing spondylitis. *Cellular Immunology*, **112**, 55–63.

Mikecz, K., Glant, T. T., Buzas, E., and Poole, A. R. (1990). Proteoglycan-induced polyarthritis and spondylitis adoptively transferred to naive (nonimmunized) BALB/c mice. *Arthritis and Rheumatism*, **33**, 866–76.

Mir-Madilessi, S. H., Taylor, J. S., and Farmer, R. G. (1985). Clinical course and evolution of erythema nodosum and pyoderma gangrenosum in chronic ulcerative colitis: a study of 42 patients. *American Journal of Gastroenterology*, **80**, 615–20.

Moll, J. M. H. (ed.) (1980). *Ankylosing spondylitis*. Churchill Livingstone, Edinburgh.

Moll, J. H. M. (1985). Inflammatory bowel disease. *Clinics of Rheumatic Diseases*, **11**, 87–113.

Moll, J. M. H. and Wright, V. (1972). An objective clinical method of measuring spinal extension. *Rheum Phys Med*, **11**, 293–312.

Moll, J. M. H. and Wright, V. (1973). Psoriatic arthritis. *Seminars in Arthritis and Rheumatism*, **3**, 55–78.

Moll, J. M. H., Haslock, I., MacRae, I., *et al.* (1974). Associations between ankylosing spondylitis, psoriatic arthritis, Reiter's disease, the intestinal arthropathies, and Behcet's syndrome. *Medicine*, **53**, 343–64.

Møller, P. (1990). Lewis (Secretor) phenotype and ankylosing spondylitis. *Scandinavian Journal of Rheumatology*, **19**, 248.

Møller, P., Berg, K., and Vinje, O. (1981). HLA phenotypes and joint affection in psoriasis, acute anterior uveitis and chronic prostatitis. *Clinical Genetics*, **19**, 266–70.

Monsen, U., Sorstad, J., Hellers, G., and Johansson, C. (1990). Extracolonic diagnoses in ulcerative colitis: An epidemiological study. *American Journal of Gastroenterology*, **85**, 711–16.

Morris, A. J., Madhock, R., Sturrock, R. D., Capell, H. A., and Mac Kenzie, J. F. (1991). Enteroscopic diagnosis of small bowel ulceration in patients receiving non-steroidal anti-inflammatory drugs. *Lancet*, **337**, 520.

Mullin, G. E., Maycon, Z. Braun-Elwert, L., *et al.* (1996). Inflammatory bowel disease mucosal biopsies have specialized lymphokine mRNA profiles. *Inflammatory Bowel Disease*, **2**, 16–26.

Murch, S. H., Lamkin, V. A., Savage, M. O., Walker-Smith, J. A., and MacDonald, T. T. (1991). Serum concentrations of tumour necrosis factor in childhood chronic inflammatory bowel disease. *Gut*, **32**, 913–7.

Murray, G. C. and Persellin, R. H. (1981). Cervical fracture complicating ankylosing spondylitis. A report of eight cases and review of the literature. *American Journal of Medicine*, **70**, 1033–41.

Naides, S. J. (1995). Viral arthritis including HIV. *Current Opinion in Rheumatology*, **7**, 337–42.

Nanagara, R., Li, F., Beutler, A., Hudson, A., and Schumacher, H. R. Jr. (1995). Alteration of *Chlamydia trachomatis* biologic behavior in synovial membranes. *Arthritis and Rheumatism*, **38**, 1410–17.

Naom, L., Lee, J., Ford, D., Bowman, S. J., Lanchbury, J. S., Haris, I., Hodgson, S. V., Easton, D., Lennard-Jones, J., and Mathew, C. G. (1996). Analysis of the contribution of HLA genes to the genetic predisposition to inflammatory bowel disease. *American Journal of Human Genetics* **59**, 266–33.

Nashel, D. J., Petrone, D. L., Ulmer, C. C., and Sliwinski, A. J. (1986). C-reactive protein: a marker for disease activity in ankylosing spondylitis and Reiter's syndrome. *Journal of Rheumatology*, **13**, 364–7.

Nasution, A. R., Mardjuadi, A., Suryadhana, N. G., *et al.* (1993). Higher relative risk of spondylarthropathies among B27 positive Indonesian Chinese than native Indonesians. *Journal of Rheumatology*, **20**, 988–90.

Nasution, A. R., Majuardi, A., *et al.* (1996). HLA-B27 subtypes and their association with ankylosing spondylitis. *Proceedings of APLAR Congress of Rheumatology*, P43.

Nasution, A. R., Mardjuadi, A., Kunmartini, S., *et al.* (1997). HLA-B27 subtypes positively and negatively associated with spondyloarthropathy. *Journal of Rheumatology*, **24**, 111–4.

Nehls, M., Pfeifer, D., Schorpp, M., Hedrich, H., and Boehm, T. (1994). New member of the winged-helix protein family disrupted in mouse and rat nude mutations. *Nature*, **372**, 103–7.

Nepom, G. T. (1990). A unified hypothesis for the complex genetics of HLA associations with IDDM. *Diabetes*, **39**, 1153–7.

Nettelnbreker, E., Koehler, L., Barthels, H., Dreses-Werringloer, U., and Zeidler, H. (1994). Persistent infection of the monocytic cell line U937 with *Chlamydia trachomatis* and expression of the 57 kD heat shock protein. In *Chlamydial infections. Proceedings of the eighth international symposium on human chlamydial infections* (ed. J. Orfila *et al.*), pp 447–50. Societa editrice eosulapio, Italy.

Neumann, V. and Wright, V. (1983). Arthritis associated with bowel disease. *Clinics in Gastroenterology*, **12**, 767–95.

Nickerson, C. L., Luthra, H. L., Savarirayan, S., and David, C. (1990). Susceptibility of HLA-B27 transgenic mice to *Yersinia enterocolitica* infection. *Human Immunology*, **28**, 382–96.

Nikkari, S. (1994). *Use of PCR in studies on microbial involvement in arthritis*. Dissertation, Department of Medical Microbiology, Turku University.

Nikkari, S., Merilahti-Palo, R., Saario, R., *et al.* (1992). Yersinia-triggered reactive arthritis. Use of polymerase chain reaction and immunocytochemical staining in the detection of bacterial components from synovial specimens. *Arthritis and Rheumatism*, **36**, 1080–6.

Nissilä, M., Lehtinen, K., Leirisalo-Repo, M., Luukkainen, R., Mutru, O., and Yli-Kerttula, U. (1988) Sulphasalazine in the treatment of ankylosing spondylitis. *Arthritis and Rheumatism*, **31**,1111–16.

Nissilä, M., Lahesmaa, R., Leirisalo-Repo, M., Lehtinen, K., Toivanen, P., and Granfors, K. (1994). Antibodies to *Klebsiella pneumoniae*, *Escherichia coli* and *Proteus mirabilis* in ankylosing spondylitis: effect of sulfasalazine treatment. *Journal of Rheumatology*, **21**, 2082–7.

Njobva, P. D., McGill, P. E., Jellis, J. E., and Pobee, J. O. M. (1997). Rheumatic disorders at a Zambian teaching hospital. *British Journal of Rheumatology*, **36**, 404–5.

Noer, H. R. (1966). An 'experimental' epidemic of Reiter's syndrome. *Journal of the American Medical Association*, **198**, 693–8.

Norton, K. I., Eichenfield, A. M., Rosh, J. R., Stern, M. T., and Hermann, G. (1993). Atypical arthropathy associated with Crohn's disease. *American Journal of Gastroenterology*, **88**, 948–52.

Norton, W. L., Lewis, D., and Ziff, M. D. (1966). Light and electron microscopic observations on the synovitis of Reiter's disease. *Arthritis and Rheumatism*, **9**, 747–57.

Noyori, K., Okamoto, R., Takagi, T., Hyodo, A., Suzuke, K., and Koshino, T. (1994). Experimental induction of arthritis in rats immunized with *Escherichia coli 0:14* lipopolysaccharide. *Journal of Rheumatology*, **21**, 484–8.

Nurminen, M., Leinonen, M., and Saikku, P. (1983). The genus-specific antigen of Chlamydia: resemblance to the lipopolysaccharide of enteric bacteria. *Science*, **220**, 1279–81.

Oates, J. K. and Hancock, J. A. H. (1959). Neurological symptoms and lesions occurring in the course of Reiter's disease. *American Journal of Medical Science*, **238**, 79.

O'Brien, W. M., Van Scott, E. J., Black, R., and Eisen, A. (1962). Clinical trial of amethopterin (methotrexate) in psoriatic and rheumatoid arthritis (preliminary report). *Arthritis and Rheumatism*, **5**, 312–16.

Obst, R., Armandola, E., *et al.* (1995). TAP polymorphism does not influence transport of peptide variants in mice and humans. *European Journal of Immunology*, **25**, 2170–6.

Odeh, M. and Oliven, A. (1992). Chlamydial infections of the heart. *European Journal of Clinical Microbiology and Infectious Disease*, **11**, 885–93.

O'Donnell, B., O'Laughlin, S., *et al.* (1993). HLA typing in Irish psoriatics. *Irish Medical Journal*, **86**, 65–8.

Oen, K. G., and Cheang, M. (1996). Epidemiology of chronic arthritis in childhood. *Seminars in Arthritis and Rheumatism*, **26**, 575–91.

Oen, K., Postl, B., Chalmers, I. M., *et al.* (1986). Rheumatic diseases in an Inuit population. *Arthritis and Rheumatism*, **29**, 65–74.

Oh, M. K., Florence, R., Brown, P. R., Richey, C. M., and Hook, E. W. (1996). PCR-based urine screening for chlamydia in females: Utility in an urban adolescent clinic setting (Abst). *Journal of Investigative Medicine*, **44**, 22A.

Oldstone, M. B. A., Nerenberg, M., Southern, P., Price, J., and Lewicki, H. (1991). Virus infection triggers insulin-dependent diabetes mellitus in a transgenic model—role of anti-self (virus) immune response. *Cell*, **65**, 319–31.

Olivieri, I., Padula, A., Pierro, A., Favaro, L., Oranges, G. S., and Ferri, S. (1995). Late onset undifferentiated spondyloarthropathy. *Journal of Rheumatology*, **22**, 899–903.

Olivieri, I., Cantini, F., and Salvarani, C. (1997). Diagnostic and classification criteria, clinical and functional assessment, and therapeutic advances for spondyloarthropathies. *Current Opinion in Rheumatology*, **9**, 284–90.

O'Mahony, S., Anderson, N., Nuki, G., and Ferguson, A. (1992). Systemic and mucosal antibodies to klebsiella in patients with ankylosing spondylitis and Crohn's disease. *Annals of the Rheumatic Diseases* **51**, 1296–300.

Omdal, R. and Husby, G. (1987). Renal affection in patients with ankylosing spondylitis and psoriatic arthritis. *Clinical Rheumatology*, **6**, 74–9.

O'Neill, T. W. and Bresnihan, B. (1992). The heart in ankylosing spondylitis. *Annals of Rheumatic Diseases*, **51**, 705–6.

O'Neill, T. W., Harrison, B. J., Yin, J. A. L., and Holt, P. J. L. (1997). Ankylosing spondylitis associated with IgA lamda chain myeloma. *British Journal of Rheumatology*, **36**, 401–2.

Østensen, M. (1992). The effect of pregnancy on ankylosing spondylitis, psoriatic arthritis, and juvenile rheumatoid arthritis. *American Journal of Reproductive Immunology*, **28**, 235–7.

Østensen, M. and Husby, G. (1990). Seronegative spondylarthritis and ankylosing spondylitis: biological effects and management of disease during pregnancy. In *Pregnancy, auto-immunity and connective tissue disorders* (ed. J. S. Scott and H. A. Bird), pp. 163–184. Oxford University Press, Oxford.

Østernsen, M., Romberg, O., and Husby, G. (1982). Ankylosing spondylitis and motherhood. *Arthritis and Rheumatism*, **25**, 140–3.

Pal, A., Hill, M. R., *et al.* (1997). Secretor status and ankylosing spondylitis. *British Journal of Rheumatology*. (In press.)

Palazzi, C., D'Amico, E., Fratelli, V., Capani, F. (1997). Chronic arthritis after genitourinary inflammation: response to quinolones. *Journal of Clinical Rheumatology* **3,** 183–4.

Palit, J., Hill, J., Capell, A., *et al.* (1990). A multicenter double-blind comparison of auranofin, intramuscular gold thiomalate and placebo in patients with psoriatic arthritis. *British Journal of Dermatology*, **29**, 280–3.

Palmiter, R. D. and Brinster, R. L. (1986). Germ-line transformation of mice. *Annual Review of Genetics*, **20**, 465–99.

Pande, I., Mackay, K., Chatfield, C., and Calin, A. (1995). The Bath Ankylosing Spondylitis Radiology Index (BASRI): a new validated approach to disease assessment. *British Journal of Rheumatology*, **34** (Suppl. 2), 37.

Pando, J. A., Yarboro, C., Ellaban, A., *et al.* (1995). Prevalence of *Chlamydia trachomatis* by PCR in the synovium of patients with early rheumatoid arthritis. *Arthritis and Rheumatism*, **38** (Suppl), S287.

Parham, P., Adams, E. J., Arnett, K. L. (1995). The origins of HLA-A,B,C polymorphism. *Immunology Review* **143**, 141–80.

Parham, P. and Ohta, T. (1996). Population biology of antigen presentation by MHC class I molecules. *Science*, **272**, 67–74.

Parham, P. (1996). Presentation of HLA Class I-derived peptides: Potential involvement in allorecognition and HLA-B27-associated arthritis. *Immunological Reviews*, **154**, 137–54.

Park, H., Schumacher, H. R., Zeiger, A. R., and Rosenbaum, J. T. (1984). Antibodies to peptidoglycan in patients with spondylarthritis: A clue to disease aetiology? *Annals of the Rheumatic Diseases*, **43**, 725–8.

Parker KC, Biddison WE, Coligan JE. (1994). Pocket mutations of HLA-B27 show that anchor residues act cumulatively to stabilize peptide binding, *Biochemistry* **33,** 7736–43.

Paronen, I. (1948). Reiter's disease. A study of 344 cases observed in Finland. *Acta Medica Scandinavica*, **131** (Suppl. 212), 1–113.

Passo, M. H., Fitzgerald, J. F., and Brandt, K. D. (1986). Arthritis associated with inflammatory bowel disease in children: relationship of joint disease to activity and severity of bowel lesion. *Digestive Diseases and Sciences*, **31**, 492–7.

Paul, W. E. and Seder, R. A. (1994). Lymphocyte responses and cytokines. *Cell*, **76**, 241–51.

Paulus, H. E., Pearson, C. M., Pitts, W. Jr. (1972). Aortic insufficiency in five patients with Reiter's syndrome. A detailed clinical and pathologic study. *American Journal of Medicine* **53,** 464–72.

Pazmany, L., Rowland-Jones, S., Huet, S., *et al.* (1992). Genetic modulation of antigen presentation by HLA-B27 molecules. *Journal of Experimental Medicine*, **175**, 361–9.

Pearlman, M. D. and McNeeley, S. G. (1992). A Review of the microbiology, immunology, and clinical implications of *Chlamydia trachomatis* infections. *Obstetrical and Gynecological Survey*, **47**, 448–61.

Pearlman, S. G., Gerber, L. H., Roberts, M., Nigra, T. P., and Barth, W. F. (1979). Photochemotherapy and psoriatic arthritis. *Annals of Internal Medicine*, **91**, 717–22.

Pearson, C. M. and Chang, Y. H. (1979). Adjuvant disease: pathology and immune reactivity. Workshop IV. Aetiopathogenetic factors in Reiter's syndrome. *Annals of Rheumatic Diseases*, **38**, (Suppl. 1), 102–10.

Pedersen, O. O. (1980). Acute anterior uveitis. *Scandanavian Journal of Rheumatology*, **32** (Suppl), 226–8.

Peeters, A. J., Van den Wall Bake, L., Van Albada-Kuipers, G. A., *et al.* (1988). IgA containing immune complexes and hematuria in ankylosing spondylitis. A prospective longitudinal study. *Journal of Rheumatology*, **15**, 1662–7.

Peeters, A. J., Van den Wall Bake, A. W. I., Daha, M. R., and Breedveld, F. C. (1990). Inflammatory bowel disease and ankylosing spondylitis associated with cutaneous vasculitis, glomerulonephritis, and circulating IgA immune complexes. *Annals of the Rheumatic Diseases*, **49**, 638–40.

Pelegri, C., Morante, M. P., Castellote, C., Franch, A., and Castell, M. (1996). Treatment with an anti-CD4 monoclonal antibody strongly ameliorates established rat adjuvant arthritis. *Clinical and Experimental Immunology*, **103**, 273–8.

Peliskova, Z., Pavelka, K. J., and Trnavsky K (1991). A placebo controlled, double-blind study of Salazopyrin-EN (SASP) in refractory reactive arthritis (ReA). *Scandinavian Journal of Rheumatology*, **80**, 45.

Pepose, J. S., Holland, G. N., and Wilhelmus, K. R. (1996). HLA-B27-associated diseases. In *Ocular infection and immunity* (ed. J. S. Pepose, G. N. Holland, and K. R. Wilhelmus), pp. 475–84. Mosby, St Louis.

Perdomo, O. J. J., Cavaillon, J. M., Huerre, M., Ohayon, H., Gounon, P., Sansonetti, P. J. (1994). Acute inflammation causes epithelial invasion and mucosal destruction in experimental Shigellosis. *Journal of Experimental Medicine*, **180**, 1307–19.

Perkins, E. S. and Folk, J. (1984). Uveitis in London and Iowa. *Ophthalmologica*, **189**, 36–40.

Peterson, M. C. (1994). Rheumatic manifestations of *Campylobacter jejuni* and *C. fetus* infections in adults. *Scandinavian Journal of Rheumatology*, **23**, 167–70.

Pfeifer, J. D., Wick, M. J., Roberts, R. L., Findlay, K., Normark, S. J., and Harding, C. V. (1993). Phagocytic processing of bacterial antigens for class I MHC presentation to T cells. *Nature*, **361**, 359–62.

Piazzini, M., Fioravanti, A., Sabadini, L., Vassalli, D., Bellisai, F., and Marcolongo, R. (1995). Laboratory and instrumental clinical study of 150 patients with arthritis. *Recenti Progressi in Medicine*, **86**, 183–8.

Pierson, D. E. (1994). Mechanisms of Yersinia entry into mammalian cells. *Molecular genetics of bacterial pathogenesis* (ed. V. L. Miller, J. B. Kaper, D. A. Portnoy, and R. R. Isberg), pp. 235–48.

Pile, K. D., Laurent, M. R., Salmond, C. E., Best, M. J., Pyle, E. A., and Moloney, R. O. (1991). Clinical assessment of ankylosing spondylitis: a study of observer variation in spinal measurements. *British Journal of Rheumatology*, **30**, 29–34.

Pinals, R. S. (1986). Arthritis associated with gluten-sensitivity entheropathy. *Journal of Rheumatology*, **13**, 201–3.

Pincus, T., Summey, J. A., Soraci Jr, S. A., Wallston, K. A., and Hummon, N. P. (1983). Assessment of patient satisfaction in activities of daily living using a modified Stanford health assessment questionnaire. *Arthritis and Rheumatism*, **26**, 1346–53.

Ploski, R., Flato, B., Vinje, O., Maksymowych, W., Forre, O., Thorsby, E. (1995). Association to HLA-DRB1*08, HLA-DPB1*0301 and homozygosity for an HLA-linked proteasome gene in juvenile ankylosing spondylitis. *Human Immunology*, **44**, 88–96.

Pope, M., Kotlarski, I., and Doherty, K. (1994). Induction of Lyt-2+ cytotoxic T lymphocytes following primary and secondary Salmonella infection. *Immunology*, **81**, 177–82.

Popert, A. J., Gill, A. J., and Laird, S. M. (1964). A prospective study of Reiter's syndrome. An interim report on the first 82 cases. *British Journal of Venereal Disease*, **40**, 160–5.

Popert, A. J., Jones, P. J., and El-Badawy, S. A. (1996). Ankylosing spondylitis: Treatment of chronic painful focal lesions with low-dose radiotherapy (Abstract). *British Journal of Rheumatology*, **35** (Suppl. 1, Abstract #302), 156.

Powis, S. J., Young, L. L., *et al.* (1993). Major histocompatibility complex-encoded ABC transporters and rat class I peptide motifs. *Transplant Proceedings*, **25**, 2752–3.

Price, R. and Gibson, T. (1986). D-Penicillamine and psoriatic arthropathy. *British Journal of Dermatology*, **25**, 228.

Prieur, A. M., Listrat, V., Dougados, M., and Amor, B. (1990). Evaluation of the ESSG and the Amor criteria for juvenile spondyloarthropathies (JSA). Study of 310 consecutive children referred to one pediatric rheumatology center. *Arthritis and Rheumatism*, **33** (Suppl.), S160.

Prieur, A. M., Listrat, V., Dougados, M., and Amor, B. (1993). Critéres de classification des spondylarthropathies chez les enfants. *Archives Francaises Pediatrie*, **50**, 379–85.

Probst, P., Hermann, E., Meyer zum Büschenfelde, K. -H., and Fleischer, B. (1993*a*). Identification of the *Yersinia enterocolitica* urease β subunit as a target antigen for human synovial T lymphocytes in reactive arthritis. *Infection and Immunity*, **61**, 4507–9.

Probst, P., Hermann, E., Meyer zum Büschenfelde, K.-H., and Fleischer, B. (1993*b*). Multiclonal synovial T cell response to *Yersinia enterocolitica* in reactive arthritis: the Yersinia 61-kDa heat-shock protein is not the major target antigen. *Journal of Infectious Diseases*, **167**, 385–91.

Pullar, T., Hunter, J. A., and Capell, H. A. (1985). Which component of Sulphasalazine is active in rheumatoid arthritis? *British Journal of Rheumatology*, **290**, 1535–8.

Purrmann, J., Zeidler, H., Bertrams, J., *et al.* (1988). HLA-antigens in ankylosing spondylitis associated with Crohn's disease. Increased frequency of the HLA phenotype B27, B44. *Journal of Rheumatology*, **15**, 1658–61.

Putterman, C. and Rubinow, A. (1993). Reactive arthritis associated with *Clostridium difficile* pseudomembranous colitis. *Seminars in Arthritis and Rheumatism*, **22**, 420–6.

Quinn, T. C. (1996). Global burden of the HIV pandemic. *Lancet*, **348**, 99–106.

Rahman, M. U., Ahmed, S., Schumacher, R., and Zeiger, A. R. (1990). High levels of antipeptidoglycan antibodies in psoriatic and other seronegative arthritides. *Journal of Rheumatology*, **17**, 621–5.

Rahman, M. U., Cheema, M. A., Schumacher, H. R., and Hudson, A. P. (1992*a*). Molecular evidence for the presence of chlamydia in the synovium of patients with Reiter's syndrome. *Arthritis and Rheumatism*, **35**, 521–9.

Rahman, M. U., Hudson, A. P., and Schumacher, H. R. (1992*b*). Chlamydia and Reiter's syndrome (reactive arthritis). *Rheumatic Disease Clinics of North America*, **18**, 67–9.

Ramirez-Solis, R. and Bradley, A. (1994). Advances in the use of embryonic stem cell technology. *Current Opinion in Biotechnology*, **5**, 528–33.

Rammensee, H., Friede, T., *et al.* (1995). MHC ligands and peptide motifs: first listing. *Immunogenetics*, **41**, 178–228.

Ramos-Remus, C., Major, P., Gomez-Vargas, A. *et al.* (1997). Temporomandibular joint osseous morphology in a consecutive sample of ankylosing spondylitis patients. *Annals of Rheumatic Diseases*, **56**, 103–7.

Rampton, D. S., Mc Neil, N. L., and Sarner, M. (1993). Analgesic ingestion and other factors preceding relapse in ulcerative colitis. *Gut*, **24**, 187–9.

Rankin, G. B. (1990). Extraintestinal and systemic manifestations of inflammatory bowel disease. *Medical Clinics of North America*, **74**, 39–50.

Rath, H. C., Herfarth, H. H., Grenther, T., *et al.* (1996*a*). Normal luminal bacteria, particularly *Bacteroides*, mediate chronic colonic, gastric, and systemic inflammation in HLA-B27 transgenic rats, *Journal of Clinical Investigation*, **98**, 945–53.

Rath, H. C., Ikeda, J. S., Herfarth, H. H., *et al.* (1996*b*). Anaerobic bacteria, especially *Bacteroides sp.,* stimulate colitis and gastritis in HLA-B27 transgenic rats. *Gastroenterology*, **110**, A998.

Reed, W. W. B. and Becker, S. W. (1960). Psoriasis and arthritis. *Archives of Dermatology*, **81**, 577–85.

Reid, G. D., Patterson, M. W. H., and Patterson, A. C. P. (1979). Aortic insufficiency in association with juvenile ankylosing spondylitis *Journal of Pediatrics*, **95**, 78–90.

Reiter, H. (1916). Über eube bisher underkannte Spirochaeteninfektion (spirochaetosis arthritica). *Deutsche Medizinische Wochenshrift*, **42**, 1535–6.

Relman, D. A., Schmidt, T. M., Mac Dermott, R. P., and Falkow, S. (1992). Identification of the uncultured bacillus of Whipple's disease. *New England Journal of Medicine*, **327**, 293–301.

Remmers, E. L., Longman, R. E., Du, Y., O'Hare, A., Cannon, G. W., Griffiths, M. M., Wilder, R. L. (1996). A genome scan localizes five non-MHC loci controlling collagen-induced arthritis in rats. *Nature Genetics*, **14**, 82–5.

Ren, E. C., Koh, W. H., Sim, D., *et al.* (1997). Possible protective role of HLA-B*2706 for ankylosing spondylitis. *Tissue Antigens*, **49**, 67–9.

Resnick, D. and Niwayama, G. (1995) Ankylosing spondylitis. In *Diagnosis of bone and joint disorders* (ed. D. Resnick), pp. 1008–74. W. B. Saunders, Philadelphia.

Reveille, J. D., Suarez, A. M., *et al.* (1994). HLA in ankylosing spondylitis: is HLA-B27 the only MHC gene involved in disease pathogenesis? *Seminars in Arthritis and Rheumatism*, **23**, 295–309.

Reveille, J., Fraser, P., Taurog, J., *et al.* (1996). HLA-B27 subtypes in African Americans with spondyloarthropathy (SpA). *Arthritis and Rheumatism*, **39**, S204.

Reveille *et al.* 1996—ch 4 p. 17.

Rice-Oxley, J. M. and Truelove, S. (1950). Complications of ulcerative colitis. *Lancet*, **1**, 607–11.

Richens, J. and McGill, P. E. (1995). The spondyloarthropathies. *Baillière's Clinical Rheumatology*, **9**, 95–109.

Rigby, A. S. and Wood, P. H. N. (1993). Observations on diagnostic criteria for ankylosing spondylitis. *Clinical and Experimental Rheumatology*, **11**, 5–12.

Riley, S. A., Mani, V., Goodman, M. J., and Lucas, S. (1990). Why do patients with ulcerative colitis relapse? *Gut*, **31**, 179–83.

Roberton, D. M., Cabral, D. A., Malleson, P. N., and Petty, R. E. (1996). Juvenile psoriatic arthritis: followup and evaluation of diagnostic criteria. *Journal of Rheumatology*, **23**, 166–70.

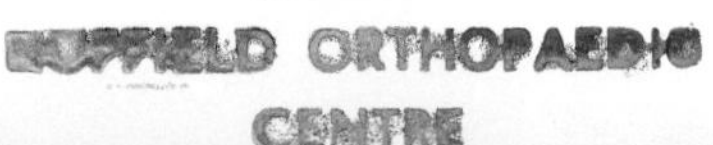

Roberts, M. E. T., Wright, V., Hill, A. G. S., and Mehra, A. C. (1976). Psoriatic arthritis. Follow-up study. *Annals of Rheumatic Diseases*, **35**, 206–12.

Roberts, R. S. (1993). Pooled outcome measures in arthritis: the pros and cons. *Journal of Rheumatology*, **20**, 566–7.

Robinson, W. P., van der Linden, S. M., Khan, M. A., *et al.* G. (1989). HLA-Bw60 increases susceptibility to ankylosing spondylitis in HLA-B27+ patients. *Arthritis and Rheumatism*, **32**, 1135–41.

Rock, K. L. (1996). A new foreign policy—MHC class I molecules monitor the outside world. *Immunology Today*, **17**, 131–7.

Rodriguez, A., Akova, Y. A., Pedroza-Seres, M., and Foster, C. S. (1996). Posterior segment ocular manifestations in patients with HLA-B27-associated uveitis. *Ophthalmology*, **101**, 1267–4.

Rojo, S., García, F., Villadangos, J. A., López de Castro, J. A. (1993). Changes in the repertoire of peptides bound to HLA-B27 subtypes and to site-specific mutants inside and outside pocket B. *Journal of Experimental Medicine* **177**, 613–20.

Romanus, H. (1953). Pelvo-spondylitis ossificans in the male. *Acta Medica Scandinavica*, **280** (Suppl.), 1.

Rook, G. A. W. and Stanford, J. L. (1992). Slow bacterial infections or autoimmunity. *Immunology Today*, **13**, 160–4.

Rosenbaum, J. T. (1981). Why HLA-B27: an analysis based on two animal models. *Annals of Internal Medicine*, **94**, 261–3.

Rosenbaum, J. T. (1989*a*). Characterization of uveitis associated with spondyloarthritis. *Journal of Rheumatology*, **16**, 792–6.

Rosenbaum, J. T. (1989*b*). Uveitis. An internist's view. *Archives of Internal Medicine*, **149**, 1173–6.

Rosenbaum, J. T. (1991). Systemic associations of anterior uveitis. *International Ophthalmology, Clinics* **31**, 131–42.

Rosenbaum, J. T. (1992). Acute anterior uveitis and spondyloarthropathies. *Rheumatic Disease Clinics of North America*, **18**, 143–51.

Rosenbaum, J. T., McDevitt, H. O., Guss, R. B., and Egbert, P. R. (1980). Endotoxin-induced uveitis in rats as a model for human disease. *Nature*, **286**, 611–13.

Rosenbaum, J. T., Theofilopoulos, A., McDevitt, H. O., *et al.* (1981). Presence of circulating immune complexes in Reiter's syndrome and ankylosing spondylitis. *Clinical Immunity and Immunopathology*, **18**, 291–7.

Rosenbaum, J. T., Tammaro, J., and Robertson, Jr., J. E. (1991). Uveitis precipitated by non-penetrating ocular trauma. *American Journal of Ophthalmology*, **112**, 392–5.

Rosenberg, A. M. (1987). Uveitis associated with juvenile rheumatoid arthritis. *Seminars in Arthritis and Rheumatism*, **16**, 158–73.

Rosenberg, A. M. and Petty, R. E. (1979) Reiter's disease in children. *American Journal of Diseases of Children*, **133**, 394–8.

Rosenberg, A. M., and Petty, R. E. (1982). A syndrome of seronegative enthesopathy and arthropathy in children. *Arthritis and Rheumatism*, **25**, 1041–7.

Rosenberg, A. M. Petty, R., Oen, K. G., and Schroeder, M. L. (1982). Rheumatic disease in Western Canadian Indian children. *Journal of Rheumatology*, **9**, 589–92.

Rosenow, E., Strimlan, C. V., Muhm, J. R., and Ferguson, R. H. (1977). Pleuropulmonary manifestations of ankylosing spondylitis. *Mayo Clinic Proceedings*, **52**, 641–9.

Rosner, I. A., Burg, C. G., Wisnieski, J. J., *et al.* (1993). The clinical spectrum of the arthropathy associated with hidradenitis suppurativa and acne conglobata. *Journal of Rheumatology*, **20**, 4.

Roth, P.E., Grosshans, E., and Bergoend, H. (1991). Psoriasis: development and fatal complications. *Annals of Dermatology and Venereology*, **118**, 97–105.

Rothova, A., van Veenedaal, M. S., Linssen, A., Glasius, E., Kijlstra, A. and de Jong, P. T. V. M. (1987). Clinical features of acute anterior uveitis. *American Journal of Ophthalmology*, **103**, 137–45.

Rothova, A., Buitenhuis, H. J., Meenken, C., *et al.* (1992). Uveitis and systemic disease. *British Journal of Ophthalmology*, **76**, 137–41.

Rothschild, B. M. and Woods, R. J. (1989). Spondyloarthropathy in gorillas. *Seminars in Arthritis and Rheumatism*, **18**, 267–76.

Rötzschke, O., Falk, K., Deres, K., Schild, H., Norda, M., Metzger, J., Jung, G., Rammensee, H.-G. (1990a). Isolation and analysis of naturally processed viral peptides as recognized by cytotoxic T cells. *Nature* **348**, 252–4.

Rötzschke, O., Falk, K., Wallny, H. J., Faath, S., Rammensee, H. G. (1990b). Characterization of naturally occurring minor histocompatibility peptides including H-4 and H-Y. *Science* **249**, 283–7.

Rötzschke, O., Falk, K., *et al.* (1994). Dominant aromatic/aliphatic C-terminal anchor in HLA-B*2702 and B*2705 peptide motifs. *Immunogenetics*, **39**, 74–7.

Roussomoustakaki, M., Satsangi, J., *et al.* (1996). Genetic markers may predict disease behaviour in patients with ulcerative colitis, *Gastroenterology*, **112**, 1845–53.

Rowland-Jones, S. L., Powis, S. H., Sutton, J., *et al.* (1993). An antigen processing polymorphism revealed by HLA-B8-restricted cytotoxic T lymphocytes which does not correlate with TAP gene polymorphism. *European Journal of Immunology*, **23**, 1999–2004.

Rowson, N. J. and Dart, J. K. (1992). Keratitis in Reiter's syndrome (letter). *British Journal of Ophthalmology*, **76**, 126.

Rubatelli, L., Fiocco, U., Cozzi, L., *et al.* (1994). Prospective sonographic and arthroscopic evaluation of proliferative knee joint synovitis. *Journal of Ultrasound Medecine*, **13**, 855–62.

Rubin, L. A., Amos, C. I., *et al.* (1994). Investigating the genetic basis for ankylosing spondylitis. Linkage studies with the major histocompatibility complex region. *Arthritis and Rheumatism*, **37**, 1212–20.

Rudwaleit, M., Pile, K. D., Burney, R., *et al.* (1994). T-cell receptor germline polymorphism is not a major contributor to ankylosing spondylitis (AS) susceptibility. *British Journal of Rheumatology*, **33** (Suppl. 1), 165.

Rudwaleit, M., Bowness, P., *et al.* (1996). The nucleotide sequence of HLA-B*2704 reveals a new amino acid substitution in exon 4 which is also present in HLA-B*2706. *Immunogenetics*, **43**, 160–2.

Russell, A. S. (1977). Arthritis, inflammatory bowel disease, and histocompatibility antigens (Editorial). *Annals of Internal Medicine*, **86**, 820–1.

Russell, A. S., Lentle, B. C., Percy, J. S., and Jackson, F. I. (1976). Scintigraphy of sacroiliac joints in acute anterior uveitis. A study of thirty patients. *Annals of Internal Medicine*, **85**, 606–8.

Russell, A. S. and Suarez-Almazor, M. E. (1992). Ankylosing spondylitis is not caused by klebsiella. *Rheumatic Disease Clinics of North America*, **18**, 95–104.

Ryan, P. J. and Fogelman, I. (1995). The bone scan: where are we now? *Seminars in Nuclear Medicine*, **25**, 76–91.

Rynes, R. O. I., Volastro, P. S., and Bartholomew, L. E. (1984). Exacerbation of B27 positive spondyloarthropathy by enteric infections. *Journal of Rheumatology*, **11**, 96–7.

Saari, R., Lahti, R., and Saari, K. M. (1982). Frequency of rheumatic diseases in patients with acute anterior uveitis. *Scandinavian Journal of Rheumatology*, **11**, 121–3.

Saario, R. and Toivanen, A. (1993). *Chlamydia pneumoniae* as a cause of reactive arthritis. *British Journal of Rheumatology*, **32**, 1112.

Sahly, H., Kekow, J., Podschun, R., Schaff, M., Gross, W. L., and Ullmann, U. (1994*a*). Comparison of the antibody responses to the 77 Klebsiella capsular types in ankylosing spondylitis and various rheumatic diseases. *Infection and Immunity*, **62**, 4838–43.

Sahly, H., Podschun, R., Sass, R., *et al.* (1994*b*). Serum antibodies to Klebsiella capsular polysaccharides in ankylosing spondylitis. *Arthritis and Rheumatism*, **37**, 754–9.

Saikku, P., Leinonen, M., Teukanen, L., *et al.* (1992). Chronic *Chlamydia pneumoniae* infection as a risk factor for coronary heart disease in the Helsinki heart study. *Annals of Internal Medicine*, **116**, 273–8.

Sairanen, E. and Tiilikainen, A. (1975). HL-A27 in Reiter's disease following shigellosis. *Scandinavian Journal of Rheumatology*, **4** (Suppl. 8), 30–11.

Sairanen, E., Paronen, I., and Mähönen, H. (1969). Reiter's syndrome: a follow-up study. *Acta Medica Scandinavica*, **185**, 57–63.

Salmi, M., Andrew, D. P., Butcher, E. C., and Jalkanen, S. (1995). Dual binding capacity of mucosal immunoblasts to mucosal and synovial endothelium in humans: dissection of the molecular mechanism. *Journal of Experimental Medicine*, **181**, 137–49.

Salmon, J. F., Wright, J. P., Bowen, R. M., and Murray, A. D. (1989). Granulomatous uveitis in Crohn's disease. *Archives Ophthalmologica*, **107**, 718–29.

Salmon, J. F., Wright, J. P., and Murray, A. D. (1991). Acute inflammation in Crohn's disease. *Ophthalmology*, **98**, 480–4.

Salvarani, C., Lo Scocco, G., Macchiono, P., *et al.* (1995). Prevalence of psoriatic arthritis in Italian psoriatic patients. *Journal of Rheumatology*, **22**, 1499–503.

Sampson, H. W. (1988*a*). Spondyloarthropathy in progressive ankylosis (*ank/ank*) mice: morphological features. *Spine*, **13**, 645–9.

Sampson, H. W. (1988*b*). Ultrastructure of the mineralizing metacarpophalangeal joint of progressive ankylosis (*ank/ank*) mice. *American Journal of Anatomy*, **182**, 257–69.

Sampson, H. W. and Davis, J. S. (1988). Histopathology of the intervertebral disc of progressive ankylosis mice. *Spine*, **13**, 650–4.

Sampson, H. W. and Trzeciakowski, J. P. (1990). Intervertebral disk mineralization in progressive ankylosis mice. *Bone and Mineral*, **10**, 71–7.

Sampson, H. W., Davis, R. W., and Dufner, D. C. (1991). Spondyloarthropathy in progressive ankylosis mice: ultrastructural features of the intervertebral disk. *Acta Anatomica*, **141**, 36–41.

Samuel, M. P., Zwillich, S. H., Thomson, G. T. D., *et al.* (1995). Fast food arthritis—a clinico-pathologic study of post-salmonella reactive arthritis. *Journal of Rheumatology*, **22**, 1947–52.

Sanmarti, R., Canete, J. D., *et al.* (1991). Comment on the article by Robinson *et al. Arthritis and Rheumatism*, **34**, 247–8.

Sansonetti, P. J. (1992). Molecular and cellular biology of *Shigella flexneri* invasiveness: from cell assay system to Shigellosis. *Current Topics in Microbiology and Immunology*, **180**, 1–19.

Sansonetti, P. J., Ryter, A., Clerc, P., Maurelli, A. T., and Mounier, J. (1986). Multiplication of Shigella flexneri within HeLa cells: Lysis of the phagocytic vacuole and plasmid-mediated contact hemolysis. *Infection and Immunity*, **51**, 461–9.

Santin, M., Mascaro, J., Nolla, J. M., Roca, G., and Badrinas, F. (1990). To the Editor: Uveitis associated with spondyloarthritis. *Journal of Rheumatology*, **17**, 854.

Sartor, R. B. (1994). Cytokines in intestinal inflammation. Pathophysiologic and clinical considerations. *Gastroenterology*, **106**, 533–9.

Sartor, R. B. (1995*a*). Microbial factors in the pathogenesis of Crohn's disease, ulcerative colitis, and experimental intestinal inflammation. In *Inflammatory bowel disease*, (4th edn) (ed. J. B. Kirsner and R. G. Shorter), pp. 96–124. Williams and Wilkins, Baltimore, MD.

Sartor, R. B. (1995*b*). The role of normal enteric bacteria and bacterial products in chronic intestinal inflammation. In *Inflammatory bowel disease* (ed. G. N. J. Tytgat, J. F. W. M.) Bartelsman, and S. J. H. van de Venter), pp. 519–28. Kluwer Academic Press, Dordrecht.

Sartor, R. B. (1995*c*). Insights into the pathogenesis of inflammatory bowel diseases provided by new rodent models of spontaneous colitis. *Inflammatory Bowel Diseases*, **1**, 64–75.

Sartor, R. B. (1995*d*). Current concepts of the etiology and pathogenesis of ulcerative colitis and Crohn's disease. *Gastroenterology Clinics of North America*, **24**, 475–508.

Sartor, R. B. and Lichtman, S. N. (1994). Mechanisms of systemic inflammation associated with intestinal injury. In *Inflammatory bowel disease: From bench to bedside*, (ed. S. R. Targan and F. Shanahan), pp. 210–29. Williams and Wilkins, Baltimore, MD.

Sartor, R. B., Cleland, D. R., Catalano, C. J., and Schwab, H. J. (1984). Serum antibody response indicates intestinal absorption of bacterial cell wall peptidoglycan. *Gastroenterology*, **88**, A1571.

Sartor, R. B., Bond, T. M., and Schwab, J. H. (1988). Systemic uptake and intestinal inflammatory effects of luminal bacterial cell wall polymers in rats with acute colonic injury. *Infection and Immunity*, **56**, 2101–8.

Sartor, R. B., Bender, D. E., Allen, J. B., *et al.* (1993). Chronic experimental enterocolitis and extraintestinal inflammation are T lymphocyte dependent. *Gastroenterology*, **104**, 775A.

Sartor, R. B., DeLa Cadena, R. A., Green, K. D., *et al.* (1996*a*). Selective kallikrein–kinin system activation in inbred rats differentially susceptible to granulomatous enterocolitis. *Gastroenterology*, **110**, 1467–81.

Sartor, R. B., Rath, H. C., Lichtman, S. N., and van Tol, E. A. F. (1996*b*). Animal models of intestinal and joint inflammation. *Baillière's Clinical Rheumatology*, **10**, 55–76.

Sartor, R. B., Rath, H. C., and Sellon, R. K. (1996*c*). Microbial factors in chronic intestinal inflammation. *Current Opinion in Gastroenterology*, **12**, in press.

Satsangi, J., Parkes, M., Louis, E., Lathrop, M., Bell, J., and Jewell, D. P. (1996). Systematic genome wide search for susceptibility genes in inflammatory bowel disease: Evidence for the involvement of non-HLA genes. *Gastroenterology*, **100**, A1009.

Saxon, A., Shanahan, F., Landers, C., Glanz, T., and Targan, S. (1990). A distinct subset of antineutrophil cytoplasmic antibodies is associated with inflammatory bowel disease. *Journal of Allergy and Clinical Immunology*, **86**, 202–10.

Sayrat, J. -H. (1992). Side effects of systemic retinoids and their clinical management. *Journal of the American Academy of Dermatology*, **27**, S23–8.

Scarpa, R., Oriente, P., Pucino, A., *et al.* (1984). Psoriatic arthritis in psoriatic patients. *British Journal of Rheumatology*, **23**, 246–50.

Scarpa, R., Oriente, P., Pucino, A., *et al.* (1988). The clinical spectrum of psoriatic spondylitis. *British Journal of Rheumatology*, **27**, 133–7.

Scarpa, R., D'Arienzo, A., Del Puente, A., *et al.* (1990). Reverse correlation between extent of colon involvement and number of affected joints in patients with ulcerative colitis. *Journal of Gastroenterology*, **85**, 331–2.

Scarpa, R., Del Puente, A., D'Arienzo, A., *et al.* (1992*a*). The arthritis of ulcerative colitis: clinical and genetic aspects. *Journal of Rheumatology*, **19**, 373–7.

Scarpa, R., Del Puente, A., di Girolamo, C., Biondi Oriente, C., and Oriente, P. (1992*b*). Interplay between environmental factors, articular involvement, and HLA–B27 in patients with psoriatic arthritis. *Annals of Rheumatic Diseases*, **51**, 78–9.

Schachter, J. (1978). Chlamydial infections. *New England Journal of Medicine*, **298**, 428–35.

Schachter, J. (1985). Overview of *Chlamydia trachomatis* infection and the requirements for a vaccine. *Reviews of Infectious Diseases*, **7**, 713–16.

Schachter, J., Marshall, J. B., Jones, J. P., Engleman, E. P., and Meyer, K. F. (1966). Isolation of bedsoniae from the joint of patients with Reiter's syndrome. *Proceedings of the Society for Experimental Biology and Medicine*, **22**, 283–5.

Schachter, J., Moncada, J., Dawson, C. R., *et al.* (1988). Nonculture methods for diagnosing chlamydial infection in patients with trachoma: A clue to pathogenesis of the disease? *Journal of Infectious Disease*, **158**, 1347–52.

Schaller, J. C. (1984). Chronic childhood arthritis and the spondylarthropathies. In *Spondylarthropathies* (ed. A. Calin), pp. 187–205. Greene and Stratton, Orlando, FL.

Schatteman, L., Mielants, H., Veys, E. M., *et al.* (1995). Gut inflammation in psoriatic arthritis: a prospective ileocolonoscopic study. *Journal of Rheumatology*, **22**, 680–3.

Scherak, O., Kolarz, G., Popp, W., Wottawa, A., Ritschka, L., and Braun, O. (1993). Lung involvement in rheumatoid factor-negative arthritis. *Scandinavian Journal of Rheumatology*, **22**, 225–8.

Schlaak, J., Hermann, E., Ringhoffer, M., *et al.* (1992). Predominance of TH1-type T helper cells in synovial fluid of patients with Yersinia-induced reactive arthritis. *European Journal of Immunology*, **22**, 2771–6.

Schlosstein, L. P., Terasaki, P. I., Bluestone, R., and Pearson, C. M. (1973). High association of an HLA antigen, W27, with ankylosing spondylitis. *New England Journal of Medicine*, **288**, 704–6.

Schmitz, E., Nettelnbreker, E., Zeidler, H., Hammer, M., Manor, E., and Wollenhaupt, J. (1993). Intracellular persistence of chlamydial major outer membrane protein, lipopolysaccharide and ribosomal RNA after non-productive infection of human monocytes with *Chlamydia trachomatis* serovar K. *Journal of Medical Microbiology*, **38**, 278–85.

Schober, von P. (1937). The lumbar vertebral column and backache. *Munchener Medizinische Wochenschrit*, **84**, 336–8.

Schorr-Lesnick, B. and Brandt, L. J. (1988). Selected rheumatologic and dermatologic manifestations of inflammatory bowel disease. *American Journal of Gastroenterology*, **83**, 216–23.

Schulz, L. C., Schaening, U., Pena, M., and Hermanns, W. (1985). Borderline-tissues as sites of antigen disposition and persistence—a unifying concept of rheumatoid inflammation. *Rheumatology-International*, **5**, 522–7.

Schulze-Koops, H., Burkhardt, H., Heesemann, J., von der Mark, K., and Emmrich, F. (1995). Characterization of the binding region for the *Yersinia enterocolitica* adhesin YadA on types I and II collagen. *Arthritis and Rheumatism*, **38**, 1283–9.

Schumacher, H. R., (1995). How micro-organisms are handled to localize to joints and within joints. *Scandinavian Journal of Rheumatology*, **24**, 199–202.

Schumacher, H. R., Cheriant, V., Sieck, M., and Clayburne, G. (1986). Ultrastructural identification of chlamydial antigens in synovial membrane in acute Reiter's syndrome. *Arthritis and Rheumatism*, **29** (Suppl. 4), S31.

Schumacher, H. R., Magge, S., Cherian, P. V., *et al.* (1988). Light and electron microscopic studies on the synovial membrane in Reiter's syndrome. *Arthritis and Rheumatism*, **31**, 937–46.

Schwab, J. H. (1993). Phlogistic properties of peptidoglycan–polysaccharide polymers from cell walls of pathogenic and normal-flora bacteria which colonize humans. *Infection and Immunity*, **61**, 4535–9.

Schwab, J. H., Anderle, S. K., Brown, R. R., Dalldor, F. G., and Thompson, R. C. (1991). Pro-and anti-inflammatory roles of interleukin-1 in recurrence of bacterial cell wall-induced arthritis in rats. *Infection and Immunity*, **59**, 4436–42.

Schwab, J. H., Brown, R. R., Anderle, S. K., and Schlievert, P. M. (1993). Superantigen can reactivate bacterial cell wall-induced arthritis. *Journal of Immunology*, **150**, 4151–9.

Schwimmbeck, P. L. and Oldstone M. B. A. (1988). Molecular mimicry between human leukocyte antigen B27 and Klebsiella. Consequences for spondyloarthropathies. *American Journal of Medicine*, **85**, 51–3.

Schwimmbeck, P. L., Yu, D. T. Y., and Oldstone, M. B. A. (1987). Autoantibodies to HLA-B27 in the sera of HLA B27 patients with ankylosing spondylitis and Reiter's syndrome. *Journal of Experimental Medicine*, **166**, 173–81.

Scofield, R. H. (1996). Etiopathogenesis and biochemical and immunologic evaluation of spondyloarthropathies. *Current Opinion in Rheumatology*, **8**, 309–15.

Scofield, R. H., Warren, W. L., Koelsch, G., and Harley, J. B. (1993). A hypothesis for the HLA-B27 immune dysregulation in spondyloarthropathy: Contributions from enteric organism, B27 structure, peptides bound by B27, and convergent evolution. *Proceedings of the National Academy of Science, USA*, **90**, 9330–4.

Scofield, R. H., Kurien, B., Gross, T., Warren, W. L., and Harley, J. B. (1995). HLA-B27 binding of peptide from its own sequence and similar peptides from bacteria: implications for spondyloarthropathies. *Lancet*, **345**, 1542–4.

Scott, W., Fishman, E., Kushman, J., *et al.* (1990). Computed tomographic evaluation of the sacroiliacal joints in Crohn's disease. *Skeletal Radiology*, **19**, 206–10.

Scutellari, P. N., Orzincolo, C., and Ceruti, S. (1993). The temporomandibular joint in pathologic conditions: rheumatoid arthritis and seronegative spondyloarthritis. *Radiology Medicine* (Torino), **86**, 456–66.

Seideman, P. (1990). Sulphasalazine treatment of psoriatic arthritis. *British Journal of Rheumatology*, **29**, 491–2.

Selby, W. S., Kater, R. M., Heap, T. R., and Galagher, N. D. (1979). Crohn's disease: a review of 122 cases. *Australian New Zealand Journal of Medicine*, **9**, 145–52.

Selin, L. K., Nahill, S. R., and Welsh, R. M. (1994). Cross-reactivities in memory cytotoxic T lymphocyte recognition of heterologous viruses. *Journal of Experimental Medicine*, **179**, 1933–43.

Sercarz, E. E., Lehmann, P. V., Ametani, A., Benichou, G., Miller, A., and Moudgil, K. (1993). Dominance and crypticity of T cell antigenic determinants. *Annual Review of Immunology*, **11**, 729–66.

Serrander, R., Magnusson, K. E., and Kihlström, E. (1986). Acute yersinia infections in man increase intestinal permeability for low molecular polyethylene glycols. *Scandinavian Journal of Infectious Diseases*, **18**, 409–13.

Service, R. F. (1994). Triggering the first line of defense. *Science*, **265**, 1522–4.

Sesztak, M., Koo, E., Farkas, V., and Weisz, M. (1995). Diagnosis and differential diagnosis of psoriatic arthritis on basis of follow-up of 215 cases. *Orvosi Hetilap*, **22**, 675–9.

Severijnen, A. J., Hazenberg, M. P., and van de Merwe, J. P. (1989*a*). Induction of chronic arthritis in rats by cell wall fragments of anaerobic coccoid rods isolated from the fecal flora of patients with Crohn's disease. *Digestion*, **39**, 118–25.

Severijnen, A. J., van Kleef, R., Hazenberg, M. P., and van de Merwe, J. P. (1989*b*). Cell wall fragments from major residents of the human intestinal flora induce chronic arthritis in rats. *Journal of Rheumatology*, **16**, 1061–8.

Severijnen, A. J., van Kleef, R., Hazenberg, M. P., and van de Merwe, J. P. (1990). Chronic arthritis induced in rats by cell wall fragments of Eubacterium species from human intestinal flora. *Infection and Immunity*, **58**, 523–8.

Shbeeb, M. I., Sunku, J., Hunder, G. G., *et al.* (1995). Incidence of psoriasis and psoriatic arthritis: a population based study [abstract]. *Arthritis & Rheumatism*, **38**, S379.

Sheehan, N. J., Slavin, B. M., Donovan, M. P., Mount, J. N., and Mathews, J. A. (1986). Lack of correlation between clinical disease activity and erythrocyte sedimentation rate, acute phase proteins or protease inhibitors in ankylosing spondyltis. *British Journal of Rheumatology*, **25**, 171–4.

Shinebaum, R., Blackwell, C. C., *et al.* (1987). Non-secretion of ABO blood group antigens as a host susceptibility factor in the spondyloarthropathies. *British Medical Journal of Clinical Research Education*, **294**, 208–10.

Shodjai-Moradi, F., Ebringer, A., and Abuljadayel, I. (1992). IgA antibody response to klebsiella in ankylosing spondylitis measured by immunoblotting. *Annals of the Rheumatic Diseases*, **51**, 233–7.

Shore, A. and Ansell, B. M. (1982). Juvenile psoriatic arthritis—an analysis of 60 cases. *Journal of Pediatrics*, **100**, 529–35.

Siegele, D. A. and Kolter, R. (1992). Life after log. *Journal of Bacteriology*, **174**, 345–8.

Sieper J. and Braun J. (1995). Pathogenesis of spondylarthropathies. Persistent bacterial antigen, autoimmunity, or both? *Arthritis and Rheumatism*, **38**, 1547–54.

Sieper, J. and Kingsley, G. S. (1996). Recent advances in the pathogenesis of reactive arthritis. *Immunology Today*, **17**, 160–3.

Sieper, J., Kingsley, G., Palacios-Boix, A., *et al.* (1991). Synovial T lymphocyte specific immune response to *Chlamydia trachomatis* in Reiter's disease. *Arthritis and Rheumatism*, **34**, 588–98.

Sieper, J., Braun, J., Brandt, J., *et al.* (1992*a*). Pathogenetic role of Chlamydia, Yersinia and Borrelia in undifferentiated oligoarthritis. *Journal of Rheumatology*, **19**, 1236–42.

Sieper, J., Braun, J., Döring, E., *et al.* (1992*b*). The aetiological role of reactive arthritis-associated bacteria in pauciarticular juvenile chronic arthritis. *Annals of Rheumatic Diseases*, **51**, 1208–14.

Sieper, J., Braun, J., Wu, P., Hauer, R., and Laitko, S. (1993*a*). The possible role of Shigella in sporadic enteric reactive arthritis. *British Journal of Rheumatology*, **32**, 582–5.

Sieper, J., Braun, J., Wu, P., and Kingsley, G. (1993*b*). T cells are responsible for the enhanced synovial cellular immune response to triggering antigen in reactive arthritis. *Clinical and Experimental Immunology*, **91**, 96–103.

Sieper, J., Wu, P., Wucherpfennig, K., and Braun, J. (1995). CD4+ T cell response to an HLA B27-derived peptide in ankylosing spondylitis. *Arthritis and Rheumatism*, **38**, S315.

Sieper, J., Kingsley, G. H., and Märker-Hermann, E. (1996). Aetiological agents and immune mechanisms in enterogenic reactive arthritis. *Baillière's Clinical Rheumatology*, **10**, 102–22.

Silman, A. J. and Hochberg, M. D. (1993). *Epidemiology of the rheumatic diseases*. Oxford University Press, Oxford.

Silveira, L. H., Gutiérrez, F., Scopelitis, E., Cuéller, M. L., Citera, G., and Espinoza, L. R. (1993). Chlamydia-induced reactive arthritis. *Rheumatic Disease Clinics of North America*, **19**, 351–62.

Simenon, G., Van Gossum, A., Adler, M., Rickaert, F., and Appelboom, T. (1990). Macroscopic and microscopic gut lesions in seronegative spondylarthropathies. *The Journal of Rheumatology*, **17**, 1491–4.

Simmons, W. A., Leong, L. Y. W., Satumtira, N., *et al.* (1996). Rat MHC-linked peptide transporter alleles strongly influence peptide binding by HLA-B27 but not B27-associated inflammatory disease. *Journal of Immunology*, **156**, 1661–7.

Simmons, W. A., Summerfield, S. G., Roopenian, D. C., Slaughter, C. A., Zuberi, A. R., Gaskell, S. J., Bordoli, R. S., Hoyes, J., Moomaw, C. R., Colbert, R. A., Leong, L. Y.-W., Butcher, G. W., Hammer, R. E., Taurog, J. D. (1997). Novel HY peptide antigens presented by HLA-B27. *Journal of Immunology* **159**, 2750–9.

Simon, A. K., Seipelt, E., Wu, P., Wenzel, B., Braun, J., and Sieper, J. (1993). Analysis of cytokine profiles in synovial T cell clones from chlamydial reactive arthritis patients: predominance of the Th1 subset. *Clinical and Experimental Immunology*, **94**, 122–6.

Simon, A. K., Seipelt, E., and Sieper, J. (1994). Divergent T-cell cytokine patterns in inflammatory arthritis. *Proceedings of the National Academy of Science, USA*, **91**, 8562–6.

Simon, D. G., Kaslow R. A., Rosenbaum, J., Kaye, R. L., and Calin, A. (1981). Reiter's syndrome following epidemic Shigellosis. *Journal of Rheumatology*, **8**, 969–73. **(6,8)**

Skurnik, M. (1995). Role of YadA in Yersinia-enterocolitica-induced reactive arthritis: a hypothesis. *Trends in Microbiology*, **3**, 318–19.

Skurnik, M. and Wolf-Watz, H. (1989). Analysis of the yopA gene encoding toe YOP1 virulence determinants of *Yersinia* spp. *Molecular Microbiology*, **3**, 517–29.

Skurnik, M., Batsford, S., Mertz, A., Schiltz, E., and Toivanen, P. (1993). The putative arthritogenic cationic 19-kilodalton antigen of *Yersinia enterocolitica* is a urease β subunit. *Infection and Immunity*, **61**, 2498–504.

Small, P. L. C., Ramakrishnan, L., and Falkow, S. (1994). Remodeling schemes of intracellular pathogens. *Science*, **263**, 637–9.

Smith, M., Gibson, R., *et al.* (1985). Abnormal bowel permeability in ankylosing spondylitis and rheumatoid arthritis. *Journal of Rheumatology*, **12**, 299–305.

Smith, R. (1992). Treatment of rheumatoid arthritis by colectomy. *Annals of Surgery*, **76**, 515–78.

Solinger, A. M. and Hess, E. V. (1993). Rheumatic diseases and AIDS: is the association real? *Journal of Rheumatology*, **20**, 678–83.

Soltis, R. D., Hasz, D., Morris, M. J., and Wilson, I. D. (1979). Evidence against the presence of circulating immune complexes in chronic inflammatory bowel disease. *Gastroenterology*, **76**, 1380–5.

Sonozaki, H., Mitsui, H., Miyanaga, Y., *et al.* (1981). Clinical features of 53 cases with pustulotic arthro-osteitis. *Annals of Rheumatic Diseases*, **40**, 547–53.

Soren, A. (1966). Joint affections in regional enteritis. *Archives of Internal Medicine*, **117**, 78–86.

Southwood, T. R. and Gaston, J. S. (1993). Evolution of synovial fluid mononuclear cell responses in a HLA B27-positive patient with Yersinia-associated juvenile arthritis. *British Journal of Rheumatology*, **32**, 845–8.

Southwood, T. R., Petty, R. E., Malleson, P. N., *et al.* (1989). Psoriatic arthritis in children. *Arthritis and Rheumatism*, **32**, 1007–13.

Soylu, M., Ersoz, T. R., Haciyakupoglu, G., and Eroglu, A. (1993). Aetiological distribution of uveitis patients in Southern Turkey. *Ocular Immunology and Inflammation*, **1**, 355–61.

Spencer Wells, R. and Parham, P. (1996). HLA class I genes: structure and diversity. In *HLA and MHC: genes, molecules and function* (ed. M. Browning and A. McMichael), pp. 77–96. BIOS Scientific Publishers Ltd, Oxford.

Stagg, A. J., Breban, M., Hammer, R. E., Knight, S. C., and Taurog, J. D. (1995*a*). Defective dendritic cell (DC) function in a HLA-B27 transgenic rat model of spondyloarthropathy (SpA). In *Dendritic cells in fundamental and clinical immunology*, Vol. 2, (ed. J. Banchereau and D. Schmitt), Plenum Press, New York.

Stagg, A. J., Breban, M. E., Knight, S. C., and Taurog, J. D. (1995*b*). Defective dendritic cell function in a HLA-B27 transgenic rat model of spondyloarthropathy. *Advances in Experimental Medicine and Biology* **378**, 557–9.

Ståhlberg, T. H., Granfors, K., Pekkola-Heino, K., Soppi, E., and Toivanen, A. (1987*a*). Immunoblotting analysis of human IgM, IgG and IgA responses to chromosomally coded antigens of *Yersinia enterocolitica* 0:3. *Acta Pathologica Microbiologica et Immunologica Scandinavica Section C*, **95**, 71–9.

Ståhlberg, T. H., Granfors, K., and Toivanen, A. (1987*b*). Immunoblot analysis of human IgM, IgG and IgA responses to plasmid-encoded antigens of *Yersinia enterocolitica* serovar O3. *Journal of Medical Microbiology*, **24**, 157–63.

Ståhlberg, T. H., Tertti, R., Wolf-Watz, H., Granfors, K., and Toivanen, A. (1987*c*). Antibody response in *Yersinia pseudotuberculosis* III infection: Analysis of an outbreak. *Journal of Infectious Diseases*, **156**, 388–91.

Stanworth, A. and Sharp, J. (1956). Uveitis and rheumatic diseases. *Annals of Rheumatic Disease*, **15**, 140–50.

Starnbach, M. N. and Bevan, M. J. (1994*a*). Cells infected with Yersinia present an epitope to class I MHC-restricted CTL. *Journal of Immunology*, **153**, 1603–11.

Starnbach, M. N., Bevan, M. J., and Lampe, M. F. (1994*b*). Protective cytotoxic T lymphocytes are induced during murine infection with *Chlamydia trachomatis*. *Journal of Immunology*, **153**, 5183–9.

Stein, C. M. and Davis, P. (1996). Arthritis associated with HIV infection in Zimbabwe. *Journal of Rheumatology*, **23**, 506–11.

Stein, C. M., Davis, P., *et al.* (1990). The spondyloarthropathies in Zimbabwe: a clinical and immunogenetic profile. *Journal of Rheumatology*, **17**, 1337–9.

Stein, H., Volpin, G., Shapira, D., Snir, E., Sterenberg, A., and Eidelman, S. (1993). Musculoskeletal manifestations of Crohn's disease. *Hospital Bulletin for Joint Diseases*, **53**, 17–20.

Steinbrocker, O., Traeger, C. H., and Batterman, R. C. (1949). Therapeutic criteria for rheumatoid arthritis. *Journal of the American Medical Association*, **140**, 659–62.

Steinson, K., Jonsdottir, I., and Valdimarsson, H. (1990). Cyclosporin A in psoriatic arthritis. An open study. *Annals of Rheumatic Diseases*, **49**, 603–6.

Stern, L., Brown, J., *et al.* (1994). Crystal structure of the human class 2 MHC protein HLA-DR1 complexed with an influenza virus peptide. *Nature*, **368**, 215–21.

Stern, R. S. (1985). The epidemiology of joint complaints in patients with psoriasis. *Journal of Rheumatology*, **12**, 315–20.

Sternberg, E. M., Hill, J. M., Chrousos, G. P., *et al.* (1989). Inflammatory mediator-induced hypothalamis–pituitary–adrenal axis activation is defective in streptococcal cell wall arthritis-susceptible Lewis rats. *Proceedings of the National Academy of Sciences, USA*, **86**, 2374–8.

Stieglitz, H. and Lipsky, P. (1993). Association between reactive arthritis and antecedent infection with *Shigella flexneri* carrying a 2-Md plasmid and encoding an HLA-B27 mimetic epitope. *Arthritis and Rheumatism*, **36**, 1387–91.

Stieglitz, H., Fosmire, S., and Lipsky, P. (1989). Identification of a 2-Md plasmid from *Shigella flexneri* associated with reactive arthritis. *Arthritis and Rheumatism*, **32**, 937–48.

Stimpson, S. A., Brown, R. R., Anderle, S. K., *et al.* (1986). Arthropathic properties of cell wall polymers from normal flora bacteria. *Infection and Immunity*, **51**, 240–51.

Stimpson, S. A., Esser, R. E., Carter, P. B., *et al.* (1987). Lipopolysaccharide induces recurrence of arthritis in rat joint previously injured by peptidoglycan–polysccharide. *Journal of Experimental Medicine*, **165**, 1688–702.

Stimpson, S. A., Dalldorf, F. G., Otterness, I. G., and Schwab, J. H. (1988*a*). Exacerbation of arthritis by IL–1 in rat joints previously injured by peptidoglycan–polysaccharide. *Journal of Immunology*, **140**, 2964–9.

Stimpson, S. A., Dalldorf, F. G., Otterness, I. G., and Schwab, J. H. (1988*b*). Pain and reactivation of arthritis induced by recombinant cytokines in rat ankles previously injured by peptidoglycan–polysaccharide. *Arthritis and Rheumatism*, **31** (Suppl. SA5), S49.

Strauss, R. E. (1988). Ocular manifestations of Crohn's disease: literature review. *Mount Sinai Journal of Medicine*, **55**, 353–6.

Suarez, A. M. and Russell, A. S. (1990). Sacroiliitis in psoriasis: relationship to peripheral arthritis and HLA–B27. *Journal of Rheumatology*, **17**, 804–8.

Summers, R. W., Switz, D. M., Session, J. T., *et al.* (1979). National cooperative Crohn's disease study: results of drug treatment. *Gastroenterology*, **77**, 847–69.

Sun, J. P., Khan, M. A., Farhat, A. Z. and Bahler, R. C. (1992). Alterations in cardiac diastolic function in patients with ankylosing spondylitis. *International Journal of Cardiology*, **37**, 65–72.

Suschke, H. J. (1992). Die behandlung der juvenilen spondylarthritis und der reactiven arthritis mit sulfasalazin. *Monats Kinderheilkunde*, **140**, 658–60.

Sutton, J., Rowland-Jones, S., *et al.* (1993). A sequence pattern for peptides presented to cytotoxic T lymphocytes by HLA B8 revealed by analysis of epitopes and eluted peptides. *European Journal of Immunology*, **23**, 447–453.

Svenungson, B. (1994). Reactive arthritis. *British Medical Journal*, **308**, 671–2.

Sweet, H. O. and Green, M. C. (1981). Progressive ankylosis, a new skeletal mutation in the mouse. *Journal of Heredity*, **72**, 87–93.

Taccetti, G., Trapani, S., Ermini, M., and Falcini, F. (1994). Reactive arthritis triggered by *Yersinia enterocolitica:* a review of 18 pediatric cases. *Clinical and Experimental Rheumatology*, **12**, 681–4.

Tacket, C., Narain, J., Sattin, R., *et al.* (1984). A multistate outbreak of infections caused by *Yersinia enterocolitica* transmitted by pasteurized milk. *Journal of the Americal Medical Association*, **251**, 483–6.

Taggart, A. J., Gardiner, P., Mc Evoy, F. M., Hopkins, R., Bird, H. A., and Wright, V. (1994). Which is the active moiety of Sulphasalazine in ankylosing spondylitis? *Arthritis and Rheumatism*, **37**, Abstr. 1159, S354.

Tamburrino, V., Monno, R., Valenza, M. A., and Numo, R. (1993). Incidence of *Yersinia enterocolitica* antibodies in patients with inflammatory joint diseases. *Clinical Rheumatology*, **12**, 354–6.

Tanigaki, N., Fruci, D., *et al.* (1994). The peptide binding specificity of HLA-B27 subtypes. *Immunogenetics*, **40**, 192–8.

Tarasova, L. N. and Grigor'eva, E. G. (1991). Syndromic uveitis in Reiter's disease. *Vestnik Oftalmologii*, **107**, 53–6.

Taurog, J. D. (1995). The role of bacteria in HLA-B27-associated reactive arthritis. *Cliniguide to Rheumatology*, **5** (issue 3), 1–8.

Taurog, J. D., Argentieri, D. C., and McReynolds, R. A. (1988*a*). Adjuvant arthritis. *Methods in Enzymology*, **162**, 339–55

Taurog, J. D., Lowen, L., Forman, J., and Hammer, R. E. (1988*b*). HLA-B27 in inbred and noninbred transgenic mice. Cell surface expression and recognition as an alloantigen in the absence of human $\beta 2$-microglobulin. *Journal of Immunology*, **141**, 4020–3.

Taurog, J. D., Maika, S. D., Simmons, W. A., Breban, M., and Hammer, R. E. (1993). Susceptibility inflammatory disease in HLA-B27 transgenic rat lines correlates with the level of B27 expression. *Journal of Immunology*, **150**, 4168–78.

Taurog, J. D., Richardson, J. A., Croft, J. T., *et al.* (1994). The germfree state prevents development of gut and joint inflammatory disease in HLA-B27 transgenic rats. *Journal of Experimental Medicine*, **180**, 2359–64.

Taurog, J. D., Satumtira, N. *et al.* (1996). Alleles of the inbred Dark Agouti (DA) rat strain are protective against inflammatory disease in HLA-B27 transgenic rats. *Arthritis and Rheumatism*, **39**, S121

Tay-Kearney, M. -L., Schwam, B. L., Lowder, C., *et al.* (1996). Clinical features and associated systemic diseases of HLA-B27 uveitis. *American Journal of Ophthalmology*, **121**, 47–56.

Taylor, H. G., Wardle, T., Beswick, E. J., and Dawes, P. T. (1991). The relationship of clinical and laboratory measurements to radiological change in ankylosing spondylitis. *British Journal of Rheumatology*, **30**, 330–5.

Taylor-Robinson, D. and Thomas, B. J. (1980). The role of Chlamydia trachomatis in genital-tract and associated diseases. *Journal of Clinical Pathology*, **33**, 205–33.

Taylor-Robinson, D., Thomas, B. J., Dixey, J., Osborn, M. F., Furr, P. M., and Keat, A. C. (1988). Evidence that *Chlamydia trachomatis* causes seronegative arthritis in women. *Annals Rheumatic Diseases*, **47**, 295–9.

Taylor-Robinson, D., Gilroy, C. B., Thomas, B. J., and Keat, A. C. S. (1992). Detection of Chlamydia trachomatis DNA in joints of reactive arthritis patients by polymerase chain reaction. *Lancet*, **340**, 81–2.

Tertti, R., Granfors, K., Lehtonen, O. -P., *et al.* (1984). An outbreak of *Yersinia pseudotuberculosis* infection. *Journal of Infectious diseases*, **149**, 245–50.

Thomas, A. F., Solomon, L., and Rabson, A. (1975). Polyarthritis associated with *Yersinia enterocolitica* infection. *South African Medical Journal*, **49**, 18–20.

Thomson, G. T. D., Johnston, J. L., Baragar, F. D., and Toole, J. W. (1990). Psoriatic arthritis and myopathy. *Journal of Rheumatology*, **17**, 395–8.

Thomson G. T. D., Chiu, B., De Rubeis, D., Falk, J., and Inman, R. D. (1992). Immunoepidemiology of post-salmonella reactive arthritis in a cohort of women. *Clinical Immunology and Immunopathology*, **64**, 227–32.

Thomson, G. T. D., Alfa, M., Orr, K., Thomson, B. R. J., and Olson, N. (1994*a*). Secretory immune response and clinical sequelae of salmonella infection in a point source cohort. *Journal of Rheumatology*, **21**, 132–7.

Thomson, G. T. D., McKibbon, C., and Inman, R. D. (1994*b*). Mesalamine therapy in Reiter's syndrome. *Journal of Rheumatology*, **21**, 570–2.

Thomson, G. T. D., DeRubeis, D. A., Hodge, M. A., Rajanayagam, C., and Inman, R. D. (1995). Post-salmonella reactive arthritis: late clinical sequelate in a point source cohort. *American Journal of Medicine*, **98**, 13–21.

Tieng, V., Dulphy, N., Boisgérault, F., Tamouza, R., Charron, D., Toubert, A. HLA-B*2707 peptide motif: Tyr C-terminal anchor is not shared by all disease-associated subtypes. *Immunogenetics*, in press.

Tiwari, J. L. and Terasaki, P. I. (ed.) (1985). *HLA and disease associations*, pp. 32–99. Springer-Verlag, New York.

Toivanen, A. and Khan, M. A. (1994). Therapeutic dilemma in ankylosing spondylitis and related spondylarthropathies. *Rheumatology Reviews*, **3**, 21–7.

Toivanen, A. and Toivanen, P. (1994). Epidemiologic aspects, clinical features, and management of ankylosing spondylitis and reactive arthritis. *Current Opinion in Rheumatology*, **6**, 354–9.

Toivanen, A. and Toivanen, P. (1995*a*). Aetiopathogenesis of reactive arthritis. *Rheumatology in Europe*, **24**, 5–8.

Toivanen, A. and Toivanen, P. (1995*b*). Epidemiologic, clinical, and therapeutic aspects of reactive arthritis and ankylosing spondylitis. *Current Opinion in Rheumatology*, **7**, 279–83.

Toivanen, A. and Toivanen, P. (1996). Reactive arthritis. *Current Opinion in Rheumatology*, **8**, 334–40.

Toivanen, A. and Toivanen, P. (1997). Reactive arthritis. *Current Opinion in Rheumatology*, **9**, 321–7.

Toivanen, A., Granfors, K., Lahesmaa-Rantala, R., Leino, R., Ståhlberg, T. and Vuento, R. (1985). Pathogenesis of yersinia-triggered reactive arthritis: immunological, Microbiological and clinical aspects. *Immunological Reviews*, **86**, 47–70.

Toivanen, A., Lahesmaa-Rantala, R., Ståhlberg, T. H., Merilahti, P. R. and Granfors, K. (1987*a*). Do bacterial antigens persist in reactive arthritis? *Clinical and Experimental Rheumatology*, **5/S-1**, 25–7.

Toivanen, A., Lahesmaa-Rantala, R., Vuento, R., and Granfors, K. (1987*b*). Association of persisting IgA response with Yersinia triggered reactive arthritis: A study of 104 patients. *Annals of the Rheumatic Diseases*, **46**, 898–901.

Toivanen, A., Yli-Kerttula, T., Luukkainen, R., Merilahti-Palo, R., Granfors, K., and Seppälä, J. (1993). Effect of antimicrobial treatment on chronic reactive arthritis. *Clinical and Experimental Rheumatology*, **11**, 301–7.

Tomfohrde, J., Silverman, A., Barnes, R., *et al.* (1994). Gene for familial psoriasis susceptibility mapped to distal end of human chromosome 17q. *Science*, **264**, 1141–5.

Tomlingson, I. W. and Jayson, M. I. (1991). Erosive Crohn's arthritis. *Journal of the Royal Society of Medicine*, **74**, 540–2.

Tomlinson, M. J., Barefoot, J., and Dixon, A. S-J. (1986). Intensive in-patient physiotherapy courses improve movement and posture of ankylosing spondylitis. *Physiotherapy*, **72**, 238–40.

Torre Alonso, J. C., Rodriguez-Perez, A., Arribas Castrillo, J. M., Ballina Garcia, J., Riestra Noriega, J. L., and Lopez Larrea, C. (1991). Psoriatric arthritis: a clinical, immunological and radiological study of 180 patients. *British Journal of Rheumatology*, **30**, 245–50.

Towner, S. R., Michet, C. J., O'Fallon, W. M., and Nelson, A. M. (1983). The epidemiology of juvenile arthritis in Rochester, Minnesota 1960–1979. *Arthritis and Rheumatism*, **26**, 1208–13.

Townsend, A. R., Gotch, F. M., *et al.* (1985). Cytotoxic T cells recognize fragments of the influenza nucleoprotein. *Cell*, **42**, 457–67

Townsend, A. R. M., Rothbard, J., Gotch, F. M., Bahadur, G., Wraith, D., McMichael, A. J. (1986). The epitopes of influenza nucleoprotein recognized by cytotoxic T lymphocytes can be defined with short synthetic peptides. *Cell* **44**, 959–68.

Tran, V. T., Auer, C., Guex-Crosier, Y., Pittet, N., and Herbort, C. P. (1994). Epidemiologic characteristics of uveitis in Switzerland. *International Ophthamology*, **18**, 293–8.

Trnavsky, K., Peliskova, Z., and Vacha, J. (1990). Sulphasalazine in the treatment of reactive arthritis. *Scandinavian Journal of Rheumatology*, **80**, 45.

Trull, A. K., Ebringer, R., Panayi, G. S., Colthorpe, D., James, D. C., and Ebringer, A. (1983). IgA antibodies to *klebsiella pneumoniae* in ankylosing spondylitis. *Scandinavian Journal of Rheumatology*, **12**, 249–53.

Trull, A. K., Ebringer, A., Panayi, G. S., Ebringer, R., and James, D. C. (1984). HLA-B27 and the immune response to enterobacterial antigens in ankylosing spondylitis. *Clinical and Experimental Immunology*, **55**, 74–80.

Tsuchiya, N., Husby, G., *et al.* (1990). Autoantibodies to the HLA-B27 sequence cross-react with the hypothetical peptide from the arthritis-associated Shigella plasmid. *Journal of Clinical Investigations*, **86**, 1193–203.

Tucker, C. R., Fowles, R. E., Calin, A., *et al.* (1982). Aortitis in ankylosing spondylitis: early detection of aortic root abnormalities with two-dimensional echocardiography. *American Journal of Cardiology*, **9**, 680–6.

Tullous, M. W., Skerhut, H. E. I., Story, J. L., *et al.* (1990). Cauda equina syndrome of long-standing ankylosing spondylitis. Case report and review of the literature. *Journal of Neurosurgery*, **73**, 441–7.

Tuori, M.-L. and Valtonen, V. (1983). An out-patient epidemic caused by *Yersinia enterocolitica* serotype 0:3. *Duodecim*, **99**, 706–11.

Tussey, L. G., Rowland-Jones, S., Zheng, T. S., *et al.* (1995). Different MHC class I alleles complete for presentation of overlapping viral epitopes. *Immunity*, **3**, 65–77.

Ugrinovic, S., Mertz, A., Braun, J., and Sieper, J. (1995). HLA-B27 restricted cytotoxic T cells specific for peptides derived from the ribosomal L23 protein of *Yersinia enterocolitica* 0:3 are found in Yersinia-arthritis patients. *Arthritis and Rheumatism*, **38**, S201.

Ugrinovic, S., Mertz, A., Wu, P., Braun, J., and Sieper, J. (1997). A single nonamer from the Yersinia 60kd heat shock protein is the target of HLA-B27 restricted CTL response in Yersinia-induced reactive arthritis. *Journal of Immunology* (in press).

Undlien, D. E., Friede, T., Rammensee, H. G., Joner, G., Dahl-Jorgensen, K., Sovik, O., Akselsen, H. E., Knutsen, I., Ronningen, K. S., Thorsby, E. (1997). HLA-encoded genetic predisposition in IDDM: DR4 subtypes may be associated with different degrees of protection. *Diabetes* **46**, 143–9.

Urban, R. G., Chicz, R. M., *et al.* (1994). A subset of HLA-B27 molecules contains peptides much longer than nonamers. *Proceedings of the National Academy of Science, USA*, **91**, 1534–8.

Utsinger, P. M. (1980). Systemic immune complex disease following intestinal bypass surgery in bypass disease. *Journal of the American Academy of Dermatology*, **2**, 488–95.

Valtonen, V. V., Leirisalo, M., Pentikäinen, P. J., *et al.* (1985). Triggering infections in reactive arthritis. *Annals of the Rheumatic Diseases*, **44**, 399–405.

Van Bleek, G. M. and Nathenson, S. G. (1990). Isolation of an endogenously processed immunodominant viral peptide from the class I H-2K^b molecule. *Nature* **348**, 213–6.

van Bohemen, C. G., Lionarons, R. J., van Bodegom, P., *et al.* (1985). Susceptibility and HLA-B27 in post-dysenteric arthropathies. *Immunology*, **56**, 377–9.

van Bohemen, C. G., Nabbe, A. J. J. M., Landheer, J. E., *et al.* (1986*a*). HLA-B27M1M2 and high immune responsiveness to *Shigella flexneri* in post-dysenteric arthritis. *Immunology Letters*, **13**, 71–4.

van Bohemen, C. G., Nabbe, A. J. J. M., The, H. S., Dekker-Saeys, A. J., and Zanen, H. C. (1986*b*). Antibodies to enterobacteriaceae in ankylosing spondylitis. *Scandinavian Journal of Rheumatology*, **15**, 143–7.

van den Broek, M. F., Van de Putte, L. B. A., and Van den Berg, W. B. (1988). Crohn's disease associated with arthritis: A possible role for cross-reactivity between gut bacteria and cartilage in the pathogenesis of arthritis. *Arthritis and Rheumatism*, **31**, 1077–9.

van den Broek, M. F., Hogervorst, E. J. M., Van Bruggen, M. C. J., Van Eden, W., Van der Zee, R., and Van den Berg, W. B. (1989). Protection against streptococal cell wall-induced arthritis by pretreatment with the 65 kD mycobacterial heat shock protein. *Journal of Experimental Medicine*, **170**, 449–66.

van den Broek, M. F., van den Langerijt, L. G., van Bruggen, M. C., Billingham, M. E., van den Berg, W. B. (1992). Treatment of rats with monoclonal anti-eD$_4$ induces long-term resistence to streptococal cell wall-induced arthritis. *European Journal of Immunology*, **22**, 57–61.

van den Heijde, D. M. F. M., van't Hof, M., van Riel, P. L. C. M., and van der Putte, L. B. A. (1993). Validity of single variables and indices to measure disease activity in rheumatoid arthritis. *Journal of Rheumatology*, **20**, 538–41.

van der Linden, S., van der Heijde, D. M. F. M. (1995). Ankylosing spondylitis and other B27 related spondylartyhropathies. *Bailliere's Clinical Rheumatology*, **9**, 355–73.

van der Linden, S. M., Valkenburg, H. A., and Cats, A. (1984*a*). Evaluation of diagnostic criteria for ankylosing spondylitis. A proposal for modification of the New York criteria. *Arthritis and Rheumatism*, **27**, 361–8.

van der Linden, S. M., Valkenberg, H. A., de Jongh, B., and Cats, A. (1984*b*). The risk of developing ankylosing spondylitis: a comparison of relatives of spondylitis patients with the general population. *Arthritis and Rheumatism*, **27**, 241–9.

van Hees, P. A. M., Van Lier, H. J. J., Van Elteren, P., *et al.* (1981). Effect of Sulphasalazine in patients with active Crohn's disease: a controlled double-blind study. *Gut*, **22**, 404–9.

van Kregten, E., Huber-Bruning, O., Vanderbroucke, J. P., and Williers, J. M. N. (1991). No conclusive evidence of an epidemiological relation between Klebsiella and ankylosing spondylitis. *Journal of Rheumatology*, **18**, 384–8.

van Patter, W. N., Bargen, J. A., Dockerty, M. B., Feldman, W. M., Mayo, C. W., and Waugh, J. M. (1954). Regional enteritis. *Gastroenterology*, **26**, 347–450.

Vargas-Alarcon, G., Garcia, A., *et al.* (1994). HLA-B allatcs and complotypes in Mexican patients with seronegative spondyloarthropathies. *Annals of Rheumatic Diseases*, **53**, 755--8.

Vasey, F. B. and Espinoza, L. R. (1984). Psoriatic arthropathy. In *Spondylarthropathies* (ed. A. Calin), pp. 151–85. Grune and Stratton, Orlando, Florida.

Vasey, F. B., Deitz, C., Fenske, N. A., Germain, B. F., and Espinoza, L. R. (1982). Possible involvement of group A streptococci in the pathogenesis of psoriatic arthritis. *Journal of Rheumatology*, **9**, 719–22.

Veale, D., Rogers, S., and Fitzgerald, O. (1994). Classification of clinical subsets in psoriatic arthritis. *British Journal of Rheumatology*, **33**, 133–8.

Veale, D., Rogers, S., and Fitzgerald, O. (1995). Immunolocalization of adhesion molecules in psoriatic arthritis, psoriatic and normal skin. *British Journal of Dermatology*, **132**, 32–8.

Verjans, G. M. G. M., van der Linden, S. M., van Eys, G. J. J. M., *et al.* (1991). Restriction fragment length polymorphism of the tumor necrosis factor region in patients with ankylosing spondylitis. *Arthritis and Rheumatism*, **34**, 486–9.

Verjans, G. M., Brinkman, B. M., *et al.* (1994). Polymorphism of tumour necrosis factor-alpha (INF-alpha) at position – 308 in relation to ankylosing spondylitics. *Clinical and Experimental Immunology*, **97**, 45–7

Viitanen, A., Arstila, T. P., Lahesmaa, R., Granfors, K., Skurnik, M., and Toivanen, P. (1991). Application of the polymerase chain reaction and immunofluorescence techniques to the detection of bacteria in yersinia-triggered reactive arthritis. *Arthritis and Rheumatism*, **34**, 89–96.

Vilar, M. J. P., Cury, S. E., Ferraz, M. B., Sesso, R., and Atra, E. (1997). Renal abnormalities in ankylosing spondylitis. *Scandinavian Journal of Rheumatology*, **26**, 19–23.

Villadangos, J. A., Galocha, B., García, F., Albar, J. P., López de Castro, J. A. (1995). Modulation of peptide binding by HLA-B27 polymorphism in pockets A and B, and peptide specificity of B*2703. *European Journal Immunology* **25**, 2370–7.

Villanueva, M. S., Fischer, P., Feen, K., and Pamer, E. G. (1994). Efficiency of MHC class I antigen processing: A quantitative analysis. *Immunity*, **1**, 479–89.

Vinje, O., Dale, K., and Moller, P. (1983). Radiographic changes, HLA-B27 and back pain in patients with psoriasis or acute anterior uveitis. *Scandanavian Journal of Rheumatology*, **12**, 219–24

Virtala, M., J. Kirveskari and Granfors, K. 1997. HLA-B27 modulates life of Salmonella in transfected L cells possibly by impaired nitric oxide production. *Infection and Immunity*, **65**, in-press.

Viscidi, R. P., Bobo, L., Hook, E. W., and Quinn, Th. C. (1993). Transmission of Chlamydia trachomatis among sex partners assessed by polymerase chain reaction. *Journal of Infectious Diseases*, **168**, 488–92.

Volkman, A. and Collins, F. M. (1975). Pathogenesis of salmonella-associated arthritis in rats. *Infection and Immunity*, **11**, 222–30.

Wagner, S. A., Peter, R. U., Adam, O., Ruzicka, T. (1993). Therapeutic efficacy of oral low-dose cyclosporin A in severe psoriatic arthritis. *Dermatology*, **186**, 62–7.

Wahl, S. M. (1991). Cellular and molecular interactions in the induction of inflammation in rheumatic diseases. In *Monoclonal antibodies, cytokines, and arthritis*, (ed. T. F. Kresina), Marcel Dekker, New York.

Wahl, S. M., Allen, J. B., Dougherty, S., *et al.* (1986). T-lymphocyte dependent evolution of bacterial cell wall induced hepatic granulomas. *Journal of Immunology*, **137**, 2199–209.

Wakefield, D. and Penny, R. (1983). Cell-mediated immune response to chlamydia in anterior uveitis: role of HLA-B27. *Clinical and Experimental Immunology*, **51**, 191–6.

Wakefield, D., Easter, J., and Penny, R. (1984). Clinical features of HLA-B27 anterior uveitis. *Australian Journal of Ophthalmology*, **12**, 1991–6.

Wakefield, D., Robinson, P., Easter, J., Graham, D., and Penny, R. (1985). Decreased chemiluminescent associated phagocytic response of peripheral blood mononuclear cells to *Chlamydia trachomatis* in patients with HLA-B27+ anterior uveitis. *British Journal of Rheumatology*, **24**, 332–9.

Wakefield, D., Buckley, R., Golding, J., *et al.* (1988). Association of complement allotype C4B2 with anterior uveitis. *Human Immunology*, **21**, 233–7.

Wakefield, D., Stahlberg, T. H., Toivanen, A., Granfors, K., and Tennant, C. (1990). Serologic evidence of Yersinia infection in patients with anterior uveitis. *Archives of Ophthalmology*, **108**, 219–21.

Wakefield, D., Breit, S. N., Clark, P., and Penny, R. (1982). Immunogenetic factors in inflammatory eye disease. Influence of HLA-B27 and alpha-1-antitrypsin phenotypes on disease expression. *Arthritis and Rheumatism*, **25**, 1431–4.

Wands, J. R., La Mont, J. T., Mann, E., and Isselbacher, K. J. (1976). Arthritis associated with intestinal-bypass procedure for morbid obesity. *New England Journal of Medicine*, **294**, 121–4.

Ward, M. E. (1988). The chlamydial developmental cycle. In *Microbiology of chlamydia* (ed. A. L. Barron), pp. 71–95. CRC Press, Boca Raton.

Ward, M. (1995). The immunobiology and immunopathology of chlamydial infections. *APMIS*, **103**, 769–96.

Warren, R. E. and Brewerton, D. A. (1980). Faecal carriage of klebsiella by patients with ankylosing spondylitis and rheumatoid arthritis. *Annals of the Rheumatic Diseases*, **39**, 37–44.

Watkins, D. I. (1995). The evolution of major histocompatibility class Igenes in primates. *Critical Reviews in Immunology*, **15**, 1–29.

Watson, P. G. and Hezleman, B. L. (1976). *The sclera and systemic disorders.* WB Saunders Company, Philadelphia.

Weinberger, H., Ropes M., Kulka J. P., *et al.* (1962). Reiter's syndrome's clinical and pathological observations. *Medicine*, **41**, 35–91.

Weiner, A. and BenEzra, D. (1991). Clinical patterns and associated conditions in chronic uveits. *American Journal of Ophthalmology*, **112**, 151–8.

Weiner, S. R., Clarke, J., Taggart, N. A., and Utsinger, P. D. (1991). Rheumatic manifestations of inflammatory bowel disease. *Seminars in Arthritis and Rheumatism*, **20**, 353–66.

Weinreich, S., Eulderink, F., Capkova, J., *et al.* (1995). HLA-B27 as a relative risk factor in ankylosing enthesopathy in transgenic mice. *Human Immunology*, **42**, 103–15.

Weiss, E. H., Schliesser, G., Kuon, W., *et al.* (1990). Copy number and presence of human beta-2 microglobulin control cell surface expression of HLA-B27 antigen in transgenic mice with a 25 kb B27 gene fragment. In *Transgenic mice and mutants in MHC research* (ed. I. K. Egorov and C. S. David), pp. 205–13. Springer-Verlag, Berlin.

Welsh, J., Avakian, H., Cowling, P., *et al.* (1980). Ankylosing spondylitis, HLA-B27 and klebsiella. I. Cross-reactivity studies with rabbit antisera. *British Journal of Experimental Pathology*, **61**, 85–91.

Wenckert, A., Kristensen, M., Eklune, A. E., *et al.* (1978). The long-term prophylatic effect of salicylazo-sulphapyridine (salazopyrin) in primary resected patients with Crohn's disease. *Scandinavian Journal of Rheumatology*, **13**, 161–7.

Wendling, D., Bidet, A., and Guidet, M. (1990). Intestinal permeability in ankylosing spondylitis. *Journal of Rheumatology* **17**, 114.

Westman, P., Partanen, J., *et al.* (1995). TAP1 and TAP2 polymorphism in HLA-B27-positive subpopulations—no allelic differences in ankylosing spondylitis and reactive arthritis. *Human Immunology*, **44**, 236–42.

Weyand, C. M. and Goronzy, J. J. (1992). Clinically silent infections in patients with oligoarthritis: Results of a prospective study. *Annals of the Rheumatic Diseases*, **51**, 253–8.

Whelan, M. A. and Archer, J. R. (1993). Chemical reactivity of an HLA-B27 thiol group. *European Journal of Immunology*, **23**, 3278–85.

Whitman, G. J. and Khan, M. A. (1989). Unusual occurrence of ankylosing spondylitis and multiple sclerosis in a black patient. *Cleveland Clinic Journal of Medicine*, **56**, 819–22.

WHO (World Health Organization) (1947). *Constitution of the World Health Organization*. WHO, Geneva.

WHO (World Health Organization) (1948). *Official records of the World Health Organization*, No. 2, pp. 100. WHO, Geneva.

Wiedermann, U., Hanson, L. A., Bremeoll, T., Kahu, H., and Dahlgren, U. I. (1995). Increased translocation of *Escherichia coli* and development of arthritis in vitamin A-deficient rats. *Infection and Immunity*, **63**, 3062–8.

Wilder, R. L. (1995). Neuroendocrine–immune system interactions and autoimmunity. *Annual Review of Immunology*, **13**, 307–38.

Wildner, G. and Thurau, S. R. (1994). Cross-reactivity between and HLA-B27-derived peptide and a retinal autoantigen peptide: a clue to major histocompatibility complex association with autoimmune disease. *European Journal of Immunology*, **24**, 2579–85.

Wilkinson, M. and Bywaters, E. G. L. (1958). Clinical features and course of ankylosing spondylitis as seen in a follow-up of 222 hospital referred cases. *Annals of Rheumatic Disease*, **17**, 209–28.

Will, R., Palmer, R., Bhalla, A. K., Ring, F., and Calin, A. (1989). Osteoporosis in early ankylosing spondylitis: a primary pathological event? *Lancet*, **2**, 1483–5.

Will, R., Amor, B., and Calin, A. (1990). The changing epidemiology of rheumatic diseases: should ankylosing spondylitis now be included? *British Journal of Rheumatology*, **29**, 299–300.

Will, R., Calin, A., and Kirwan, J. (1992). Increasing age at presentation with ankylosing spondylitis. *Annals of Rheumatic Diseases*, **52**, 340–2.

William, G. H. (1989). Hope for the humblest? The role of self-help in chronic illness: the case of ankylosing spondylitis. *Sociology of Health and illness*, **11**

Williams, H. C. and DuVivier, A. W. (1991). Etretinate and AIDS-related Reiter's syndrome. *British Journal of Dermatology*, **124**, 389–92.

Williams, N. S. (1989). Restorative proctocolectomy is the first choice elevative surgical treatment for ulcerative colitis. *British Journal of Surgery*, **76**, 1109–10.

Williams, R., Harrison, H. R., Tempest, B., *et al.* (1989). Chlamydial infection and arthritis. *Journal of Rheumatology*, **16**, 846 (letter).

Willkens, R. F., Arnett, F. C., Bitter, T., *et al.* (1981). Reiter's syndrome: evaluation of preliminary criteria for definite disease. *Arthritis and Rheumatology*, **24**, 844–9.

Winblad, S. (1970). Yersiniainfektioner hos människan. *Medicinisk Årbog*, **13**, 244–58.

Winblad, S. (1975). Arthritis associated with *Yersinia enterocolitica* infections. *Scandinavian Journal of Infectious Diseases*, **7**, 191–5.

Winrow, V. R., Mojdehi, G. M., Ryder, S. D., Rhodes, J. M., Blake, D. R., and Rampton, D. S. (1993). Stress proteins in colorectal mucosa: Enhanced expression in ulcerative colitis. *Digestive Diseases and Sciences*, **38**, 1994–2000.

Wollenhaupt, J. and Zeidler, H. (1990*a*). Chlamydia-induced arthritis. *EULAR Bulletin*, **3**, 72–7.

Wollenhaupt, J. and Zeidler, H. (1990*b*). Die Chlamydien-induzierte Arthritis. *Med Welt*, **41**, 346–53.

Wollenhaupt, H. J., Schneider, C., Zeidler, H., Krech, T., and Kuntz, B. M. E. (1989*a*). Klinische und serologische Charakterisierung der Chlamydien-induzierten Arthritis. *Deutsche Medizinische Wochenschrift*, **114**, 1949–54.

Wollenhaupt, J., Bialowons, A., and Zeidler, H. (1989*b*). Verlauf der Chlamydien-induzierten Arthritis (CIA): Ergebnisse einer Follow-up-Studie. *Aktuelle Rheumatologie*, **14**, 225 (Abstract).

Wollenhaupt, H. J., Krech, T., Schneider, C., and Zeidler, H. (1989*c*). Specific serum IgA-antibodies in Chlamydia-induced arthritis. *Zeitschrift für Rheumatologie*, **48**, 86–88, **14**, 225. (Abstract).

Wollenhaupt, H. J., Schmitz, E., and Zeidler, H. (1990). Chlamydien-induzierte Arthritis: Diagnose–Verlauf–Therapie. *Wiener Medizinische Wochenschrift*, **12**, 302–6.

Wollenhaupt, J., Kolbus, F., Weiggbbrodt, H., Schneider, C., Krech, T., and Zeidler, H. (1995). Manifestations of Chlamydia induced arthritis in patients with silent versus symptomatic urogenital chlamydial infection. *Clinical and Experimental Rheumatology*, **13**, 453–8.

Wong, E. S., Hooten, T. M., Hill, C. C., *et al.*. (1988). Clinical and microbiological features of persistent or recurrent non-gonococcal urethritis in men. *Journal of Infectious Diseases*, **158**, 1098–101.

Woodrow, J. C. and Eastmond, C. J. (1978). HLA-B27 and the genetics of ankylosing spondylitis. *Annals of Rheumatic Diseases*, **37**, 504–8.

Wordsworth, B. P. and Mowat, A. G. (1986). A review of 100 patients with ankylosing spondylitis with particular reference to socio-economic effects. *British Journal Rheumatology*, **25**, 175–80,

Wordsworth, P. (1995). Genes and arthritis. *British Medical Bulletin*, **51**, 249–66.

Wordsworth, P., Pile, K. D., *et al.* (1992). HLA heterozygosity contributes to susceptibility to rheumatoid arthritis. *American Journal of Human Genetics*, **51**, 585–91.

Wright, V. (1956). Psoriasis and arthritis. *Annals of Rheumatic Diseases*, **15**, 348–56.

Wright, V. (1959). Rheumatism and psoriasis. A re-evaluation. *American Journal of Medicine*, **27**, 454–62.

Wright, V. (1978*a*). Seronegative polyarthritis. A unified concept. *Arthritis and Rheumatism*, **21**, 618–33.

Wright, V. (1978*b*). In *Copeman's textbook of the rheumatic diseases*. (ed. J. T. Scott), p. 553. Churchill Livingstone, London.

Wright, V. (1980). Relationships between ankylosing spondylitis and other spondarthritides. In *Ankylosing Spondylitis* (ed. J. M. H. Moll). Churchill Livingstone, Edinburgh.

Wright, V. and Moll, J. M. H. (1976*a*). *Seronegative polyarthritis*. North Holland Publishing Company, Amsterdam.

Wright, V. and Moll, J. M. H. (1976*b*). Psoriatic arthritis. In *Seronegative polyarthritis*, No. **16**, pp. 169–235. North Holland, Amsterdam.

Wright, V. and Watkinson, G. (1959). The arthritis of ulcerative colitis. *Medicine*, **38**, 243–59.

Wright, V. and Watkinson, G. (1965*a*). The arthritis of ulcerative colitis. *British Medical Journal*, **2**, 670–5.

Wright, V. and Watkinson, G. (1965*b*). Sacro-illitis and ulcerative colitis. *British Medical Journal*, **2**, 675–80.

Wucherpfennig, K. W. and Strominger, J. L. (1995). Molecular mimicry in T cell-mediated autoimmunity: viral peptides activate human T cell clones specific for myelin basic protein. *Cell*, **80**, 695–705.

Wucherpfennig, K. W. & Strominger, J. L. (1995). Selective binding of self peptides to disease-associated major histocompatibility complex (MHC) molecules: a mechanism for MHC-linked susceptibility to human autoimmune diseases. *Journal of Experimental Medicine* **181**, 1597–601.

Wuorela, M., Jalkanen, S., Toivanen, P., and Granfors, K. (1993). Yersinia lipopolysaccharide is modified by human monocytes. *Infection and Immunity*, **61**, 5261–70.

Wuorela, M., Jalkanen, S., Toivanen, P., and Granfors, K. (1996). Epression of MHC class II molecules on human monocytes is regulated independently from each other after phagocytosis of bacteria. *Scandinavian Journal of Immunology*, **43**, 39–46.

Wynn Parry, C. B. (19??). Management of ankylosing spondylitis. *Proceedings of the Royal Society of Medicine*, **59**, 619–20.

Wynn Parry, C. B. (1974). Rehabilitation of the inflammatory arthropathies. *Proceedings of the Royal Society of Medicine*, **67**, 494–5.

Wynn Parry, C. B. and Deary K. J. (1980). Physical measureas in rehabilitations. In *Ankylosing spondylitis* (ed. J. Moll), Churchill Livingstone, London.

Yahia, B., Dave, U., Keat, A., and Forbes, A. (1996). Arthropathy in inflammatory bowel disease (IBD): An under-estimated problem? *Gastroenterology*, **110**, A1048.

Yamada, T., Sartor, R. B., Marshall, S., Specian, R. D., and Grisham, M. B. (1993). Mucosal injury and inflammation in a model of chronic granulomatous colitis. *Gastroenterology*, **104**, 759–71.

Yamaguchi, A., Tsuchiya, N., Mitsui, H., *et al.* (1995). Association of HLA-B39 with HLA-B27-negative ankylosing spondylitis and pauciarticular juvenile rheumatoid arthritis in Japanese patients. *Arthritis and Rheumatism*, **38**, 1672–7.

Yanagisawa, H., Hammer, R. E., Taurog, J. D., and Richardson, J. A. (1995). Characterization of psoriasiform and alopecic skin lesions in HLA-B27 transgenic rats. *American Journal of Pathology*, **147**, 955–64.

Yao, Z., Kimura, A., Hartung, K., *et al.* (1993). Polymorphism to the DQA1 promoter region (QAP) and DRB1, QAP, DQA1, DQB1 haplotypes in systemic lupus erythematosus. *Immunogenetics*, **38**, 421–9.

Yin, Z., Braun, J., Neure, L., Wu, P., *et al.* (1997) Crucial role of Interleukin-10/interleukin-12 balance in the regulation of the type 2T helper cytokine response in reactive arthritis. *Arthritis and Rheumatism* (in press).Yli-Kerttula, T., Tertti, R., and Toivanen, A. (1995). Ten-year follow up study of patients from a *Yersinia pseudotuberculosis* III outbreak. *Clinical and Experimental Rheumatology*, **13**, 333–7.

Yli-Kerttula, U. I. and Vilpulla, A. H. (1988). Reactive salpingitis. In *Reactive Arthritis* (ed. A. Toivanen and P. Toivanen), pp. 125–31. CRC Press, Boca Raton.

Young, A. C. M., Zhang, W., Sacchettini, J. C., Nathenson, S. G. (1994). The three-dimensional structure of H-2D^b at 2.4 Å resolution: implications for antigen determinant selection. *Cell* **76**, 39–50.

Youssef, P. P., Bertouch, J. V., and Jones, P. D. (1992). Successful treatment of human immunodeficiency virus-associated Reiter's syndrome with sulfasalazine. *Arthritis and Rheumatism*, **35**, 723–4.

Yssel, H., Shanafelt, M. -C., Soderberg, C., Schneider, P., Anzola, J., and Peltz, G. (1991). *B. Burgdorferi* activates TH1-like T cell subset in Lyme arthritis. *Journal of Experimental Medicine*, **174**, 593–601.

Yui Yip, S. (1984). The prevalence of psoriasis in the mongoloid race. *Journal of the American Academy of Dermatology*, **10**, 965–8.

Zapanta, M., Aldo-Benson, M., Biegel, A., and Madura, J. (1979). Arthritis associated with jejunoileal bypass: Clinical and immunologic evaluation. *Arthritis and Rheumatism*, **22**, 74–7.

Zeidler, H. (1992). Chlamydia-induced arthritis. Clinical features, diagnosis and therapy. In *Rheumatology state of the art* (ed. G. Balint *et al.*), pp. 49–62. Elsevier, London. **(7)**

Zeidler, H. and Wollenhaupt, J. (1991). Chlamydia-induced arthritis: the clinical spectrum, serology and prognosis. In *HLA-B27 + spondyloarthropathies* (ed. P. E. Lipsky and J. D. Taurog), pp. 175–87. Elsevier, London.

Zeidler, H., Werdier, D., Klauder, A., *et al.* (1987). Undifferentiated arthritis and spondylarthropathy as a challenge for prospective follow-up. *Clinical Rheumatology*, **6**, (Suppl. 2), 112–20.

Zeidler, H., Mau, W., and Khan, M. A. (1992). Undifferentiated spondyloarthropathies. *Rheumatology Disease Clinics of North America*, **18**, 187–202.

Zen-Yoji, H., Maruyama, T., Sakai, S., Kimura, S., Mizuno, T., and Momose, T. (1973). An outbreak of enteritis due to *Yersinia enterocolitica* occurring at a junior high school. *Japanese Journal of Microbiology*, **17**, 220–2.

Zhang, Y., Gripenberg-Lerche, C., Soderstrom, K-O., *et al.* (1996). Antribiotic prophylaxis and treatment of reactive arthritis. *Arthritis and Rheumatism*, **39**, 1238–43.

Zinkernagel, R. M., Cooper, S., Chambers, J., Lazzarini, R. A., Hengarter, H., and Arnheiter, H. (1990). Virus-induced autoantibody response to a transgenic viral antigen. *Nature*, **345**, 68–71.

Zinkernagel, R. M. (1993). Immunity to viruses. In *Fundamental immunology* (ed. W. Paul), pp. 1211–50. Raven Press, New York.

Zinkernagel, R. M. and Doherty, P. C. (1979). MHC-restricted cytotoxic T cells: studies on the biological role of polymorphic major transplantation antigens determining T-cell restriction-specificity, function, and responsiveness. *Advances in Immunology*, **27**, 51–177.

Zwillich, S. H. and Ritchlin, C. T. (1991). Olsalazine in Reiter's syndrome. *Journal of Rheumatology*, **21**, 2169–70.

Zychlinsky, A., Prevost, M. C., and Sansonetti, P. J. (1992). *Shigella flexneri* induces apoptosis in infected macrophages. *Nature*, **358**, 167–9.

Index